MW01483108

THE INFECTIOUS ETIOLOGY OF CHRONIC DISEASES

Defining the Relationship, Enhancing the Research, and Mitigating the Effects

Workshop Summary

Stacey L. Knobler, Siobhán O'Connor, Stanley M. Lemon,
Marjan Najafi, *Editors*

Forum on Microbial Threats

Board on Global Health

INSTITUTE OF MEDICINE
OF THE NATIONAL ACADEMIES

THE NATIONAL ACADEMIES PRESS
Washington, D.C.
www.nap.edu

THE NATIONAL ACADEMIES PRESS   500 Fifth Street, NW   Washington, DC 20001

NOTICE: The project that is the subject of this report was approved by the Governing Board of the National Research Council, whose members are drawn from the councils of the National Academy of Sciences, the National Academy of Engineering, and the Institute of Medicine.

Support for this project was provided by the U.S. Department of Health and Human Services' National Institutes of Health, Centers for Disease Control and Prevention, and Food and Drug Administration; U.S. Agency for International Development; U.S. Department of Defense; U.S. Department of State; U.S. Department of Veterans Affairs; U.S. Department of Agriculture; American Society for Microbiology; Burroughs Wellcome Fund; Ellison Medical Foundation; Pfizer; GlaxoSmithKline; and The Merck Company Foundation. The views presented in this report are those of the editors and attributed authors and are not necessarily those of the funding agencies.

This report is based on the proceedings of a workshop that was sponsored by the Forum on Microbial Threats. It is prepared in the form of a workshop summary by and in the name of the editors, with the assistance of staff and consultants, as an individually authored document. Sections of the workshop summary not specifically attributed to an individual reflect the views of the editors and not those of the Forum on Microbial Threats. The content of those sections is based on the presentations and the discussions that took place during the workshop.

International Standard Book Number 0-309-08994-8 (Book)
International Standard Book Number 0-309-52673-6 (PDF)
Library of Congress Control Number: 2004107939

Additional copies of this report are available from the National Academies Press, 500 Fifth Street, NW, Lockbox 285, Washington, DC 20055; (800) 624-6242 or (202) 334-3313 (in the Washington metropolitan area); Internet, http://www.nap.edu.

For more information about the Institute of Medicine, visit the IOM home page at: **www.iom.edu.**

The serpent has been a symbol of long life, healing, and knowledge among almost all cultures and religions since the beginning of recorded history. The serpent adopted as a logotype by the Institute of Medicine is a relief carving from ancient Greece, now held by the Staatliche Museen in Berlin.

COVER: The background for the cover of this workshop summary is a photograph of a batik designed and printed specifically for the Malaysian Society of Parasitology and Tropical Medicine. The print contains drawings of various parasites and insects; it is used with the kind permission of the Society.

"Knowing is not enough; we must apply.
Willing is not enough; we must do."
—Goethe

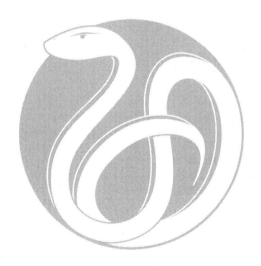

INSTITUTE OF MEDICINE
OF THE NATIONAL ACADEMIES

Adviser to the Nation to Improve Health

THE NATIONAL ACADEMIES
Advisers to the Nation on Science, Engineering, and Medicine

The **National Academy of Sciences** is a private, nonprofit, self-perpetuating society of distinguished scholars engaged in scientific and engineering research, dedicated to the furtherance of science and technology and to their use for the general welfare. Upon the authority of the charter granted to it by the Congress in 1863, the Academy has a mandate that requires it to advise the federal government on scientific and technical matters. Dr. Bruce M. Alberts is president of the National Academy of Sciences.

The **National Academy of Engineering** was established in 1964, under the charter of the National Academy of Sciences, as a parallel organization of outstanding engineers. It is autonomous in its administration and in the selection of its members, sharing with the National Academy of Sciences the responsibility for advising the federal government. The National Academy of Engineering also sponsors engineering programs aimed at meeting national needs, encourages education and research, and recognizes the superior achievements of engineers. Dr. Wm. A. Wulf is president of the National Academy of Engineering.

The **Institute of Medicine** was established in 1970 by the National Academy of Sciences to secure the services of eminent members of appropriate professions in the examination of policy matters pertaining to the health of the public. The Institute acts under the responsibility given to the National Academy of Sciences by its congressional charter to be an adviser to the federal government and, upon its own initiative, to identify issues of medical care, research, and education. Dr. Harvey V. Fineberg is president of the Institute of Medicine.

The **National Research Council** was organized by the National Academy of Sciences in 1916 to associate the broad community of science and technology with the Academy's purposes of furthering knowledge and advising the federal government. Functioning in accordance with general policies determined by the Academy, the Council has become the principal operating agency of both the National Academy of Sciences and the National Academy of Engineering in providing services to the government, the public, and the scientific and engineering communities. The Council is administered jointly by both Academies and the Institute of Medicine. Dr. Bruce M. Alberts and Dr. Wm. A. Wulf are chair and vice chair, respectively, of the National Research Council.

www.national-academies.org

FORUM ON MICROBIAL THREATS

MICHAEL OSTERHOLM, Director, Center for Infectious Disease Research and Policy and Professor, School of Public Health, University of Minnesota, Minneapolis

GEORGE POSTE, Director, Arizona BioDesign Institute, Arizona State University, Tempe

GARY ROSELLE, Program Director for Infectious Diseases, VA Central Office, Veterans Health Administration, Department of Veterans Affairs, Washington, DC

JANET SHOEMAKER, Director, Office of Public Affairs, American Society for Microbiology, Washington, DC

P. FREDRICK SPARLING, J. Herbert Bate Professor Emeritus of Medicine, Microbiology, and Immunology, University of North Carolina, Chapel Hill

Liaisons

YVES BERGEVIN, Department of Child and Adolescent Health and Development, World Health Organization, Geneva, Switzerland

ENRIQUETA BOND, President, Burroughs Wellcome Fund, Research Triangle Park, North Carolina

EDWARD McSWEEGAN, National Institute of Allergy and Infectious Diseases, National Institutes of Health, Bethesda, Maryland

Staff

STACEY KNOBLER, Director, Forum on Microbial Threats

MARJAN NAJAFI, Research Associate

KATHERINE OBERHOLTZER, Research Assistant

Reviewers

All presenters at the workshop have reviewed and approved their respective sections of this report for accuracy. In addition, this workshop summary has been reviewed in draft form by independent reviewers chosen for their diverse perspectives and technical expertise, in accordance with procedures approved by the National Research Council's Report Review Committee. The purpose of this independent review is to provide candid and critical comments that will assist the Institute of Medicine (IOM) in making the published workshop summary as sound as possible and to ensure that the workshop summary meets institutional standards. The review comments and draft manuscript remain confidential to protect the integrity of the deliberative process.

The Forum and IOM thank the following individuals for their participation in the review process:

Paul Eke, Centers for Disease Control and Prevention, Chamblee, Georgia

Charlotte Gaydos, Johns Hopkins University School of Medicine, Baltimore, Maryland

Julie Parsonnet, Stanford University School of Medicine, Palo Alto, California

David Relman, Veterans Administration Palo Alto Health Care System, Palo Alto, California

Donald Silberberg, University of Pennsylvania School of Medicine, Philadelphia

The review of this report was overseen by **Melvin Worth, M.D.**, Scholar-in-Residence, National Academies, who was responsible for making certain that an independent examination of this report was carried out in accordance with institutional procedures and that all review comments were carefully considered. Responsibility for the final content of this report rests entirely with the editors and individual authors.

Preface

The Forum on Microbial Threats was created in 1996 in response to a request from the Centers for Disease Control and Prevention and the National Institutes of Health. The goal of the Forum is to provide structured opportunities for representatives from academia, industry, professional and interest groups, and government to examine and discuss scientific and policy issues that are of shared interest and that are specifically related to research and prevention, detection, and management of emerging infectious diseases. In accomplishing this task, the Forum provides the opportunity to foster the exchange of information and ideas, identify areas in need of greater attention, clarify policy issues by enhancing knowledge and identifying points of agreement, and inform decision makers about science and policy issues. The Forum seeks to illuminate issues rather than resolve them directly; hence, it does not provide advice or recommendations on any specific policy initiative pending before any agency or organization. Its strengths are the diversity of its membership and the contributions of individual members expressed throughout the activities of the Forum.

ABOUT THE WORKSHOP

The belief that many long-recognized chronic diseases are infectious in origin goes back to the mid-nineteenth century, when cancer was studied as a possible infectious disease. In the 1950s and 1960s, much biomedical research was directed, unsuccessfully, at the identification of microorganisms purportedly causing a variety of chronic diseases. In recent years the picture has begun to change. One chronic disease after another has been linked, in some cases definitively, to an infectious etiology (e.g., peptic ulcer disease with *Helicobacter pylori,* cervical cancer with several human papillomaviruses, Whipple's disease with *Tropheryma whippeli,* Lyme arthritis and neuroborreliosis with *Borrelia burgdorferi,* AIDS with HIV). Evidence implicating microorganisms as etiologic agents of chronic diseases with substantial mortality and morbidity impact, including atherosclerosis and cardiovascular disease, diabetes mellitus, inflammatory bowel disease, and a variety of neurological and neuropsychiatric diseases, continues to mount.

Emerging infectious diseases are conceptualized as either newly identified or appreciated illnesses, conditions, or well-recognized diseases that are newly attributed to infection. Now, scientists are beginning to believe that a substantial portion of chronic diseases may actually be associated with infection.

In an effort to identify cross-disciplinary aspects of the challenge of infectious etiologies of chronic diseases, including inflammatory syndromes and cancer, the Institute of Medicine's Forum on Microbial Threats hosted a two-day workshop on October 21–22, 2002. The workshop, Linking Infectious Agents and Chronic Diseases, explored the factors that drive infectious etiologies of chronic diseases to prominence, and sought to identify more broad-based strategies and research programs that need to be developed. The goals of the workshop were to:

1. Review the range of pathogenic mechanisms and diversity of etiologic microbes and chronic diseases, including inflammatory syndromes and cancer;

2. Explore trends, advances, and gaps in collaborative research on diagnostic technologies, and their integration into epidemiologic studies and surveillance;

3. Identify chronic diseases and syndromes that warrant further investigation;

4. Identify research needed to clarify the etiologic agents and pathogenic mechanisms involved in chronic diseases, screening for multiple potential agents of the same outcome, and considering that one microbe might induce multiple syndromes;

5. Identify the principal bottlenecks and opportunities to detect, prevent, and mitigate the impact of chronic diseases on human health against the overall backdrop of emerging infections;

6. Consider the benefits and risks of early detection and prevention of chronic diseases caused by infectious agents.

The issues pertaining to these goals were addressed through invited presentations and subsequent discussions, which highlighted ongoing programs and actions taken, and also identified the most vital needs in this important area.

ORGANIZATION OF WORKSHOP SUMMARY

This workshop summary report is prepared for the Forum membership in the name of the editors, with the assistance of staff and consultants, as a collection of individually authored papers. Sections of the workshop summary not specifically attributed to an individual reflect the views of the editors and not those of the Forum on Microbial Threats' sponsors or the Institute of Medicine (IOM). The contents of the unattributed sections are based on the presentations and discussions that took place during the workshop.

The workshop summary is organized within chapters as a topic-by-topic description of the presentations and discussions. Its purpose is to present lessons from relevant experience, delineate a range of pivotal issues and their respective problems, and put forth some potential responses as described by the workshop participants. The Summary and Assessment chapter discusses the core messages that emerged from the speakers' presentations and the ensuing discussions. Chapters 1 through 4 begin with overviews provided by the editors, followed by authored papers that reflect the topics and findings of the authors' workshop presentations. Chapter 1 presents case studies of infectious agents that have been shown to be associated with chronic diseases. Chapter 2 illustrates implications for developing countries where many infectious diseases remain endemic. Chapter 3 describes methodologies currently used in this area of research. Chapter 4 presents strategies to prevent and mitigate the impact of chronic diseases caused by infectious agents. Appendix A presents the workshop agenda. Appendix B is a list of information resources that review the relationship between infections and chronic diseases. Appendix C presents Forum member and speaker biographies.

Although this workshop summary provides an account of the individual presentations, it also reflects an important aspect of the Forum philosophy. The workshop functions as a dialogue among representatives from different sectors and presents their beliefs on which areas may merit further attention. However, the reader should be aware that the material presented here expresses the views and opinions of those participating in the workshop and not the deliberations of a formally constituted IOM study committee. These proceedings summarize only what participants stated in the workshop and are not intended to be an exhaustive exploration of the subject matter.

ACKNOWLEDGMENTS

The Forum on Microbial Threats and the IOM wish to express their warmest appreciation to the individuals and organizations who gave valuable time to provide information and advice to the Forum through their participation in the workshop.

The Forum is indebted to the IOM staff who contributed their time and efforts in planning and executing the workshop and the production of this workshop summary. On behalf of the Forum, we gratefully acknowledge the efforts led by Stacey Knobler, director of the Forum, and Marjan Najafi, research associate, coeditors of this report, who dedicated much effort and time to developing this workshop's agenda, and for their thoughtful and insightful approach and skill in translating the workshop proceedings and discussion into this workshop summary. We would also like to thank the following Academies staff and consultants for their valuable contributions to this activity: Rob Coppock, Tom Burroughs, Carlos Orr, Jennifer Bitticks, Bronwyn Schrecker, Sally Stanfield, Rachel Marcus, Beth Gyorgy, Patricia Cuff, Katherine Oberholtzer, and Laura Sivitz.

Finally, the Forum also thanks sponsors that supported this activity. Financial support for this project was provided by the U.S. Department of Health and Human Services' National Institutes of Health, Centers for Disease Control and Prevention, and Food and Drug Administration; U.S. Agency for International Development; U.S. Department of Defense; U.S. Department of State; U.S. Department of Veterans Affairs; U.S. Department of Agriculture; American Society for Microbiology; Burroughs Wellcome Fund; Ellison Medical Foundation; Pfizer; GlaxoSmithKline; and The Merck Company Foundation. The views presented in this workshop summary are those of the editors and workshop participants and are not necessarily those of the funding organizations.

Adel A.F. Mahmoud, *Chair*
Stanley M. Lemon, *Vice-Chair*
Forum on Microbial Threats

Contents

APPENDIXES

Summary and Assessment

The belief that infectious agents may cause certain chronic diseases can be traced to the mid-19th century, when cancer was studied as a possible infectious disease. This effort met with little success. In the 1950s and 1960s, much more biomedical research was directed, again unsuccessfully, at the identification of microorganisms purported to cause a variety of chronic diseases. In recent years, however, the picture has begun to change. A number of chronic diseases have now been linked, in some cases definitively, to an infectious etiology: peptic ulcer disease with *Helicobacter pylori*, cervical cancer with several human papillomaviruses, Whipple's disease with *Tropheryma whipplei*, Lyme arthritis and neuroborreliosis with *Borrelia burgdorferi*, AIDS with the human immuno-deficiency virus, liver cancer and cirrhosis with hepatitis B and C viruses, to name a few. Indeed, evidence continues to mount implicating microorganisms as etiologic agents of chronic diseases that have substantial morbidity and mortality, including atherosclerosis and cardiovascular disease, type 1 diabetes, inflammatory bowel disease, and a variety of neurological diseases. The proven and suspected roles of microbes does not stop with physical ailments; infections are increasingly being examined as associated causes of or possible contributors to a variety of serious, chronic neuropsychiatric disorders and to developmental problems, especially in children.

It also has become apparent that multiple pathogens sometimes interact in causing chronic diseases or rendering them more virulent. For example, people who have concomitant infection with hepatitis C virus and the organism that causes schistosomiasis—as many individuals do in some developing countries—often develop schistosomiasis much more rapidly than do people who are not

1

coinfected. Exploring such pathogen interactions and their effects on the immune system represent rapidly burgeoning areas of scientific interest.[1]

This report summarizes a two-day workshop held by the Institute of Medicine's Forum on Microbial Threats on October 21–22, 2002, to address this rapidly evolving field. Invited experts presented research findings on a range of recognized and potential chronic sequelae of infections, as well as on diverse pathogenic mechanisms leading from exposure to chronic disease outcomes. Cancers, cardiovascular disease, demyelinating syndromes, neuropsychiatric diseases, hepatitis, and type 1 diabetes were among the conditions addressed. Participants explored factors driving infectious etiologies of chronic diseases of prominence, identified difficulties in linking infectious agents with chronic outcomes, and discussed broad-based strategies and research programs to advance the field. Table S-1 lists the infectious agents and associated diseases discussed in this report.

Emerging infectious diseases are conceptualized either as newly identified or appreciated infectious illnesses and conditions, or as previously recognized syndromes that are newly attributed to infection. Some scientists now believe that a substantial portion of chronic diseases may be causally linked to infectious agents. Just as the germ theory opened the way for numerous discoveries about the sources of acute infections, changing ideas about the nature of both infectious diseases and chronic diseases, coupled with the advent of powerful new laboratory techniques, are leading to novel claims concerning the infectious origins of chronic diseases.

DEFINING THE RELATIONSHIP

The traditional standards for establishing a microbial or bacterial cause of disease are those that were developed for acute infections. Known as "Koch's postulates," they state that the causal organism must be:

1. present in diseased tissue;
2. isolated and grown in pure culture outside the animal host;
3. shown to induce the same disease when injected into a healthy animal; and
4. isolated from the experimentally inoculated animal in pure culture and shown to be the same as the original agent.

---

[1]It should be clearly noted throughout this summary report that the nature of the evidence for causality of a chronic disease from an infectious agent varies considerably. Each of the cases reviewed here represents a wide spectrum of the nature of the relationship between the infectious agent and the chronic disease. In some cases, the links are definitive (e.g., human papillomavirus and cervical cancer). In other cases, the relationship has only recently been investigated with little more than suspected associations from preliminary data (e.g., enteroviruses and Type I diabetes).

TABLE S-1 Possible Infectious Etiologies for Chronic Diseases Discussed at the Workshop

Infectious Agent	Chronic Disease/Condition	Chapter
Human papillomavirus	Cervical cancer	1
Hepatitis B virus	• Liver cancer	
	• Cirrhosis	1
Chlamydia pneumoniae	Atherosclerosis	1
Vaccinia virus	Postinfectious encephalomyelitis or acute disseminated encephalomyelitis (ADEM)	1
JC virus	Progressive multifocal leucoencephalopathy (PML)	1
Various viruses	Multiple sclerosis	1
Enteroviruses	Type I diabetes mellitus	1
Toxoplasma gondii	Schizophrenia	1
Herpes Simplex virus Type 2	Schizophrenia	1
Jaagsiekte sheep retrovirus (JSRV)	Ovine pulmonary adenocarcinoma	1
Propionibacterium acnes	• Chronic inflammatory acne	
	• Other chronic diseases	1
Cryptosporidiosis and intestinal helminthic infections	Disability consequences including growth shortfalls, fitness and cognitive impairment	2
Helminthic infections	Epilepsy	2
Plasmodium falciparum	Epilepsy	2
Treponema pallidum	Congenital syphilis	2
Toxoplasma gondii	Congenital toxoplasmosis	2
Maternal rubella virus	Congenital rubella	2
Perinatal HIV	Developmental disabilities	2
Perinatal herpes viruses	Neurodevelopmental disabilities	2
Plasmodium falciparum	• Cognitive development	
	• Childhood anemia	2
Haemophilus influenzae Type B meningitis	Nervous system impairment	2
Japanese encephalitis virus	Neuropsychiatric sequelae	2
Measles virus	Developmental disabilities	2
Poliovirus	Paralysis	
Chlamydia trachomatis	Trachoma	
Human T-cell lymphotropic virus Type 1	• Adult T-cell leukemia/lymphoma	2
	• Autoimmune disorders	
	• Infections associated with immunosuppression	
Human herpes virus Type 8	Kaposi's sarcoma	3
Borna disease virus	Neurodevelopmental disorders	3
Hepatitis C virus and *Schistosoma mansoni* interaction		2
HIV and *Plasmodium falciparum* interaction		2

In almost all cases, identifying and confirming an infectious cause of a chronic disease using Koch's postulates is complicated by several factors, including:

* Disease etiology may be multifactorial, including environmental, host genetic, and microbial genomic factors. Michael Dunne (Chapter 1) surveys a number of pathogens proposed to contribute to atherosclerosis and cardiovascular disease. *Chlamydia pneumoniae*, cytomegalovirus, and herpes simplex virus are among the suggested bacterial and viral pathogens, with the greatest body of evidence surrounding *C. pneumoniae*. Yet in all of these cases, when these agents are considered in the context of well-established risk factors for cardiovascular disease—family history, high-fat diet, inactivity—it is less clear how much infection would truly contribute to the condition and the outcome. Eduardo Franco (Chapter 1) describes the association that has been found between human papillomavirus and cervical cancer. Even years after discovery of this link, however, questions remain about the roles of cofactors, as only some of the many people infected develop malignancy.

* Microorganisms may act in a hit-and-run fashion, striking and then disappearing from the host by the time the disease process becomes apparent. This form of attack appears to be the case in Reiter's syndrome, Guillain-Barré syndrome, and rheumatic heart disease. As another example, Robert Yolken and Fuller Torrey (Chapter 1) report that a retrospective study of schizophrenics found that their mothers' blood at the time of birth exhibited elevated IgG, IgM, and certain cytokines, suggesting that an ongoing inflammatory process may possibly be associated with *Toxoplasma* infection. Antibodies directed against endogenous retroviruses, including Herv-W, have also been found at elevated levels. Infection in the perinatal period may have set the stage for later neurological disease, although there may be little or no evidence of active infection at the time of diagnosis.

* Acute, chronic, latent, or recurrent infections may be involved in pathogenesis, and coinfections may play a critical role in disease manifestation. Richard Johnson (Chapter 1) describes postinfectious encephalomyelitis in which patients develop fever, become obtunded, and develop multifocal neurological signs several days after resolution of an acute rash caused by a virus. This is an example of an acute systemic disease with a postinfectious immune response leading to demyelination within the central nervous system. In other cases, a long period of active viral replication may precede the onset of disease. William Mason (Chapter 1) reports that the risk of developing chronic hepatitis B virus infection is greater than 90 percent when a person is infected at birth or in early childhood, but drops to less than 10 percent when a person is infected as an adult. In such chronic infections, the risk of fatal liver disease (cirrhosis or liver cancer) rises to approximately 25 percent, with a 30 year to 50 year interval between the onset of the infection and the consequent pathological outcome. A similar picture

occurs with hepatitis C virus infection, although in this case there is virus persistence when the infection occurs in adulthood. Viral infections may also be latent at the time of diagnosis. For example, there are several viruses for which patients with multiple sclerosis (MS) exhibit higher antibody levels than control patients. Johnson reports on one study which revealed that 23 percent of MS patients had antibodies to two or more viruses present within their central nervous systems, with one patient presenting with 11 viruses. It is not yet clear whether infection(s) triggers MS or whether elevated markers of infection are secondary to the underlying inflammatory processes of the disease. Such findings emphasize the complexity of directly attributing chronic disease to one or more specific infectious agents.

  • Detecting and/or isolating microbes that are present in a variety of tissues may pose significant technical difficulties. Current methods to identify novel or rare microorganisms may be inadequate. During the workshop, David Persing reported on the deficiencies and weaknesses of conventional methods for identifying and subtyping microorganisms. However, newer molecular technology, such as broad-range amplification of ribosomal targets directly from tissue or culture, can complement conventional systems, and these tools have helped in identifying several new species and pathogenic subtypes. For example, the infectious agent strongly suspected of causing Whipple's disease remained elusive for years. Applying broad-range polynuclear chain reaction techniques enabled scientists to amplify and categorize the etiologic *Tropheryma whipplei* bacterium. Patrick Moore (Chapter 3) recounts the development of a technique called representational difference analysis to identify Kaposi's sarcoma-associated herpesvirus as a cause of AIDS-associated Kaposi's sarcoma. These discoveries exemplify the diligent effort required to move from identification of a new DNA sequence to confirming causality in a specific disease. During the workshop, Persing also described the potential for gene expression arrays (microarrays), proteomics, and other technologies to identify patterns of host response to an infection(s) that might explain the pathogenic processes from exposure to chronic disease and lead to the development of diagnostic tools for these entities. Phylogenetic analysis can relate new pathogens for which there are no effective diagnostic assays to known agents through conserved epitopes and other properties, facilitating the evaluation of new infectious causes of disease.

Given the various reasons why it may often prove difficult to satisfy Koch's postulates in linking a particular infectious agent to a particular chronic disease, alternative sets of criteria may need to be developed for determining causation. Such criteria must take into account the more complex relationships that are being observed between microbial agents and chronic disease, and they likely will require collection of more challenging types of experimental data, especially molecular data, that can help clarify discrete causal links. Toward this goal, several promising avenues of research are being pursued, including extending various genetic technologies and modifying animal and cell culture models of human disease to make them more immediately relevant to microbial disease causation.

Ensuing discussions highlighted gaps in scientific knowledge and in the translation of research data to health care interventions for both well-accepted and more speculative causal associations. Participants noted the complexity of these issues, as well as the importance of strengthening the critical linkages among clinicians, researchers, epidemiologists, and public health officials.

IMPLICATIONS FOR DEVELOPING COUNTRIES

Chronic diseases are a leading health issue in economically established countries, and they take a significant toll in developing countries as well. Human T-cell lymphotropic virus type 1 infection and hepatitis C-schistosomiasis coinfection demonstrate the impact of progressive chronic infections that already disproportionately affect developing regions. During the next 20 years, chronic diseases are expected to become even more important in economically developing regions, as the types of chronic conditions currently found primarily in industrialized nations spread to other regions. Not only will changing economics, demographic shifts with lower childhood mortality, and changing lifestyles drive this trend, but migration from rural to urban areas and into previously uninhabited ecosystems may expose populations to new infectious agents that underlie chronic disease. Both newly identified and well-recognized infectious etiologies of chronic disease, including infections known to enter a chronic state, such as tuberculosis and malaria, will acquire increasing importance to domestic and global health. These associations also will create serious burdens in addition to the chronic infection. Richard Guerrant (Chapter 2) relates that enteric and parasitic infections, often marked by diarrhea and contributing to malnutrition, can have long-term consequences, impairing development and cognitive abilities as well as general health. Once again, coinfections and common acute infections are likely to loom large and may represent an under-recognized source of chronic pathology. Attending to the challenges imposed by chronic diseases will be difficult in strained healthcare systems that have limited research capacity and that already are overwhelmed by the myriad of acute health problems in developing regions.

OBSTACLES AND OPPORTUNITIES FOR FRAMING THE RESEARCH: PRIORITIES FOR THE FUTURE

Human disease is a function of the environment in which people live and of their genetic susceptibility to infection or its outcome. People live in concert with a variety of microbial agents that may or may not cause disease, depending on an individual's exposure and surrounding environment and the genetic background on which these are superimposed. When chronic disease stems from infectious disease, the situation is even more complex, because it may be difficult to ascertain the precise timing of infection (which may have happened well in the past) or the exact nature of the pathogen.

Scientifically sound data on the infectious etiologies of chronic diseases must derive from new technologies and the optimization of existing assays. The research must be guided by epidemiologic insights gained from well-designed studies of disease in human populations and from the application of sophisticated surveillance systems to detect and monitor diseases and pathogens. Standardization and reproducibility will be essential. Selection of appropriate cases and controls is imperative, with the use of systematic case studies or experimental designs when this is not possible. Prospective cohort studies should incorporate appropriate surveillance and be capable of detecting outbreaks of infection as well as identifying recently infected individuals. Throughout all, researchers will need to employ comparable definitions of infection and of the chronic disease being explored. To develop enough human capital for these endeavors, it will be necessary to attract more scientists to the relevant fields and provide more training in attendant epidemiological and scientific areas.

Overcoming these obstacles will require the concentrated efforts of researchers from a variety of disciplines, including epidemiology, clinical medicine, molecular biology, and pathology, among others. It also will require harnessing new analytical tools and approaches that have emerged recently, and continue to emerge, from molecular biology, genomics, and biotechnology. One of the most fruitful technologies centers on the ability to detect and manipulate nucleic acid molecules in microorganisms, thus creating a powerful means for identifying previously unknown microbial pathogens and for studying the host-pathogen relationship. Other new tools being employed include broad-range polymerase chain reaction and representational difference analysis, both of which have played key roles in linking numerous pathogens with chronic diseases. Equipped with these and other advanced tools, researchers are becoming better able to move beyond the limitations of Koch's postulates and to link infectious agents with chronic diseases more precisely and with greater confidence than ever before. In addition, researchers are developing sophisticated approaches for exploring the interplay of genetic and environmental factors in the causation of a number of important developmental behavioral disorders.

Participants also identified a number of general characteristics of a comprehensive and coordinated effort that would enhance efforts both to identify links between infectious microorganisms and chronic diseases and to develop and implement interventions to minimize their health consequences. For example, they noted need to develop prototypes and standards to guide this work. Standardized case definitions are needed to facilitate research as well as the clinical diagnosis of infection (active, persistent, or latent) and the chronic syndromes or outcomes that result from it. Laboratory assays need to be adopted that are uniform in terms of sensitivity, specificity, and reproducibility. High-throughput assays meeting similar standards will be key to the study of large cohorts and populations. Without such tools, it will be difficult to interpret the significance of clinical studies and to relate the results of one study to those of another.

Research coupled with appropriate public health activities will facilitate the linkage of existing and newly designed databases, and ensure the quality surveillance and epidemiologic studies needed to better characterize infectious and chronic diseases by their population distribution and potential associations. Many settings will demand expensive longitudinal investigations or the study of new, prospective cohorts to complement case-control or cross-sectional investigations. Additional observations can be made by conducting follow-up and look-back studies using infectious disease and chronic disease surveillance systems and by following outbreak cohorts or recently infected individuals. Longitudinal studies may prove particularly valuable given that rapid advances in the field may dictate that we might not know today which pieces of evidence will be needed in the future. Detecting and confirming causal associations will require study of both larger cohorts and better-defined at-risk populations.

A number of specific populations should receive particular attention, including people who move from rural areas into cities, both in the developing and the developed world. Studies are needed to see whether such movements redefine an individual's risk for a chronic outcome based on infections that they bring with them or susceptibility to new infections that they previously had not encountered.

To provide effective clinical interventions, continued studies are needed to define temporal relationships between infections and disease—that is, what stage of infection determines outcome. Studies also are needed to clarify at which stage infection must be prevented or treated in order to minimize or eliminate chronic sequelae. It will be important to determine the expected benefit of actions, to ensure that the benefits will outweigh any possible risks.

The improvement of both prevention and treatment for chronic diseases will require a better understanding of their natural history, especially the earliest stages. To generate such knowledge, clinicians should be encouraged to identify patients who have recently developed or who seem to be developing a suspect chronic disease, to systematically collect a range of clinical specimens, to follow the course of the disease, and to identify telltale clinical features early.

Better animal models are also needed to explore and understand the potential infectious causes of chronic illness. Diseases occurring in animals should be explored to better understand the potential paradigms of causal relationships. Animal models do not necessarily mimic human pathogenic processes, but examination of the similarities and differences between various models and human diseases can be extremely informative. Additionally, more effort should be devoted to teaching health professionals about their value and their limitations. Psychiatric modeling with animals may present an especially ripe area for probing a variety of important questions, yet many practitioners in the field are not accustomed to working with such models. Basic tools, such as species-specific immunologic reagents and diagnostics, must be developed to take advantage of this potentially valuable approach. Similarly, the sensitivity and specificity of reagents for human specimens must be verified when translating animal research to people.

Issues related to informed consent and human specimen collections and repositories take on new dimensions given these demands. The potential for developing new and improved diagnostic and analytical technologies that identify new targets for chronic disease prevention strategies is very real. However, it is impossible to know how specimens collected today may be used in the future. There is widespread concern that current regulations and guidelines are too complex, too uncertain, or too restrictive for the meaningful sharing of data. Parties from government, academia, and private funding agencies must collaborate to develop a standard method of gaining patients' consent, gathering identifying information, and being able to use such information in the future. Current consent strategies typically do not allow specimens and data to be used for unforeseen purposes. Further complicating this issue are new state and federal laws regarding the safeguarding and transfer of health-related information among professionals and institutions, and stricter interpretation of long-standing regulations related to informed consent.

The complexity of this field calls for an examination of whether the scientific community is optimally organized to address these issues and whether its various components communicate effectively. The community also should mount a concerted effort to identify gaps in current knowledge about the etiology of chronic diseases, pinpoint what needs to be done to close those gaps, chart the obstacles that stand in the way, and then identify and provide the necessary financial resources (monetary and human) to drive progress. Cross-disciplinary and multidisciplinary approaches will be of critical importance, and the problems created by specialization and programmatic stove-piping should be addressed explicitly. Veterinary researchers, clinical researchers, basic scientists, and epidemiologists need to work together as teams. An increasingly large share of future research will likely involve either groups of investigators from a variety of disciplines or groups of institutions working collaboratively. In many cases, these large projects will include a multinational component to ensure that sufficient attention is paid to multiracial, multiethnic, and multicultural differences.

There are many precedents for developing investigator collaborations, interdisciplinary consortia, and partnerships among academics and public health officials, but such endeavors are not necessarily easy and may not come naturally. Both top-down and bottom-up strategies are appropriate for engaging the various scientific disciplines required for this work. By setting appropriate guidelines, funding agencies can play a major role in driving the formation of such interdisciplinary research teams. Steps have been taken toward this end, but these promising efforts need to be nurtured to ensure continued cooperation.

OPPORTUNITIES TO PREVENT AND MITIGATE THE IMPACT OF CHRONIC DISEASES CAUSED BY INFECTIOUS AGENTS

Documentation of an association between a specific infectious agent and one or more of the high-morbidity, high-mortality chronic diseases that consume most health care resources in economically developed countries would have widespread clinical and public health implications. The significance also would be felt in developing countries, since chronic diseases already are consuming increasing proportions of their available health-related resources—and the threat they face from such diseases continues to grow apace. The benefits to be derived from detecting and preventing causal infections, and from discontinuing interventions against unproven causal agents, could be substantial. Workshop participants also noted the potentially high impact of addressing less common chronic conditions for which a preventable infection is the major cause.

Achieving these potential gains will hinge on several issues. Importantly, it will be necessary to be able to identify causal links and their temporal relationships while minimizing the risks of interventions against unproven etiologies. With this scientifically sound information, new strategies can target the critical point along the path from infection to chronic disease at which interventions might avoid or mitigate illness and disability.

Linking one or more highly prevalent chronic conditions to infection with a specific virus or bacteria might enable physicians to use vaccines and/or antibiotics to prevent or cure the condition, thus eliminating the need for health workers to rely on nonspecific therapies aimed at mitigating the symptoms of the condition. A classic example is immunization with hepatitis B vaccine. The introduction of this vaccine into universal childhood immunization programs has reduced the incidence of hepatocellular carcinoma in some regions of the world where this was previously one of the most common types of malignancy. There is a strong possibility that the new sciences of genomics and proteomics will help to detect the relevant antigens and to advance our understanding of both host immunity to these pathogens and the process of disease pathogenesis. Such knowledge will certainly open new strategies for therapy and prevention. Better approaches to optimizing vaccine antigens also are being developed, and advances in the field of vaccinology should promote such efforts.

Improved coordination among basic and clinical scientists, pathologists, and epidemiologists will be critical to accomplishing these goals. Priorities for these networks and collaborative teams are the development and application of:

- standardized case definitions (to be used in defining both infection and disease outcomes);
- new and adequate specimen collections associated with pedigreed databases;

- appropriate epidemiologic design; and
- comparable methods of analysis that can be applied across a field of study.

The Forum discussions emphasized two major themes: (1) the need to define the nature and scope of future research that will balance global efforts targeting various chronic disease syndromes, and (2) the need to develop a coordinated and systematic strategy to maximize resource use and overcome the inherent technologic and epidemiologic challenges, as well as the organizational barriers, that now impede progress in this field.

CONCLUSION

The substantial burden posed by chronic diseases of likely infectious etiology demands global attention and action. Evidence continues to mount implicating microorganisms as important etiologic agents of chronic diseases that contribute substantially to morbidity and mortality. However, the identification and confirmation of infectious causes of chronic diseases is complicated by several problems, including frequent multifactor causation for many of these diseases and differences in the environmental background and genetic composition of different populations. Recently developed molecular and immunological techniques offer new approaches to addressing the technical barriers. However, improved coordination among basic and clinical scientists, pathologists, and epidemiologists also will be critical to progress. Standardization of case definitions and analytical assays combined with sound epidemiologic design will help, as will the development of broad, new strategies for creating carefully pedigreed specimen collections and disease registries. Although the task is daunting, taking the practical and pragmatic pathways described above could clarify many of the uncertain relationships between infectious agents and chronic diseases.

Siobhán O'Connor, M.D., M.P.H.
Assistant to the Director of the
  National Center for Infectious
  Diseases, Centers for Disease
  Control and Prevention
Clinical Assistant Professor,
  Emory University School of Medicine

Stanley M. Lemon, M.D.
Vice-Chair, Forum on Microbial Threats
Dean, School of Medicine, University of
  Texas Medical Branch

1

Defining the Relationship: An Examination of Infectious Agents Associated with Chronic Diseases

OVERVIEW

Chronic diseases cause 70 percent of all deaths in the United States. Yet the factors that cause many of these conditions have been poorly understood until recently. Advances in numerous detection and diagnostic techniques have revealed that several chronic illnesses result from infectious agents. For example, the human papillomavirus causes more than 90 percent of cervical cancers. The hepatitis B virus accounts for more than 60 percent of liver cancer. The Epstein-Barr virus produces in people simultaneously infected with malaria a cancer known as Burkitt's lymphoma, a leading cause of childhood cancer deaths globally. The bacterium Helicobacter pylori has been linked to a number of disorders, including duodenal ulcers, gastric cancer, and certain types of lymphomas.

Other connections between infections and chronic diseases are suspected, but not proven. Epstein-Barr virus, for example, has been found in patients with Hodgkin's disease and with aggressive breast cancers. Multiple sclerosis acts suspiciously like an infection, with patients experiencing high antibody levels as well as exacerbations and remissions. Juvenile-onset diabetes may arise when a Coxsackie B enterovirus elicits an immune response that damages the pancreas.

Identifying and confirming an infectious cause of a chronic disease is complicated by several factors:

- in some cases, microorganisms may act in a hit-and-run fashion, being undetectable by the time the disease process becomes apparent (e.g., Reiter's syndrome, Guillian-Barré syndrome, rheumatic heart disease);
- infection may be in a persistent state at the time of diagnosis;

13

- acute, chronic, or recurrent infections may be involved in pathogenesis;
- detection and culture of microbes in a variety of tissues may be difficult;
- a number of factors, including environmental and genetic (host and microbe) factors, may be involved in the disease etiology; and
- adequate methods may be lacking to identify novel or rare microorganisms.

The case studies presented in this chapter were chosen to provide insight into the range of research under way in the field. The chronic diseases covered represent the full spectrum of those that have been linked in some degree, from "clearly proven" to "suspected," with infectious agents; they are caused by a variety of microorganisms; and their association with disease is supported variously by laboratory and epidemiological studies. Although other diseases and studies might have been included, some limits were imposed by time constraints and the availability of speakers.

Eduardo Franco reviewed the evidence that human papillomavirus (HPV) infection is a cause of cervical cancer. HPV infection precedes lesion development and appears to be necessary for cervical cancer to occur. This is one of the first examples in which an infectious agent has been identified to be necessary for cancer development. This causal relationship was revealed through the use of improved diagnostic tools that enabled more accurate identification of HPV. As the role of infection by certain types of HPV is better elucidated as the cause of cervical cancer, HPV testing in cervical cancer screening programs becomes an important part of a primary prevention strategy. Another component of this strategy may be increased use of a recently developed vaccine. Clinical studies indicate that the new HPV 16 VLP vaccine was 100 percent effective in preventing acquisition of persistent infection with HPV 16, and was 90 percent effective in preventing any incident HPV 16 infection, transient or persistent. Immunization against HPV may have greatest value in developing countries, where 80 percent of the global burden of cervical cancer occurs each year.

William Mason presented the association between hepatitis B virus infection and liver disease. Infection with the virus remains a worldwide problem, with more than 350 million people chronically infected. Although a vaccine has been available for the past 20 years, its high cost prevents universal vaccination. Current research, therefore, has focused on the development of effective therapies to cure those individuals chronically infected with the virus. Mason described the research presently being conducted in a number of animal model systems, including the woodchuck. Along with clinical studies, these models have been able to characterize infections and evaluate therapies, as well as better elucidate the difficulties of treating chronic infections with nucleoside analogs.

Michael Dunne described the relationship between infection and cardiovascular disease. There is a tight association between hypercholesterolemia and atherosclerosis; recent research has examined how inflammation within the plaque accumulated on arterial walls might drive atherosclerosis. Several pathophysiologic hypotheses have been formulated:

1. Local infection might lead through a variety of pathways to arterial wall atherogenic effects.
2. Local infection might produce a systemic inflammatory mediator that travels to the atherosclerotic plaque and produces expression of adhesion molecules along the endothelium, foam cell formation, and other proinflammatory reactions.
3. Local infection might produce bacteremia or viremia from a variety of pathogens that infect the arterial wall and induce those same inflammatory changes.

There is a long list of potential causes: *Chlamydia pneumoniae*, cytomegalovirus, various dental disease organisms, *H. pylori*, and herpes simplex virus. Anything leading to increased foam cell function in the plaque is a potential culprit. This is an example where many different etiologic causes or multiple causes might be involved in the same chronic condition either individually, synergistically, or multifactorially.

Richard Johnson reviewed the various ways that viral infections are associated with demyelinating diseases in animals and humans, including such direct routes as oligodendrocytes or Schwann cells causing demyelination through cell lysis or alteration of cell metabolism; virus-induced immune-mediated reactions, such as incorporation of myelin antigens into the virus envelope or modification of antigenicity of myelin membranes; and viral disruption of regulatory mechanisms of the immune system. Human demyelinating diseases with known viral etiology include postinfectious encephalomyelitis, acute disseminated encephalomyelitis, and progressive multifocal leucoencephalopathy. A viral cause for multiple sclerosis has been postulated for more than 100 years, and epidemiologic studies support this supposition and clearly show an environmental factor. In addition, several studies show multiple sclerosis patients to have elevated levels of various antiviral antibodies compared to controls.

Mark Pallansch discussed some of the difficulties in addressing the association of chronic diseases with infectious diseases, using diabetes and enteroviruses as examples. Type 1 diabetes is clearly a multifactorial disease: there is both a clear genetic predisposition and an autoimmune component. The major manifestation is the loss of beta cells in the pancreas and the associated loss of capacity to produce insulin. There are more than 65 different enteroviruses, which include the most common human viral infections. All individuals may have multiple infections every year with at least one of these viruses. Because the standard enterovirus diagnostics are extremely labor-intensive, efforts are being made to develop diagnostic tools based on reverse transcriptase-polymerase chain reaction (RT-PCR). A semi-nested PCR method is available to determine presence or absence of enteroviruses, but ways of identifying specific enteroviruses remain to be developed using this technology.

Robert Yolken and Fuller Torrey examined associations between infectious agents and schizophrenia. Epidemiologic studies indicate that environmental events during fetal development and early infancy may contribute to the risk of schizophrenia in some individuals. Yolken and Torrey hypothesized that most cases of schizophrenia are caused by infections and other environmental events occurring in genetically susceptible individuals. The activation of endogenous retroviruses within the central nervous system may possibly be one of several mechanisms by which infections can lead to the disease. If this is the case, then medications controlling these infections could play a major role in treating schizophrenia.

Hung Fan examined evidence from an animal model supporting the possibility that an infectious agent may be involved in human lung adenocarcinoma. Ovine pulmonary adenocarcinoma (OPA) is a contagious lung cancer of sheep. Tumor samples from animals with OPA consistently contain exogenous jaagsiekte sheep retrovirus (JSRV), which has an envelope gene with oncogenic potential. JSRV-induced OPA is histologically very similar to human adenocarcinoma. The lack of association of this cancer with tobacco smoking, together with the disease's increasing incidence, suggests the possibility of viral involvement.

David Persing discussed the pathogenesis of acne, a dermatologic inflammatory disease unique to humans and the most common dermatological complaint of adolescents and young adults. In addition to the role played by the bacteria *Propionibacterium acnes* in the development of the inflammatory acne lesion, Persing explained how *P. acnes* has been implicated as a source of heart valve infections, postoperative implant infections, and prostheses failure. Recently *P. acnes* has been implicated as a possible cause of chronic inflammation in sciatica. Persing described his approaches to developing a vaccine for acne that could also benefit other *P. acnes*-related chronic diseases.

Studies in each of these areas are advancing our understanding of the role that infections play in chronic diseases. But the path from suspecting a microorganism to proving its association with a specific disease can be long. The discovery that *H. pylori* can cause duodenal ulcer disease is often cited as case in point of both the hurdles and the rewards. The medical establishment in the United States and worldwide remained skeptical of this link for years. Finally, the evidence became overwhelming, and the discovery is credited with galvanizing research for the entire field of infection and chronic disease. Medical treatment also has evolved accordingly, with therapies shifting from surgery to blocking hyperacidity and, ultimately, to the use of antibiotics directed against *H. pylori*.

THE ROLE OF VIRUSES IN ONCOGENESIS: HUMAN PAPILLOMAVIRUSES AND CERVICAL CANCER AS A PARADIGM

*Eduardo L. Franco, M.P.H., Dr.P.H.**
Departments of Oncology and Epidemiology,
McGill University, Montreal, Canada

Like other malignant neoplasms of humans, cervical cancer is a disease with multifactorial causes and long latency. Unlike most other cancers, however, in which multiple environmental, biologic, and lifestyle determinants contribute independently or jointly to carcinogenesis, cervical cancer has been shown to have a central causal agent, human papillomavirus (HPV) infection, whose contribution to the risk of the disease is much greater than that of any other recognized determinant (IARC, 1995). Recently, there has been much attention to the fact that it is virtually impossible to find cervical carcinoma specimens devoid of traces of HPV DNA, which strongly suggests that HPV infection could be a necessary cause for this malignancy (Franco et al., 1999a; Walboomers et al., 1999). If this is really the case, then it would be a first in cancer research; no human cancer has yet been shown to have a necessary cause, so clearly identified. Some of the well-studied models in cancer causation, such as tobacco smoking in lung cancer and chronic hepatitis B in liver carcinoma, are among the strongest epidemiologic associations that one can find, but they do not represent causal relations that are necessary. Lung cancers may occur in people who never smoked and had only minimal exposure to environmental tobacco smoke, frequently as a result of exposure to occupation-related carcinogens, and liver cancer may occur in individuals who never had hepatitis B, e.g., via aflatoxin exposure or hepatitis C.

The implications of this finding are substantial and have spawned new approaches to preventing cervical cancer on two fronts: (i) via screening for HPV infection as the biological surrogate that reveals asymptomatic cervical cancer precursor lesions and (ii) via primary immunization against HPV infection to prevent the onset of such precursor lesions. While there is now intense research in these two fronts the debate still continues concerning issues related to the etiologic mechanism whereby HPV infection initiates cervical carcinogenesis. This brief overview addresses the epidemiologic characteristics of HPV infection and cervical cancer and the recent progress using new approaches to preventing cervical cancer.

*The author's research on the epidemiology of HPV infection and prevention of cervical cancer is funded by grants from the Canadian Institutes of Health Research (CIHR) and from the U.S. National Institutes of Health.

Global Importance of Cervical Cancer

Cervical cancer is one of the most common malignant diseases of women. In the US each year there are approximately 12,800 new cases of invasive cervical cancer with 4,600 deaths due to this disease (Ries et al., 2000). On average during the last decade, an estimated 371,000 new cases of invasive cervical carcinoma were diagnosed annually worldwide, representing nearly 10 percent of all female cancers. Its incidence is the third among women, after breast and colorectal cancer (Parkin et al., 1999). The highest risk areas are in Central and South America, Southern and Eastern Africa, and the Caribbean, with average incidence rates around 40 per 100,000 women per year. While risk in western Europe and North America is considered relatively low at less than 10 new cases annually per 100,000 women, rates are 10 times higher in some parts of Northeastern Brazil, where the cumulative lifetime risk can approach 10 percent (Muir et al., 1987).

Every year, an estimated 190,000 deaths from cervical cancer occur worldwide, with over three-fourths of them in developing countries, where mortality from this disease is the highest among deaths caused by neoplasms (Pisani et al., 1999). Less than 50 percent of women affected by cervical cancer in developing countries survive longer than five years whereas the 5-year survival rate in developed countries is about 66 percent (Pisani et al., 1999). Moreover, cervical cancer generally affects multiparous women in the early post-menopausal years. In high-fertility developing countries these women are the primary source of moral values and education for their children. The premature loss of these mothers has important social consequences for the community.

Emergence of HPV Infection as the
Main Etiologic Factor in Cervical Cancer

Prominent among the risk factors for cervical cancer is the role of two measures of sexual activity, namely number of sexual partners and age at first intercourse (Herrero, 1996), and also the sexual behavior of the woman's male partners (Brinton et al., 1989a). The consistency of the sexually-transmitted disease model for cervical neoplasia led much of the laboratory and epidemiologic research in attempting to identify the putative microbial agent or agents acting as etiologic factor. Research conducted during the late 1960s and 1970s attempted to unveil an etiologic role for the Herpes simplex viruses (HSV). Although HSV was proven to be carcinogenic, in vitro and in vivo clinical studies eventually demonstrated that only a fraction of cervical carcinomas contained traces (viral DNA) of HSV infection and epidemiologic studies failed to demonstrate that the association between HSV and cervical cancer was the primary causal element (Franco, 1991).

In the 1980s, a solid research base emerged implicating HPV infection as the sexually-transmitted cause of cervical cancer and its precursors. In 1995, the International Agency for Research on Cancer at the World Health Organization (WHO), in its monograph series of carcinogenicity evaluation classified HPV types 16 and 18 as carcinogenic to humans, HPV types 31 and 33 as probably carcinogenic, and other HPV types (except 6 and 11) as possibly carcinogenic (IARC, 1995). This classification was conservatively made on the basis of the available published evidence until 1994. Subsequent research has permitted a more inclusive grouping of genital HPV types on the basis of the presumed oncogenic potential. HPV types 16, 18, 31, 33, 35, 39, 45, 51, 52, 56, 58, 59, and 68 are considered to be of high oncogenic risk because of their frequent association with cervical cancer and cervical intraepithelial neoplasia (CIN), the precursor, pre-invasive lesion stage. The remaining genital types, e.g., HPV types 6, 11, 42–44, and some rarer types are considered of low or no oncogenic risk (Bosch et al., 1995). The latter types may cause subclinical and clinically visible benign lesions known as flat and acuminate condylomata, respectively.

Today, it is well established that infection with high oncogenic risk HPV types is the central causal factor in cervical cancer (IARC, 1995; Koutsky et al., 1992; Nobbenhuis et al., 1999). Relative risks for the association between HPV and cervical cancer are in the 20–70 range, which is among the strongest statistical relations ever identified in cancer epidemiology. Both retrospective and prospective epidemiologic studies have demonstrated the unequivocally strong association between viral infection and risk of malignancy, both as CIN or invasive disease (Bosch et al., 2002). Table 1-1 shows that HPV infection satisfies nearly all of standard causal criteria in chronic disease epidemiology. However, not all infections with high risk HPVs persist or progress to cervical cancer, thus suggesting that, albeit necessary, HPV infection is not sufficient to induce this disease; other factors, environmental or host-related, are also involved. Among these co-factors are: smoking (Ho et al., 1998a), high parity (Brinton et al., 1989b), use of oral contraceptives (Moreno et al., 2002), diets deficient in vitamins A and C (Potischman and Brinton, 1996), and genetic susceptibility traits, such as specific HLA alleles and haplotypes (Maciag et al., 2000) and polymorphisms in the p53 gene (Makni et al., 2000). Understanding the role of these cofactors is the subject of much ongoing research on the natural history of HPV infection and cervical cancer (see Figure 1-1).

Human Papillomaviruses

HPVs are small, double-stranded DNA viruses of approximately 55 nanometers (nm) with an icosahedral protein capsid containing 72 capsomers. The genome is circular and contains 7500–8000 base pairs (bp). HPVs have the following characteristics:

- ~8 kilobase (kb) DNA virus from Papillomaviridae family
- Species- and tissue-specific

TABLE 1-1 Causality Criteria in HPV and Cervical Cancer

Causal Criterion	Degree of Evidence	Findings
Strength of the association	++	Relative risks among the highest in cancer epidemiology
Consistency	++	Association confirmed in multiple epidemiologic studies
Temporality	+	Infection precedes lesion development
Biological gradient	+	Viral persistence and viral load affect disease risk in dose-dependent manner
Coherence	++	Epidemiology does not conflict with molecular pathogenesis data
Biological plausibility	++	Overwhelming body of evidence from laboratory studies
Experimental evidence	+	HPV vaccination reduces short-term risk of cervical cancer precursor lesions
Necessary factor?	+	HPV DNA found in virtually all cervical cancers

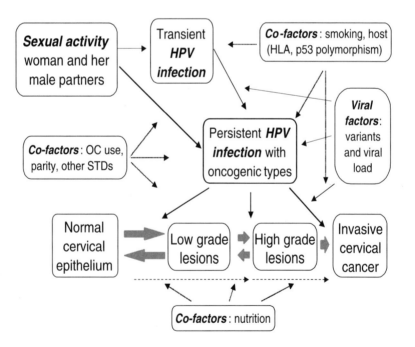

FIGURE 1-1 Etiologic model in cervical carcinogenesis showing the primary role of HPV infection, its relation with sexual activity, and the putative role of cofactors.

- Cannot be cultivated
- Over 150 genotypes identified, of which more than 40 infect the anogenital tract
- High risk (oncogenic) types: 16, 18, 31, 33, 35, 39, 45, 51, 52, 56, 58, 59, 68
- Induces both benign (caused by low risk types) and malignant (caused by high risk types) diseases
- Two major viral oncogenes: E6 (binds to p53) and E7 (binds to retinoblastoma [Rb] protein)

Taxonomically, papillomaviruses used to be a subfamily in the Papovaviridae family but are now grouped independently as a family, the Papillomaviridae. As infectious agents, they are highly specific to their respective hosts. Different HPVs are classified as types on the basis of DNA sequence homology in the E6, E7, and L1 genes. More than 150 different HPV types have been catalogued so far (zur Hausen, 2000).

The epithelial lining of the anogenital tract is the target for infection by over 40 different mucosotropic HPV types. Clinical, subclinical, and latent HPV infections are the most common sexually-transmitted viral diseases today (Cox, 1995). Latent genital HPV infection can be detected in 5 to 40 percent of sexually active women of reproductive age (IARC, 1995). In most cases, genital HPV infection is transient or intermittent (Hildesheim et al., 1994; Ho et al., 1998b; Moscicki et al., 1998; Franco et al., 1999b; Liaw et al., 2001); the prevalence is highest among young women soon after the onset of sexual activity and falls gradually with age, possibly as a reflection of accrued immunity and decrease in sexual activity (meaning a decrease in number of sexual partners).

The carcinogenic mechanism following HPV infection involves the expression of two major viral oncogenes, E6 and E7, which produce proteins that interfere with tumor suppressor genes controlling the cell cycle. Once viral DNA becomes integrated into the host's genome, E6 and E7 become upregulated. While E7 complexes with the cell growth regulator Rb protein, causing an uncontrolled cell proliferation (Chellappan et al., 1992), the binding of E6 to p53 protein promotes the degradation of the latter, thus exempting the deregulated cell to undergo p53-mediated control (Thomas et al., 1996). The degradation of p53 by E6 leads to loss of DNA repair function and prevents the cell from undergoing apoptosis. The infected cell can no longer stop further HPV-related damages and becomes susceptible to additional mutations and genomic instability. Interestingly, the effect of the E6 and E7 proteins on p53 and Rb has been shown to occur only with high-risk HPVs but not with low-risk HPVs (Dyson et al., 1989).

Persistent HPV Infection as the
Precursor Event in Cervical Carcinogenesis

Most women who engage in sexual activity will probably acquire HPV infection over a lifetime. As mentioned above, the vast majority of these infections will be transient with only a small proportion becoming persistent. We have found in our ongoing cohort study of Brazilian women that only 35 percent of the subjects who were infected at enrollment retain their infections after 12 months, with the mean duration being affected by the viral oncogenic potential (see Figure 1-2). Infections with oncogenic HPVs tend to last longer on average (13.5 months) than those with non-oncogenic types (8.2 months) (Franco et al., 1999b). A substantial increase in risk of CIN (see Figure 1-3) and cancer exists for women who develop persistent, long-term infections with oncogenic HPV types (Koutsky et al., 1992; Ho et al., 1998b; Nobbenhuis et al., 1999; Ylitalo et al., 2000; Moscicki et al., 2001; Schlecht et al., 2001).

There is currently great interest in defining persistent infection and in obtaining additional markers of pathogenesis for predictive purposes. Studies of viral load and intratypic variation of HPVs indicate that persistent infections tend to

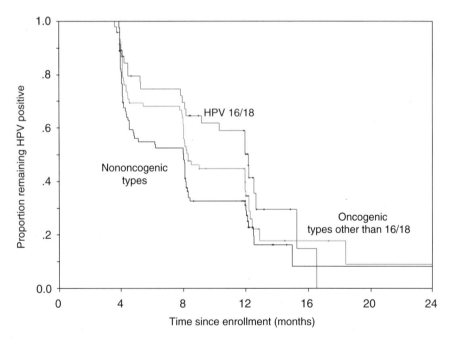

FIGURE 1-2 Actuarial curves showing clearance of prevalent HPV infection according to type present at enrollment in a cohort study of asymptomatic women presenting for cervical cancer screening.
SOURCE: Adapted from Franco et al. (1999b).

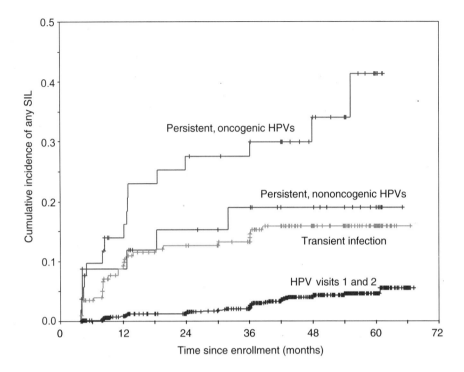

FIGURE 1-3 Actuarial curves showing the cumulative incidence of cervical squamous intraepithelial lesions (SIL) according to HPV infection in the first two visits in a cohort study of asymptomatic women presenting for cervical cancer screening.
SOURCE: Adapted from Schlecht et al. (2001).

yield higher viral loads than transient ones (Caballero et al., 1999) and those with non-European variants of HPVs 16 and 18 tend to be associated with higher risk of CIN as compared with those caused by European variants (Villa et al., 2000).

Defining viral persistence is critical because trials of HPV vaccine efficacy rely on the reduction of the risk of persistent infection as one of the primary outcomes. Similarly, concerning screening of cervical cancer by HPV testing, a main drawback is the low positive predictive value of a single test because of the relatively high prevalence of latent HPV infections in the population, particularly among young women. The predictive value would increase substantially if testing were to rely on repeated samplings, about 6 months apart, because of the aforementioned high prognostic value of persistent positivity. However, population screening cannot rely on repeated testing to be cost-effective and realistic as a public health measure. It would be highly desirable if one could, with a single HPV test, collect enough ancillary information on the virus and on the host that would allow determining whether or not a single instance of HPV positivity is likely to represent a persistent infection.

HPV Testing in Cervical Cancer Screening

Detection of HPV DNA in cervical specimens using a commercially available assay has been shown to have greater sensitivity but somewhat lower specificity to detect CIN and cervical cancer as compared with the conventional Pap cytology (Cuzick et al., 2000). This makes HPV testing a suitable alternative to the latter in screening programs in middle- and high-income countries where centralized laboratory resources are available. The costs associated with an increased number of women to be referred for colposcopy (because of the HPV test's higher false positive rate as compared to cytology) will likely be offset by the increased screening interval that could later be recommended if HPV testing is eventually used to replace cytology screening. The Pap test's low sensitivity forces screening programs to recommend repeat tests frequently to ensure that lesions will not be missed. In the US, fear of malpractice litigation has led to a conservative recommendation of annual Pap smears by many professional groups. Combination testing of Pap cytology and HPV testing has the potential to allow extending screening intervals (for women who are negative in both tests) to as long as 5 years, although this is yet to be proven a safe alternative in long-term follow-up studies.

Primary Prevention by HPV Vaccination

Two main types of HPV vaccines are currently being developed: prophylactic vaccines to prevent HPV infection and associated diseases, and therapeutic vaccines to induce regression of precancerous lesions or remission of advanced cervical cancer. DNA-free virus-like particles (VLP) synthesized by self-assembly of fusion proteins of the major capsid antigen L1 induce a strong humoral response with neutralizing antibodies. VLPs are thus the best candidate immunogen for HPV vaccine trials. Protection seems to be type-specific so that production of VLPs for a variety of high oncogenic risk types will be required. Such vaccines are already under evaluation in safety and efficacy trials in different populations and are sponsored by pharmaceutical companies and by the National Institutes of Health (Schiller, 1999). The preliminary results of one such a trial were extremely promising (Koutsky et al., 2002). It indicated that an HPV 16 VLP vaccine was 100 percent effective in preventing acquisition of persistent infection with HPV 16 and 90 percent effective in preventing any incident HPV 16 infection, transient or persistent. As a noteworthy secondary finding was the fact that all HPV 16-associated CIN cases occurred in the non-vaccinated group. Immunization against HPV may have greatest value in developing countries, where 80 percent of the global burden of cervical cancer occurs each year and where Pap screening programs have been largely ineffective.

Conclusions

During the last 20 years, the concerted effort among virologists, epidemiologists, and clinical researchers has helped to elucidate the role of infection by certain types of HPV as the necessary cause of cervical cancer. This has opened new frontiers for preventing a disease that is responsible for substantial morbidity and mortality, particularly among women living in resource-poor countries. Research on two prevention fronts has already begun in several populations in the form of preliminary trials assessing the efficacy of HPV vaccines and of studies of the value of HPV testing in cervical cancer screening (see Figure 1-4). Progress on both counts is very promising. While the benefits of vaccination against HPV infection as a cervical cancer prevention tool are at least a decade into the future, the potential benefits of HPV testing in screening for this disease can be realized now in most populations.

Primary prevention of cervical cancer can also be achieved through prevention and control of genital HPV infection. Health promotion strategies geared at a change in sexual behavior targeting all sexually-transmitted infections of public health significance can be effective in preventing genital HPV infection (Franco et al., 2001). Although there is consensus that symptomatic HPV infection (genital warts) should be managed via treatment, counseling, and partner notification, active case-finding of asymptomatic HPV infection is currently not recommended

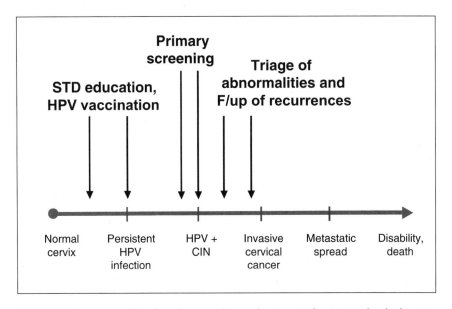

FIGURE 1-4 Opportunities for primary and secondary preventive approaches in the natural history of cervical cancer.

as a control measure. Further research is needed to determine the effectiveness of such a strategy and the significance of such infections concerning a woman's subsequent cancer risk.

Research on HPVs has progressed at a fast pace and has reached a volume of nearly 1,000 annual publications in Medline. The HPV-cervical cancer model has become a paradigm of progress in cancer research and among neoplastic diseases with infectious roots. After 20 years, we have reached the point where preventing cervical cancer via vaccination against HPV infection is in the foreseeable future. It would be disastrous, however, if countries relaxed their cervical cancer screening programs in anticipation of a successful HPV vaccine. Existing cytology-based screening programs that seem to work need to be constantly assessed for quality and coverage. Ongoing research on the efficacy and cost-effectiveness of HPV testing as a mass screening tool will help countries decide on the best approach for secondary prevention of cervical cancer and will probably lead to reduced morbidity and mortality from this disease.

REFERENCES

Bosch FX, Manos MM, Muñoz N, Sherman M, Jansen AM, Peto J, Schiffman MH, Moreno V, Kurman R, Shah KV. 1995. Prevalence of human papillomavirus in cervical cancer: a worldwide perspective. International biological study on cervical cancer (IBSCC) Study Group. *Journal of the National Cancer Institute* 87:796–802.

Bosch FX, Lorincz A, Munoz N, Meijer CJ, Shah KV. 2002. The causal relation between human papillomavirus and cervical cancer. *Journal of Clinical Pathology* 55:244–265.

Brinton LA, Reeves WC, Brenes MM, et al. 1989a. The male factor in the etiology of cervical cancer among sexually monogamous women. *International Journal of Cancer* 44:199–203.

Brinton LA, Reeves WC, Brenes MM, Herrero R, de Britton RC, Gaitan E, Tenorio F, Garcia M, Rawls WE. 1989b. Parity as a risk factor for cervical cancer. *American Journal of Epidemiology* 130:486–496.

Caballero OL, Trevisan A, Villa LL, Ferenczy A, Franco EL. 1999. High viral load is associated with persistent HPV infection and risk of cervical dysplasia. 17th International Papillomavirus Conference, Charleston, SC.

Chellappan S, Kraus VB, Kroger B, Munger K, Howley PM, Phelps WC, Nevins JR. 1992. Adenovirus E1A, simian virus 40 tumor antigen, and human Papillomavirus E7 protein share the capacity to disrupt the interaction between transcription factor E2F and the retinoblastoma gene product. *Proceedings of the National Academy of Sciences* 89:4549–4553.

Cox JT. 1995. Epidemiology of cervical intraepithelial neoplasia: the role of human papillomavirus. *Baillière's clinical obstetrics and gynaecology* 9:1–37.

Cuzick J, Sasieni P, Davies P, Adams J, Normand C, Frater A, van Ballegooijen M, van den Akker-van Marle E. 2000. A systematic review of the role of human papilloma virus (HPV) testing within a cervical screening programme: summary and conclusions. *British Journal of Cancer* 83:561–565.

Dyson N, Howley PM, Munger K, Harlow ED. 1989. The human papilloma virus-16 E7 oncoprotein is able to bind to the retinoblastoma gene product. *Science* 243:934–937.

Franco EL. 1991. Viral etiology of cervical cancer: a critique of the evidence. *Reviews of Infectious Diseases* 13:1195–1206.

Franco EL, Rohan TE, Villa LL. 1999a. Epidemiologic evidence and human papillomavirus infection as a necessary cause of cervical cancer. *Journal of the National Cancer Institute* 91:506–511.

Franco EL, Villa LL, Sobrinho JP, Prado JM, Rousseau MC, Desy M, Rohan TE. 1999b. Epidemiology of acquisition and clearance of cervical human papillomavirus infection in women from a high-risk area for cervical cancer. *The Journal of Infectious Diseases* 180:1415–1423.

Franco EL, Duarte-Franco E, Ferenczy A. 2001. Cervical cancer: epidemiology, prevention, and role of human papillomavirus infection. *Canadian Medical Association Journal* 164:1017–1025.

Herrero R. 1996. Epidemiology of cervical cancer. *Journal of the National Cancer Institute Monographs* 21:1–6.

Hildesheim A, Schiffman MH, Gravitt PE, Glass AG, Greer CE, Zhang T, Scott DR, Rush BB, Lawler P, Sherman ME, et al. 1994. Persistence of type-specific human papillomavirus infection among cytologically normal women. *The Journal of Infectious Diseases* 169:235–240.

Ho GY, Kadish AS, Burk RD, Basu J, Palan PR, Mikhail M, Romney SL. 1998a. HPV 16 and cigarette smoking as risk factors for high-grade cervical intra-epithelial neoplasia. *International Journal of Cancer* 78:281–285.

Ho GY, Bierman R, Beardsley L, Chang CJ, Burk RD. 1998b. Natural history of cervicovaginal papillomavirus infection in young women. *New England Journal of Medicine* 338:423–428.

IARC Working Group. 1995. Human papillomaviruses. IARC Monographs on the evaluation of carcinogenic risks to humans. Vol. 64. Lyon: International Agency for Research on Cancer.

Koutsky LA, Holmes KK, Critchlow CW, Stevens CE, Paavonen J, Beckmann AM, DeRouen TA, Galloway DA, Vernon D, Kiviat NB. 1992. A cohort study of the risk of cervical intraepithelial neoplasia grade 2 or 3 in relation to papillomavirus infection. *New England Journal of Medicine* 327:1272–1278.

Koutsky LA, Ault KA, Wheeler CM, Brown DR, Barr E, Alvarez FB, Chiacchierini LM, Jansen KU. 2002. A controlled trial of a human papillomavirus type 16 vaccine. *New England Journal of Medicine* 347:1645–1651.

Liaw KL, Hildesheim A, Burk RD, Gravitt P, Wacholder S, Manos MM, Scott DR, Sherman ME, Kurman RJ, Glass AG, Anderson SM, Schiffman M. 2001. A prospective study of human papillomavirus (HPV) type 16 DNA detection by polymerase chain reaction and its association with acquisition and persistence of other HPV types. *The Journal of Infectious Diseases* 183:8–15.

Maciag PC, Schlecht NF, Souza PS, Franco EL, Villa LL, Petzl-Erler ML. 2000. Major histocompatibility complex class II polymorphisms and risk of cervical cancer and human papillomavirus infection in Brazilian women. *Cancer Epidemiology, Biomarkers and Prevention* 9:1183–1191.

Makni H, Franco EL, Kaiano J, Villa LL, Labrecque S, Dudley R, Storey A, Matlashewski G. 2000. p53 polymorphism in codon 72 and risk of human papillomavirus-induced cervical cancer: effect of inter-laboratory variation. *International Journal of Cancer* 87:528–533.

Moreno V, Bosch FX, Munoz N, Meijer CJ, Shah KV, Walboomers JM, Herrero R, Franceschi S. 2002. Effect of oral contraceptives on risk of cervical cancer in women with human papillomavirus infection: the IARC multicentric case-control study. *Lancet* 359:1085–1092.

Moscicki AB, Shiboski S, Broering J, Powell K, Clayton L, Jay N, Darragh TM, Brescia R, Kanowitz S, Miller SB, Stone J, Hanson E, Palefsky J. 1998. The natural history of human papillomavirus infection as measured by repeated DNA testing in adolescent and young women. *The Journal of Pediatrics* 132:277–284.

Moscicki AB, Hills N, Shiboski S, Powell K, Jay N, Hanson E, Miller S, Clayton L, Farhat S, Broering J, Darragh T, Palefsky J. 2001. Risks for incident human papillomavirus infection and low-grade squamous intraepithelial lesion development in young females. *Journal of the American Medical Association* 285:2995–3002.

Muir C, Waterhouse J, Mack T, et al. 1987. Cancer incidence in five continents, Vol. V. IARC Scientific Publications No. 88. Lyon: International Agency for Research on Cancer.

Nobbenhuis MA, Walboomers JM, Helmerhorst TJ, Rozendaal L, Remmink AJ, Risse EK, van der Linden HC, Voorhorst FJ, Kenemans P, Meijer CJ. 1999. Relation of human papillomavirus status to cervical lesions and consequences for cervical-cancer screening: a prospective study. *Lancet* 354:20–25.

Parkin DM, Pisani P, Ferlay J. 1999. Estimates of the worldwide incidence of 25 major cancers in 1990. *International Journal of Cancer* 80:827–841.

Pisani P, Parkin DM, Bray F, Ferlay J. 1999. Estimates of the worldwide mortality from 25 cancers in 1990. *International Journal of Cancer* 83:18–29.

Potischman N and Brinton LA. 1996. Nutrition and cervical neoplasia. *Cancer Causes and Control* 7:113–126.

Ries LAG, Eisner MP, Kosary CL, Hankey BF, Miller BA, Clegg L, Edwards BK, eds. 2000. SEER Cancer Statistics Review: 1973-1997. Bethesda, MD: National Cancer Institute.

Schiller JT. 1999. Papillomavirus-like particle vaccines for cervical cancer. *Molecular Medicine Today* 5:209–215.

Schlecht NF, Kulaga S, Robitaille J, Ferreira S, Santos M, Miyamura RA, Duarte-Franco E, Rohan TE, Ferenczy A, Villa LL, Franco EL. 2001. Persistent human papillomavirus infection as a predictor of cervical intraepithelial neoplasia. *Journal of the American Medical Association* 286:3106–3114.

Thomas M, Matlashewski G, Pim D, Banks L. 1996. Induction of apoptosis by p53 is independent of its oligomeric state and can be abolished by HPV-18 E6 through ubiquitin mediated degradation. *Oncogene* 13:265–273.

Villa LL, Sichero L, Rahal P, Caballero O, Ferenczy A, Rohan T, Franco EL. 2000. Molecular variants of human papillomavirus types 16 and 18 preferentially associated with cervical neoplasia. *The Journal of General Virology* 81:2959–2968.

Walboomers JM, Jacobs MV, Manos MM, Bosch FX, Kummer JA, Shah KV, Snijders PJ, Peto J, Meijer CJ, Munoz N. 1999. Human papillomavirus is a necessary cause of invasive cervical cancer worldwide. *The Journal of Pathology* 189:12-9.

Ylitalo N, Josefsson A, Melbye M, Sorensen P, Frisch M, Andersen PK, Sparen P, Gustafsson M, Magnusson P, Ponten J, Gyllensten U, Adami HO. 2000. A prospective study showing long-term infection with human papillomavirus 16 before the development of cervical carcinoma in situ. *Cancer Research* 60:6027–6032.

zur Hausen H. Papillomaviruses causing cancer: evasion from host-cell control in early events in carcinogenesis. 2000. *Journal of the National Cancer Institute* 92:690–698.

CHRONIC HEPATITIS B VIRUS INFECTIONS

William Mason, Ph.D.
Fox Chase Cancer Center, Philadelphia, PA

Human hepatitis B virus (HBV) is a small, enveloped virus, with a partially double-stranded, relaxed circular DNA genome of 3.3 kilobase pairs. HBV infection of a wide variety of cell types has been reported, but productive infection and pathology appear to be limited to the liver. Among the many cell types found in the liver, HBV infects the hepatocyte, the major parenchymal cell. Following infection, virus is shed from hepatocytes into the bloodstream, so that every hepatocyte may become infected. During the peak of an infection, titers of virus in the blood may reach 10^{10} per cubic centimeter. Infection of hepatocytes is not typically cytopathic, and the liver pathology results from the immune response to the infected cells. Depending on the strength of the immune response, infections may be either transient or chronic. Transient infections generally resolve in fewer than 6 months, while chronic infections may be lifelong.

Hepatitis B Virus Replication

HBV replication in the liver occurs by reverse transcription (Seeger and Mason, 2000; Summers and Mason, 1982). When a hepatocyte is infected, the viral DNA genome is transported to the nucleus, where it is converted from a relaxed circular DNA to a covalently closed circular form (cccDNA), which serves as the template for viral mRNA synthesis. Though the coding capacity of HBV is limited, it is still capable of encoding three envelope proteins, a nucleocapsid protein, a transcriptional transactivator, and a reverse transcriptase (RT). Encoding of the reverse transcriptase, the largest HBV protein, requires almost the entire viral genome. (To facilitate this, the reverse transcriptase is encoded in different translational reading frames than the other viral gene products, so that overlapping reading frames can be utilized.) mRNA for the RT is, in fact, slightly greater than genome length, with a terminal redundancy of 220 base pairs (bp). When this mRNA is translated, the RT binds near to the 5′ end of its own message. This RNA/RT complex is then packaged into viral nucleocapsids, where the RT transcribes the RNA into DNA, using one of its own tyrosine resides to prime DNA synthesis (Weber et al., 1994; Zoulim and Seeger, 1994a). Following completion of reverse transcription, the RT then synthesizes most, but not all of the second DNA strand, to recreate the partially double stranded virion DNA. Prior to completion of the second strand, nucleocapsids are packaged into viral envelopes by budding into the endoplasmic reticulum, and virions are exported from the cell. Since cccDNA lacks a replication origin, new cccDNA must be created through the reverse transcription pathway (Tuttleman et al., 1986). Early after infection, and probably after division of an infected hepatocyte, extra cccDNA is synthesized, maintaining the copy number at 5 to 50 per cell. cccDNA appears to be stable in non-dividing hepatocytes (Moraleda et al., 1997), but it is unclear how efficiently cccDNA survives through mitosis.

Transmission

Transmission is parenteral, requiring exposure to the blood or blood-contaminated materials of infected individuals. The most common mode of exposure leading to chronic infection occurs at birth when the mother is chronically infected, or during the first year of life. During this period, the risk of an infection becoming chronic is at least 90 percent. In contrast, the risk of chronic infection in adults is greater than 10 percent. According to the CDC, the most common exposure risks in adults in the United States are sexual activity (50 percent of cases) and intravenous drug abuse (15 percent of cases).

Public Health Issues

Prevalence

The case fatality rate in adults due to acute hepatitis is about 1 percent. Individuals with chronic infection, typically acquired in childhood, have a ~25 percent risk of premature death due to either liver cancer or cirrhosis, both resulting from the persistent liver damage associated with infection. According to WHO, there are now 350 million chronically infected individuals worldwide. Of these, 60 million are expected to die prematurely of liver cancer or cirrhosis, at a rate of approximately 1 million per year (5,000 per year in the United States). This does not account for new cases, which will continue to accumulate in the coming decades.

Vaccines

A vaccine comprised of the viral envelope proteins has been available for over 20 years. Due in part to high cost, universal vaccination was not initially feasible in many parts of the world, but lower cost vaccines have subsequently come into use. Universal vaccination of school children is now in effect in the United States. In some parts of the world, especially in Africa and regions of Asia, chronic infection rates exceed 5–10 percent of the population, but vaccination has not yet been economically feasible in all of these areas, even with low-cost vaccines. Although attempts are under way to address this problem (Kane, 2003), for various reasons of cost and delivery, HBV is likely to remain a major public health problem. On top of this problem there is evidence for vaccine escape mutants (He et al., 2001; Torresi et al., 2002; Wilson et al., 2000). Though these do not yet seem to be a major public health problem, they remain a concern even for the large pool of individuals that have already received the current vaccine. In addition, about 5 percent of vaccinated individuals fail to produce a measurable antibody response, suggesting that they also remain at risk for HBV infection.

Current Research

A major goal of current research has thus been the development of therapies to cure chronically infected individuals. A problem in achieving this is that hepatocytes comprise a self-renewing population with a low turnover rate, and this population often appears to be 100 percent infected. This same barrier is confronted and overcome during immune clearance of transient infections, though it remains controversial how the virus is actually destroyed (Guidotti et al. 1999; Guo et al., 2000; Jilbert et al., 1992; Kajino et al., 1994; Thimme et al., 2003). However, in chronic carriers, the immune system is usually unable to mount such a response, especially in those infected as children. Some hope for better immunotherapies has however been sustained by the fact that interferon alpha administration induces virus loss in about 20–30 percent of carriers (Hoofnagle and Lau, 1997), typically those with adult-acquired infections. In addition, some carriers experience spontaneous loss of the virus in association with a flare of liver disease. In both instances, clearance is probably due to activation of the same set of immune responses that are active in clearance of transient infections. Key issues now are how this clearance is carried out, whether it requires destruction of all of the infected hepatocytes, if the immune system has the capacity to cure an infected hepatocyte, and if it can be induced in carriers that have failed to respond to interferon therapy with virus clearance.

Treatment

Another approach to treatment of chronic infections is administration of nucleoside analog inhibitors of the HBV reverse transcriptase. Lamivudine was approved by the U.S. Food and Drug Administration (FDA) in 1998 and has been shown in clinical trials to have a treatment success rate similar to interferon alpha (Perrillo, 2002). A significant problem with lamivudine is the emergence of drug-resistant variants of HBV as therapy continues past a year. Another nucleoside, adefovir dipivoxil, recently received FDA approval and to date drug-resistant variants have not been reported. Moreover, this drug retains activity against lamivudine-resistant HBV (Delaney et al., 2001). However, at doses higher than used for HBV carriers, nephrotoxicity has been observed (Tanji et al., 2001). It may be that nephrotoxicity will become a problem in HBV therapy due to a cumulative effect if carriers require treatment indefinitely. A number of other nucleoside analogs are now in Phase II trials. If these compounds are not toxic during long-term administration, and if viral multi-drug resistance does not develop, it should be possible to eliminate over time the viral cccDNA that maintains a cellular infection by a combination of dilution and hepatocyte death. Achieving this would also allow a critical test of the hypothesis that curing a chronic infection would significantly reduce the risk of death due to cirrhosis, which seems likely, and due to liver cancer, which is difficult to predict, because liver cancer may occur in a liver that appears relatively healthy histologically.

Research Models

HBV research generally reflects public health concerns. How can chronic infections be cured? Will eliminating the virus reduce the risk of liver cancer and premature death from liver disease? What is the mechanism of carcinogenesis? (It is speculated that immune-mediated chronic injury, insertional mutagenesis, and viral proteins all may play a role.) These questions have been investigated using clinical samples and a number of model systems.

Woodchucks are naturally infected with woodchuck hepatitis virus (WHV)

(Summers et al., 1978), which is closely related to HBV and, like HBV, induces liver cancer (but not cirrhosis) during a chronic infection (Popper et al., 1987). Similarly, domestic ducks are infected with duck hepatitis B virus (DHBV), a more distant relative of HBV (Mason et al., 1980; Zhou, 1980). Unlike HBV and WHV, chronic DHBV infection has not been associated with either cirrhosis or liver cancer, possibly because of a lower antiviral immune response in carriers. HBV transgenic mice have been powerful tools for studying certain aspects of the antiviral immune response (Guidotti and Chisari, 2001), even though these mice do not support a complete HBV infection cycle (Tang and McLachlan, 2002). On occasion, chimpanzees, which are susceptible to HBV, have been used to address research issues (Guidotti et al., 1999; Thimme et al., 2003).

Among the model systems, the duck has been heavily used to understand the virus life cycle at the molecular level, to study the biology of infection, and to characterize antiviral therapies, primarily with nucleoside analogs. The woodchuck model has been less used to study molecular biology issues, but has been employed extensively in the development of antiviral therapies and in characterization of the link between chronic infection and liver cancer. An unresolved issue arose in the latter studies. It was found that liver cancer in woodchucks is almost always associated with transcriptional activation of N-myc2 expression in the liver by insertion of viral enhancer sequences (Fourel et al., 1994; Wei et al., 1992). Contrary to expectation, insertional activation of N-myc2 does not appear to be a correlate of liver cancer in HBV carriers. Indeed, with a few rare exceptions, it remains unclear if the frequent sporadic integration of viral DNA that characterizes an infection has a role in most liver cancers that occur in individuals chronically infected with HBV (Dejean et al., 1986; Gozuacik et al., 2001).

The HBV transgenic mouse, in contrast to the natural infection models, has been most heavily used to demonstrate the effects of immune cytokines, such as interferons alpha and gamma, on viral replication intermediates. It was found that cytokines can induce the rapid clearance of viral proteins, RNAs, and DNAs from mouse hepatocytes (Guidotti and Chisari, 2001). These observations seem likely to provide part of the explanation for how virus replication is shut down during the clearance of transient HBV infections.

Though the relationship to natural infections is still unclear, a number of studies have shown that mice carrying the HBV transcriptional activator, X, as a transgene, are at increased risk of developing liver cancer (Kim et al., 1991; Madden et al., 2001; Terradillos et al., 1997). These data suggest that X is in fact a viral oncogene, but clinical evidence to support this conclusion is still lacking, and it is difficult to address this issue in the woodchuck model, because X is needed to establish a productive infection (Chen et al., 1993; Zoulim and Seeger, 1994b).

In addition to characterizing infections and therapies, the animal models have also provided, along with clinical studies, a better understanding of the difficulties of treating chronic infections with nucleoside analogs. From such studies, it has been determined that cccDNA can persist in the liver for months, and probably years, even when virus DNA synthesis is effectively inhibited (Colonno et al., 2001; Foster et al., 2003; Luscombe et al., 1996; Mason et al., 1994; Zhu et al., 2001). Persistence of cccDNA may be attributable to two factors: 1) an inherent stability within non-dividing hepatocytes, and 2) the relatively low turnover (perhaps a few percent per day) of hepatocytes in most carriers. Studies with animal models have also established that the mutation rate of the viruses is quite high, with a single-base mutation prevalence of about 10^{-4} (Pult et al., 2001). Thus, drug-resistant variants, especially those requiring only one or two base changes, are likely to be present at the start of therapy. The primary factors needed for subsequent emergence of drug-resistant variants are the time required for the hepatocyte population to become susceptible to spread of virus (e.g., for loss of super-infection resistance), the prevalence of a drug-resistant virus at the start of therapy, and its growth rate (Zhang and Summers, 2000). In practice, emergence of mutants can take from months to several years, the variation probably reflecting additional factors, including the effect of nucleoside therapy on the antiviral immune response of the host (Boni et al., 2001).

Outlook

Discovery of an effective HBV vaccine in the 1960s (Blumberg, 1977) led to the hope that HBV would be eliminated, or at least substantially reduced in the human population within the then foreseeable future. This still remains mostly a hope. Two objectives still need to be fulfilled, universal vaccination (Kane, 2003), and development of an effective therapy for chronic infection. Even though not everyone will be protected using the current vaccine, most would be, and the carrier incidence should decline substantially, first among the young. The goal of complete elimination seems unlikely without major advances in the treatment and elimination of chronic infections, particularly treatments that are rapid acting and cost-effective.

REFERENCES

Blumberg BS. 1977. Australia antigen and the biology of hepatitis B. *Science* 197:17–25.
Boni C, Penna A, Ogg GS, Bertoletti A, Pilli M, Cavallo C, Cavalli A, Urbani S, Boehme R, Panebianco R, Fiaccadori F, Ferrari C. 2001. Lamivudine treatment can overcome cytotoxic T-cell hyporesponsiveness in chronic hepatitis B: new perspectives for immune therapy. *Hepatology* 33:963–971.
Chen HS, Kaneko S, Girones R, Anderson RW, Hornbuckle WE, Tennant BC, Cote PJ, Gerin JL, Purcell RH, Miller RH. 1993. The woodchuck hepatitis virus X gene is important for establishment of virus infection in woodchucks. *Journal of Virology* 67:1218–1226.
Colonno RJ, Genovesi EV, Medina I, Lamb L, Durham SK, Huang ML, Corey L, Littlejohn M, Locarnini S, Tennant BC, Rose B, Clark JM. 2001. Long-term entecavir treatment results in sustained antiviral efficacy and prolonged life span in the woodchuck model of chronic hepatitis infection. *The Journal of Infectious Diseases* 184:1236–1245.

Dejean A, Bougueleret L, Grzeschik KH, Tiollais P. 1986. Hepatitis B virus DNA integration in a sequence homologous to v-erb-A and steroid receptor genes in a hepatocellular carcinoma. *Nature* 322:70–72.

Delaney WE, Edwards R, Colledge D, Shaw T, Torresi J, Miller TG, Isom HC, Bock CT, Manns MP, Trautwein C, Locarnini S. 2001. Cross-resistance testing of antihepadnaviral compounds using novel recombinant baculoviruses which encode drug-resistant strains of hepatitis B virus. *Antimicrobial Agents and Chemotherapy* 45:1705–1713.

Foster WK, Miller DS, Marion PL, Colonno RJ, Kotlarski I, Jilbert AR. 2003. Entecavir therapy combined with DNA vaccination for persistent duck hepatitis B virus infection. *Antimicrobial Agents and Chemotherapy* 47:2624–2635.

Fourel G, Couturier J, Wei Y, Apiou F, Tiollais P, Buendia MA. 1994. Evidence for long-range oncogene activation by hepadnavirus insertion. *The European Molecular Biology Organization Journal* 13:2526–2534.

Gozuacik D, Murakami Y, Saigo K, Chami M, Mugnier C, Lagorce D, Okanoue T, Urashima T, Brechot C, Paterlini-Brechot P. 2001. Identification of human cancer-related genes by naturally occurring Hepatitis B Virus DNA tagging. *Oncogene* 20:6233–6240.

Guidotti LG and Chisari FV. 2001. Noncytolytic control of viral infections by the innate and adaptive immune response. *Annual Review of Immunology* 19:65–91.

Guidotti LG, Rochford R, Chung J, Shapiro M, Purcell R, Chisari FV. 1999. Viral clearance without destruction of infected cells during acute HBV infection. *Science* 284:825–829.

Guo JT, Zhou H, Liu C, Aldrich C, Saputelli J, Whitaker T, Barrasa MI, Mason WS, Seeger C. 2000. Apoptosis and regeneration of hepatocytes during recovery from transient hepadnavirus infections. *Journal of Virology* 74:1495–1505.

He C, Nomura F, Itoga S, Isobe K, Nakai T. 2001. Prevalence of vaccine-induced escape mutants of hepatitis B virus in the adult population in China: a prospective study in 176 restaurant employees. *Journal of Gastroenterology and Hepatology* 16:1373–1377.

Hoofnagle JH and Lau D. 1997. New therapies for chronic hepatitis B. *Journal of Viral Hepatitis* 4:41–50.

Jilbert AR, Wu TT, England JM, Hall PM, Carp NZ, O'Connell AP, Mason WS. 1992. Rapid resolution of duck hepatitis B virus infections occurs after massive hepatocellular involvement. *Journal of Virology* 66:1377–1388.

Kajino, K., A. R. Jilbert, J. Saputelli, C. E. Aldrich, J. Cullen, and W. S. Mason. 1994. Woodchuck hepatitis virus infections: very rapid recovery after a prolonged viremia and infection of virtually every hepatocyte. *Journal of Virology* 68:5792–5803.

Kane MA. 2003. Global control of primary hepatocellular carcinoma with hepatitis B vaccine: The contributions of research in Taiwan. *Cancer Epidemiology, Biomarkers & Prevention* 12:2–3.

Kim CM, Koike K, Saito I, Miyamura T, Jay G. 1991. HBx gene of hepatitis B virus induces liver cancer in transgenic mice. *Nature* 351:317–320.

Luscombe C, Pedersen J, Uren E, Locarnini S. 1996. Long-term ganciclovir chemotherapy for congenital duck hepatitis B virus infection in vivo: Effect on intrahepatic-viral DNA, RNA, and protein expression. *Hepatology* 24:766–773.

Madden CR, Finegold MJ, Slagle BL. 2001. Hepatitis B virus X protein acts as a tumor promoter in development of diethylnitrosamine-induced preneoplastic lesions. *Journal of Virology* 75:3851–3858.

Mason WS, Seal G, Summers J. 1980. Virus of Pekin ducks with structural and biological relatedness to human hepatitis B virus. *Journal of Virology* 36:829–836.

Mason WS, Cullen J, Saputelli J, Wu TT, Liu C, London WT, E Lustbader, Schaffer P, O'Connell AP, Fourel I, Aldrich CE, Jilbert AR. 1994. Characterization of the antiviral effects of 2′ carbodeoxyguanosine in ducks chronically infected with duck hepatitis B virus. *Hepatology* 19:398–411.

Moraleda G, Saputelli J, Aldrich CE, Averett D, Condreay L, Mason WS. 1997. Lack of effect of antiviral therapy in nondividing hepatocyte cultures on the closed circular DNA of woodchuck hepatitis virus. *Journal of Virology* 71:9392–9399.

Perrillo RP. 2002. How will we use the new antiviral agents for hepatitis B? *Current Gastroenterology Reports* 4:63–71.

Popper H, Roth L, Purcell RH, Tennant BC, Gerin JL. 1987. Hepatocarcinogenicity of the woodchuck hepatitis virus. *Proceedings of the National Academy of Sciences* 84:866–870.

Pult I, Abbott N, Zhang YY, Summers JW. 2001. Frequency of spontaneous mutations in an avian hepadnavirus infection. *Journal of Virology* 75:9623–9632.

Seeger C and Mason WS. 2000. Hepatitis B virus biology. *Microbiology and Molecular Biology Reviews* 54:51–68.

Summers J and Mason WS. 1982. Replication of the genome of a hepatitis B-like virus by reverse transcription of an RNA intermediate. *Cell* 29:403–415.

Summers J, Smolec JM, Snyder R. 1978. A virus similar to human hepatitis B virus associated with hepatitis and hepatoma in woodchucks. *Proceedings of the National Academy of Sciences* 75:4533–4537.

Tang H and McLachlan A. 2002. Avian and mammalian hepadnaviruses have distinct transcription factor requirements for viral replication. *Journal of Virology* 76:7468–7472.

Tanji N, Tanji K, Kambham N, Markowitz GS, Bell A, D'Agati VD. 2001. Adefovir nephrotoxicity: possible role of mitochondrial DNA depletion. *Human Pathology* 32:734–740.

Terradillos O, Billet O, Renard CA, Levy R, Molina T, Briand P, Buendia MA. 1997. The hepatitis B virus X gene potentiates c-myc-induced liver oncogenesis in transgenic mice. *Oncogene* 14:395–404.

Thimme R, Wieland S, Steiger C, Ghrayeb J, Reimann KA, Purcell RH, Chisari FV. 2003. CD8(+) T cells mediate viral clearance and disease pathogenesis during acute hepatitis B virus infection. *Journal of Virology* 77:68–76.

Torresi J, Earnest-Silveira L, Civitico G, Walters TE, Lewin SR, Fyfe J, Locarnini SA, Manns M, Trautwein C, Bock TC. 2002. Restoration of replication phenotype of lamivudine-resistant hepatitis B virus mutants by compensatory changes in the "fingers" subdomain of the viral polymerase selected as a consequence of mutations in the overlapping S gene. *Virology* 299:88–99.

Tuttleman JS, Pourcel C, Summers J. 1986. Formation of the pool of covalently closed circular viral DNA in hepadnavirus-infected cells. *Cell* 47:451–460.

Weber M, Bronsema V, Bartos H, Bosserhoff A, Bartenschlager R, Schaller H. 1994. Hepadnavirus P protein utilizes a tyrosine residue in the TP domain to prime reverse transcription. *Journal of Virology* 68:2994–2999.

Wei Y, Fourel G, Ponzetto A, Silvestro M, Tiollais P, Buendia MA. 1992. Hepadnavirus integration: mechanisms of activation of the N-myc2 retrotransposon in woodchuck liver tumors. *Journal of Virology* 66:5265–5276.

Wilson JN, Nokes DJ, Carman WF. 2000. Predictions of the emergence of vaccine-resistant hepatitis B in The Gambia using a mathematical model. *Epidemiology and Infection* 124:295–307.

Zhang YY and Summers J. 2000. Low dynamic state of a viral competition in a chronic avian hepadnavirus infection. *Journal of Virology* 74:5257–5265.

Zhou YZ. 1980. A virus possibly associated with hepatitis and hepatoma in ducks. *Shanghai Medical Journal* 3:641–644.

Zhu Y, Yamamoto T, Cullen J, Saputelli J, Aldrich CE, Miller DS, Litwin S, Furman PA, Jilbert AR, Mason WS. 2001. Kinetics of hepadnavirus loss from the liver during inhibition of viral DNA synthesis. *Journal of Virology* 75:311–322.

Zoulim F and Seeger C. 1994a. Reverse transcription in hepatitis B viruses is primed by a tyrosine residue of the polymerase. *Journal of Virology* 68:6–13.

Zoulim F and Seeger C. 1994b. Woodchuck hepatitis virus X protein is required for viral infection in vivo. *Journal of Virology* 68:2026–2030.

INFECTIOUS AGENTS AND CARDIOVASCULAR DISEASE

Michael Dunne, M.D.
Pfizer Global Research and Development, New London, CT

Atherosclerosis remains the most significant threat to the health of individuals living in the United States and Europe. Myocardial infarctions, strokes, peripheral vascular disease and premature deaths constitute an enormous burden on the healthcare systems of these regions every year. Risk factors for atherosclerosis have been identified and interventions targeting these risks have helped mitigate its impact. The clinical sequelae of atherosclerosis remain significant, however, justifying continued research efforts to enhance the value of available interventions as well as identify presently unappreciated risk factors.

Examination of an atherosclerotic plaque reveals pools of cholesterol under a fibrous cap and the infiltration of monocytes and T cells at its margins. This concentration of white blood cells within the plaque is consistent with an ongoing inflammatory process, influenced by factors not yet fully understood. One such influence may be infection.

That infection may play a role in atherosclerosis was first suggested over one hundred years ago with the finding that acute infection with *Bacillus typhosus* resulted in fatty sclerotic changes in the arterial wall (Gilbert and Lion, 1889; Nieto, 1998). Interest in the role of infection in atherosclerosis was renewed with the observation that patients with coronary artery disease were more likely than matched controls to have an elevated antibody titer to *Chlamydia pneumoniae* (Saikku et al., 1988). Since that observation, a number of additional associations have been identified. The chain of events linking infections to the development of atherosclerosis is outlined in Figure 1-5. A local infection may lead to an arterial response through two different routes. First, local infection may trigger the systemic release of various proinflammatory mediators, including cytokines, bacterial lipopolysaccharide, heat shock proteins, immune complexes and, possibly, activated, but uninfected, mononuclear cells. These mediators move through the systemic circulation and incite an immune response in the arterial wall. This response may include the upregulation of receptors on the endothelial cell surface, enhancement of transendothelial migration of inflammatory cells, or activation of white blood cells already existing within the plaque. These activated WBCs may oxidize LDL cholesterol or release proteinases, which then act to destabilize the overlying fibrous cap of the atheroma.

The second route by which infection may result in progression or initiation of an atherosclerotic lesion involves the dissemination of organisms from local sites of infection directly to the arterial wall itself. The organisms may traffic to the site within an infected monocyte, attach and then diapedese through the endothelial cell layer, taking advantage of secondary host defense mechanisms to

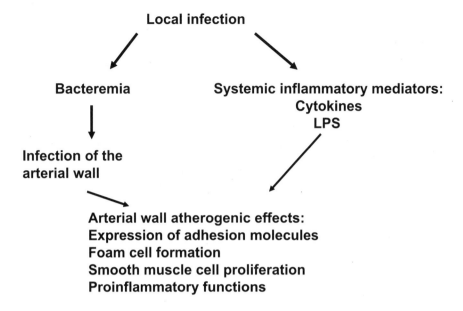

FIGURE 1-5 Pathways through which local infection can lead to atherogenesis.

infect distal tissue. Once at the site, the organisms could drive a local inflammatory process or, in addition, infect other cells within the arterial wall.

A number of potential pathogens have been associated with atherosclerosis (Danesh, 1999). The strength of the association varies with the organism but is based on seroepidemiologic studies, histopathologic evidence of disease, animal model data and various pathophysiologic associations. Among possible viral pathogens are cytomegalovirus and herpes simplex (Nieto, 1999; Dunne, 2000). Among bacterial pathogens are various dental organisms, *Helicobacter pylori*, and *Mycoplasma pneumoniae*. The most significant amount of preclinical and clinical investigation, however, has focused on *C. pneumoniae*; as an example of the types of evidence that can implicate a potential infectious pathogen driving some component of the atherosclerotic process, these data will be reviewed in more detail.

C. Pneumoniae and Atherosclerosis Seroepidemiologic Studies

Since the initial study that identified an association between elevated *C. pneumoniae* antibody titers and the prevalence of coronary artery disease, over thirty additional studies have been performed and multiple review articles published. These studies used different antibody detection assays with different titer cutoffs, different case definitions of coronary artery disease, and were performed in different geographic regions. Overall, it appears that elevated antibody titers to *C. pneumoniae* are associated with a three-fold increase in the likelihood of having coronary artery disease. The association identified in seroepidemiologic studies using titers to predict the incidence, distinct from the prevalence, of heart disease, however, only variably detect an association and, when positive, only in the range of a 20–40 percent increased risk (Dunne, 2000). While the implications of these different findings are being evaluated, the main value of these seroepidemiologic studies may be the attention they have brought to the potential for any association at all.

Histopathology

The next series of studies involve histopathologic examinations of the atheromatous plaque. In the first 15 studies reported in the literature which were conducted in the United States and Europe, approximately 45 percent of the total of 574 samples examined were found to contain evidence of *C. pneumoniae* by either immunohistochemistry, electron microscopy, *in situ* polymerase chain reaction (PCR) or, rarely, culture. The primary criticism of these studies has focused on the lack of standardization of the assay techniques but, given the bulk of the observations from these and subsequent studies, it seems likely that this pathogen can be found in the plaque.

Because antibody titers merely suggest historical exposure to the pathogen, there has been recent interest in the use of PCR to identify individuals that may have an active infection with *C. pneumoniae*. PCR has been used to assess both histopathologic specimens and circulating white blood cells. In four published papers, patients with a history of coronary artery disease were more likely than controls to have *C. pneumoniae* identified in circulating monocytes by PCR (Dunne, 2000). In a fifth paper, the incidence was not significantly different but the *C. pneumoniae* rRNA copy number was higher in patients with heart disease (Berger et al., 2000). Of interest, the proportion of individuals with PCR positive cells in these studies ranged from 9 to 60 percent in the patients with heart disease and 2 to 46 percent in the controls. While this range of exposure may be explained by epidemiologic influences, technical concerns about assay methodologies remain and efforts at standardization have been initiated (Dowell et al., 2001). When the technical concerns have been addressed, it will also be important to understand why otherwise normal individuals have evidence of this pathogen circulating in what should be a sterile space.

Animal Models

In addition to serologic and histologic evidence associating *C. pneumoniae* and atherosclerosis, a number of animal models have been established. Evidence that *C. pneumoniae* can either initiate or accelerate the atherosclerotic lesion has come from work with both mice (NIH/s, ApoE-deficient, and LDL-receptor knock-out strains) and New Zealand White rabbits. These animals generally need to consume a high cholesterol diet in order to develop observable changes, though it is possible, in one of the rabbit models, to observe effects without an atherogenic diet (Fong et al., 1999). In the LDL receptor knockout mouse, intranasal inoculation with the *C. pneumoniae* AR39 strain twice monthly for six months was performed prior to sacrifice of the animals. Uninfected mice fed a high cholesterol diet had a lesion area index (defined as the size of a digitized image of the lesion divided by the aorta luminal surface and multiplied by one hundred) of 18, while infected animals given a high cholesterol diet had an index of 42. This 130 percent increase in lesion size suggests that infection with chlamydia can accelerate the growth of an atherosclerotic plaque (Hu et al., 1999).

There are limitations to the interpretation of animal models of atherosclerosis. In some of these models the atherosclerotic lesions observed are consistent with a very early pathologic process that does not mirror the lesions responsible for causing human disease. The atherosclerotic lesions in these models generally do not rupture or lead to clinical disease in the animal. While these data do support the potential for a contribution of chlamydia to lipid accumulation at the site, they do not provide conclusive evidence that infection will lead to plaque rupture.

Chlamydia Pathogenesis and Atherogenesis

A fourth line of persuasive evidence comes from similarities in the pathophysiology of *C. pneumoniae* infection and atherogenesis. The generation of an atherosclerotic plaque is generally felt to be a chronic process. To the extent that a chlamydia infection, in addition to any acute effects, has a chronic component to its pathophysiology, an association with atherosclerosis can be more easily defended. The demonstration that chlamydia may exist in a persistent state may serve to explain the latent nature of a chlamydia infection.

Chlamydia exists as elementary bodies in the environment. Upon entry into a host cell the elementary body undergoes a series of transformations that allow it ultimately to replicate. At this stage it is referred to as a reticulate body. After cell division, it again reverts to an elementary body and is released from the host cell. If, however, host cell conditions are not favorable, chlamydia will not progress through cell division and instead moves into what has been referred to as a persistent state, appearing morphologically as a large, aberrant form (Beatty et al., 1994). The organism has been found to persist in cell culture in this state for prolonged periods of time and, in vitro, to be relatively refractory to antibiotic therapy.

While evidence for a persistent state has not been established in clinical specimens, it remains possible that chlamydia could contribute to a chronic condition by remaining relatively dormant, while still influencing the condition of the host cell. A series of experiments (Zhong et al., 1999; 2000), has offered some insights as to why a chronically infected host cell is not destroyed by the immune system. It appears that chlamydia can selectively inhibit IFN-gamma-inducible MHC class I and II expression and thereby evade antigen presentation on the cell surface. Inhibition of this process by bacterial protein synthesis inhibitors such as chloramphenicol suggests that it is dependent on chlamydial protein synthesis.

Clinically latent infections have been demonstrated with a number of chlamydia species. The blinding eye disease trachoma has occurred decades after exposure to either *C. trachomatis* or *C. pneumoniae*. Infertility can result from chronic infection of the upper genital tract with *C. trachomatis*, a process that can take place over years. *C. pneumoniae* has also been isolated from the respiratory tract long after resolution of an acute infection.

Atherosclerosis is now considered to be an inflammatory disease (Ross, 1999). The association of *C. pneumoniae* with atherogenesis is supported by the possibility that *C. pneumoniae* contributes to this inflammation. Based on data from animal models, and supported by the PCR examinations of circulating white blood cells and histologic examinations of atherosclerotic tissue, a respiratory tract infection could lead to dissemination of *C. pneumoniae* in monocytes. These monocytes release factors that enhance the likelihood of endothelial infection with chlamydia (Lin et al., 2000). Once infected, the endothelial cells could affect the local arterial environment in three ways. Transendothelial migration of the monocytes is enhanced (Molestina et al., 1999). The infected endothelial cells release tissue factor and platelet aggregation inhibitor, which leads to enhanced coagulability at the site. And thirdly, mitogenic factors are released through an NF-Kβ related mechanism, leading to smooth muscle cell proliferation (Miller et al., 2000). This triad, subendothelial monocyte accumulation, hypercoagulability at the site of the atheroma and smooth muscle cell proliferation, is the hallmark of an atherosclerotic plaque and, as such, provides further support for a contribution of local *C. pneumoniae* infection to this inflammatory state.

Clinical Trials with Antibiotics

Even with continued gaps in our understanding of the association between infection and atherosclerosis, the significance of coronary artery disease as an unmet medical need has driven interest in conducting antibiotic intervention studies. Based on the various supportive data discussed thus far, a number of clinical trials designed to investigate the role of antibiotic intervention in reducing the incidence of atherosclerotic disease have been initiated. There is certainly more work that needs to be done preclinically, including additional studies outlining the role of *C. pneumoniae* in atherogenesis, improving the capabilities around diagnostic testing, understanding the influence of antibiotics, alone or in combination, on chlamydia replication, further exploring animal models of in vivo pathogenesis, and better defining the lifecycle of chlamydia, and specifically the persistent state.

There are a number of challenges to studying the use of antibiotics in clinical coronary artery disease. While several risk factors for coronary artery disease are already well established, the relationship between these risk factors and *C. pneumoniae* infection has not been fully examined. As such associations become better known, the use of these risk factors as selection criteria may become useful. Clinical studies will need to address this problem of multiple competing risks even while the appropriateness of controlling for these factors in any statistical analyses, or selecting the target group of patients to treat, remains open to debate.

Many questions remain regarding antimicrobial activity within the plaque. While there is clinical evidence that patients with either genitourinary tract or respiratory tract infections due to chlamydia can have the clinical course of their disease positively impacted by antibiotic intervention, it remains unknown whether antibiotic treatment will affect either the replication or pathogenicity of chlamydia infections in the atherosclerotic plaque. It may not be possible to either document infection at the arterial site or substantiate a positive microbiologic outcome. There remain concerns that to the extent that cells contain chlamydia in the persistent state, it may not be possible to fully eradicate the organism. Standard in vitro testing may be inadequate to fully address this issue, given that the contribution of the immune system to clearance of infected cells is not measured.

Specific concerns about the design of clinical trials also exist. The appropriate patient population to treat is not clear. If *C. pneumoniae* is the target organism, patient selection criteria specific to the organism could be useful. Antibody titers are a crude estimate of previous exposure but may not be adequate to select those patients actively infected. As identification of infection within the atheroma is not presently possible, surrogates of active infection are needed. Perhaps, in the future, there will be a role for the measurement of *C. pneumoniae* DNA in circulating white blood cells. As is typical with cardiovascular studies of coronary artery disease, the event rates are typically low. Selection of patients likely to have a primary event is critical to ensuring that any treatment effect can be observed. Setting the sample size is made difficult by not having any estimate of the potential treatment effects; in order to avoid missing a potential effect, efficacy rates may need to be assumed to be low. These two issues require that definitive studies be large in order to have sufficient statistical power to determine treatment effects. Interpretation of the results from smaller studies is consequently more problematic.

The results of ongoing clinical trials will be best able to answer questions that are focused on the merits of the antibiotic intervention in the specific population of patients enrolled, and focused on the prespecified endpoints. The results will be compelling to the extent that the studies are adequately powered and the chosen endpoints are clinically relevant. The ongoing trials are less likely to be able to define the mechanism of action underlying any observed treatment effect.

Pre- and post-treatment measurement of such inflammatory indices as C-reactive protein, cytokines, fibrinogen and tissue factor could be performed, but determining whether any changes are a direct result of immune specific activity or an indirect result of reducing the burden of organisms may be problematic.

A number of antibiotic intervention studies have been initiated. The antibiotics used have been either macrolides, doxycycline or a fluoroquinolone, given the in vitro activity of classes of drugs against *C. pneumoniae*. Of the completed studies, the two earliest reported promising results, both with short-term therapies, but the small sample size of these trials precludes any definitive conclusions (see Table 1-2). In general, the trial design has varied such that no two are the same. They have focused on primary or secondary prevention, different antibiotic

TABLE 1-2 Clinical Trials with Antibiotics for Primary and Secondary Prevention of Atherosclerosis Diseases

Study	Population	N	Antibiotic	Endpoint	Outcome
St. George's (Gupta et al., 1997)	Post-MI	80	Azithromycin	Heart Disease[a]	Event rate: 8% vs. 28%
ROXIS (Gurfinkel et al., 1997)	CAD	200	Roxithromycin	Heart Disease[a]	Event rate: 1% vs. 10%
CROAATS (Reiner, 2002)	Post-MI	234	Azithromycin	Heart Disease[a]	Event rate: 7.0% vs. 5.2%
ACADEMIC (Anderson et al., 1999)	CAD	300	Azithromycin	Heart Disease[a]	Hazard ratio: 0.89 (0.51, 1.61)
ANTIBIO (Zahn et al., 2003)	Acute MI	892	Roxithromycin	Heart Disease[a]	Event rate: 25% vs. 21%
ISAR-3 (Neumann et al., 2001)	Angioplasty	1010	Roxithromycin	Restenosis	Hazard ratio: 1.08 (0.92, 1.26)
Macrolide for PAD (Wiesli et al., 2002)	Peripheral artery disease	40	Roxithromycin	Interventions for claudication	Event rate: 20% vs. 45%

[a]Some combination of either recurrent MI, hospitalization for angina, coronary artery intervention, stroke, or death.

interventions, different durations of therapy, different cardiovascular endpoints and different manifestations of atherosclerosis at baseline. This variability in study design is a consequence of many of the issues noted above and is to be expected at this early stage of the development of a potential new intervention strategy. Results of future study designs that incorporate data-driven refinements in patient selection, duration of dosing and choice of antibiotic will be required before a complete assessment of the value of antibiotic intervention can be made.

Conclusion

Atherosclerosis is an inflammatory disease. That infection may serve as a root cause of this inflammation is supported by a number of different lines of evidence. At present, the most compelling data support the role of *C. pneumoniae* through pathogens, such as cytomegalovirus and dental organisms, should not be discounted. The macrophage is a critical component in the pathway to atherosclerotic inflammation. To the extent that an infectious process activates a macrophage, either in the local arterial milieu or at a distant site, there is the potential for that macrophage to stimulate both local lipid accumulation and the instability that presages plaque rupture. Given the burden that coronary artery disease imparts on the healthcare system and on society in general, efforts to both understand the role of infection in atherogenesis, and to develop targeted intervention strategies, should continue apace.

REFERENCES

Anderson JL, Muhlestein JB, Carlquist J, Allen A, Trehan S, Nielson C, Hall S, Brady J, Egger M, Horne B, Lim T. 1999. Randomized secondary prevention trial of azithromycin in patients with coronary artery disease and serological evidence for Chlamydia pneumoniae infection: the azithromycin in coronary artery disease: elimination of myocardial infection with chlamydia (ACADEMIC) study. *Circulation* 99:1540–1547.

Beatty WL, Morrison RP, Byrne GI. 1994. Persistent chlamydiae: from cell culture to a paradigm for chlamydial pathogenesis. *Microbiological Reviews* 58:686–699.

Berger M, Schroder B, Daeschlin G, Schneider W, Busjahn A, Buchalow I, Luft FC, Haller H. 2000. Chlamydia pneumoniae DNA in non-coronary atherosclerotic plaques and circulating leokocytes. *Journal of Laboratory and Clinical Medicine* 136:194–200.

Danesh J. 1999. Coronary heart disease, Helicobacter pylori, dental disease, Chlamydia pneumoniae, and cytomegalovirus: meta-analyses of prospective studies. *American Heart Journal* 138:S434–437.

Dowell SF, Peeling RW, Boman J, Carlone GM, Fields BS, Guarner J, Hammerschlag MR, Jackson LA, Kuo CC, Maass M, Messmer TO, Talkington DF, Tondella ML, Zaki SR. 2001. Standardizing Chlamydia pneumoniae assays: recommendations from the Centers for Disease Control and Prevention (USA) and the Laboratory Centre for Disease Control (Canada). *Clinical Infectious Diseases* 33:492–503.

Dunne M. 2000. The evolving relationship between Chlamydia pneumoniae and atherosclerosis. *Current Opinion in Infectious Diseases* 13(6):583–591.

Fong IG, Chiu B, Viira E, Jang D, Fong MW, Peeling R, Mahony JA. 1999. Can an Antibiotic (macrolide) prevent Chlamydia pneumoniae-induced atherosclerosis in a rabbit model? *Clinical and Diagnostic Laboratory Immunology* 6:891–894.

Gilbert A and Lion G. 1889. Artérites infectieuses expérimentales. *Comptes Rendus Hebdomadaires des Séances et Mémoires de la Société de Biologie.* 41:583–584.

Gupta S, Leatham EW, Carrington D, Mendall MA, Kaski JC, Camm AJ. 1997. Elevated Chlamydia pneumoniae antibodies, cardiovascular events, and azithromycin in male survivors of myocardial infarction. *Circulation* 96:404–407.

Gurfinkel EG, Bozovich G, Daroca A, Beck E, Mautner B. 1997. Randomised trial of roxithromycin in non-Q-wave coronary syndromes: ROXIS Pilot Study. ROXIS Study Group. [comment]. *Lancet* 350:404–407.

Hu H, Pierce GN, Zhong G. 1999. The atherogenic effects of chlamydia are dependent on serum cholesterol and specific to Chlamydia pneumoniae. *Journal of Clinical Investigation* 103:747–753.

Lin TM, Campbell LA, Rosenfeld ME, Kuo CC. 2000. Monocyte-endothelial cell coculture enhances infection of endothelial cells with Chlamydia pneumoniae. *Journal of Infectious Diseases* 181:1096–1100.

Miller SA, Selzman CH, Shames BD, Barton HA, Johnson SM, Harken AH. 2000. Chlamydia pneumoniae activates nuclear factor kappaB and activator protein 1 in human vascular smooth muscle and induces cellular proliferation. *Journal of Surgical Research* 90:76–81.

Molestina RE, Miller RD, Ramirez, JA Summersgill JT. 1999. Infection of human endothelial cells with Chlamydia pneumoniae stimulates transendothelial migration of neutrophils and monocytes. *Infection & Immunity* 67:1323–1330.

Neumann FA, Kastrati A, Miethke T, Pogatsa-Murray G, Mehilli J, Valina C, Jogethaei N, da Costa CP, Wagner H. Schomig. A. 2001. Treatment of Chlamydia pneumoniae infection with roxithromycin and effect on neointima proliferation after coronary stent placement (ISAR-3): a randomised, double-blind, placebo-controlled trial. *Lancet* 357:2085–2089.

Nieto FJ. 1998. Infections and atherosclerosis: new clues from and old hypothesis? *American Journal of Epidemiology* 48:937–948.

Nieto FJ. 1999. Viruses and atherosclerosis: a critical review of the epidemiologic evidence. *American Heart Journal* 138:S453–460.

Reiner Z. 2002. Azithromycin in the secondary prevention of adverse cardiovascular events in C. pneumoniae-positive post myocardial infarction patients (CROAATS). Paper presented at the Sixth International Conference on the Macrolides, Azalides, Streptogramins, Ketolides, and Oxazolidinones, Bologna, Italy, January 23-25, 2002.

Ross R. 1999. Atherosclerosis—an inflammatory disease. [comment]. *New England Journal of Medicine* 340:115–126.

Saikku P, Leinonen M, Mattila K, Ekman MR, Nieminen MS, Makela PH, Huttunen JK, Valtonen V. 1988. Serological evidence of an association of a novel Chlamydia, TWAR, with chronic coronary heart disease and acute myocardial infarction. *Lancet* 2:983–986.

Wiesli P, Czerwenka W, Meniconi A, Maly F, Hoffman U, Vetter W, Schulthess G. 2002. Roxithromycin treatment prevents progression of peripheral arterial occlusive disease in Chlamydia pneumoniae seropositive men: a randomized, double-blind, placebo-controlled trial. *Circulation* 105:2646–2652.

Zahn R, Schneider S, Frilling B, Seidl K, Tebbe U, Weber M, Gottwik M, Altmann E, Seidel F, Rox J, Hoffler U, Neuhaus KL, Senges J. Working Group of Leading Hospital Cardiologists. 2003. Antibiotic therapy after acute myocardial infarction: a prospective randomized study. *Circulation* 107:1253–1259.

Zhong G, Fan T, Lui L. 1999. Chlamydia inhibits interferon gamma-inducible major histocompatibility complex class II expression by degradation of upstream stimulatory factor 1. *Journal of Experimental Medicine* 189:1931–1938.

Zhong G, Liu L, Fan T, Fan P, Ji H. 2000. Degradation of transcription factor RFX5 during the inhibition of both constitutive and interferon gamma-inducible major histocompatibility complex class I expression in chlamydia-infected cells. *Journal of Experimental Medicine* 191:1525–1534.

DEMYELINATING DISEASES

Richard T. Johnson, M.D.
Johns Hopkins University, Baltimore, MD

Viral infections cause a variety of demyelinating diseases in animals and humans. Demyelinating diseases are defined as disorders of the central or peripheral nervous system with destruction of myelin and *relative* preservation of axons. Other histopathological features do not alter the definition; oligodendrocytes or Schwann cells may or may not be affected, astrocytosis and gliosis may or may not be prominent, and inflammation may or may not be present. All of these features have been described in virus-induced demyelinating disorders. The pathogenesis of the demyelination is different with different infections; these mechanisms range from direct infection and lysis of oligodendrocytes to immune destruction of myelin or supporting cells by cell-mediated immune responses, antibody, or cytokines (see Box 1-1). Many studies of virus-induced demyelinat-

---

Box 1-1
Possible Mechanisms of Virus-Induced Demyelination

1. Direct viral effects
   - Virus infection of oligodendrocytes or Schwann cells causing demyelination through cell lysis or an alternation in cell metabolism
   - Myelin membrane destruction by virus or viral products

2. Virus-induced immune-mediated reactions
   - Antibody and/or cell-mediated reactions to viral antigens on cell membranes
   - Sensitization of host to myelin antigens
     o Breakdown of myelin by infection with introduction into the circulation (epitope spreading)
     o Incorporation of myelin antigens into virus envelope
     o Modification of antigenicity of myelin membranes
   - Cross-reacting antigens between virus and myelin proteins (molecular mimicry)
   - Cytokine and /or protease-mediated demyelination (innocent bystander effect)

3. Viral disruption of regulatory mechanisms of the immune system

---

SOURCE: Johnson (1998).

ing diseases have been pursued in hopes of discovering a role of viruses in multiple sclerosis, but this goal remains elusive.

Animal Models

Animal viruses can produce acute, chronic, and relapsing/remitting demyelinating central nervous system diseases in their natural or experimental hosts (see Table 1-3). The best model for human postinfectious encephalomyelitis (acute disseminated encephalomyelitis), however, is not a viral infection but experimental autoimmune encephalomyelitis (EAE) induced by injection of myelin proteins with Freund's adjuvant. The latency, clinical disease, pathology and immunological features of these two diseases are similar.

Progressive multifocal leucoencephalopathy (PML) in macaque monkeys

TABLE 1-3 Animal Models of Demyelinating Diseases

Virus Family	Virus	Host Animal	Proposed Mechanism
Papoavirus	SV40	Monkeys	Opportunistic infection of oligodendrocytes in immunodeficient animals
Coronavirus	Mouse Hepatitis Virus	Mice Rats	Persistent oligodendrocyte infection and probable humoral immune responses
Picornaviruses	Theiler's virus	Mice	Persistent infection of oligodendrocytes and macrophages and immune responses
	Encephalomyocarditis	Mice	?
Rhabdovirus	Chandipura Vesicular stomatitis virus	Mice Mice	Cell-mediated immune responses
Togavirus	Semiliki Forest virus Venezuelan equine encephalitis virus	Mice Mice	Neuronal infection and immune mediated demyelination
	Ross River virus	Mice	Direct lysis of oligodendrocytes
Paramyxovirus	Canine distemper virus	Dogs	Predominantly astrocytic infection with probable indirect demyelination
Lentivirus	Visna virus	Sheep	Macrophage and monocyte infection with cytokine-mediated demyelination
	Caprine arthritis-encephalitis virus	Goats	

SOURCE: Johnson (1998).

caused by SV40 virus is the animal equivalent of PML in man caused by the related JC virus. As in the human disease, the disease evolves in latently infected animals when other infections or illnesses cause immunodeficiencies. Four naturally occurring infections in their native hosts have been the most widely studied models of virus-induced demyelination. Theiler's virus, a picornavirus, and JHM virus, a murine coronavirus, were both originally recovered from paralyzed mice; canine distemper, a morbillivirus closely related to measles virus, has long been recognized to cause demyelination in a subacute encephalitis called "old dog disease"; and visna virus, a natural retrovirus infection of sheep, causes relapsing and remitting disease with multifocal demyelinating lesions after a long incubation period. Visna and a related caprine lentivirus (caprine arthritis-ecephalitis virus) best simulate multiple sclerosis, but they have not been widely exploited because of the need to use sheep or goats as the experiment animals. In these lentivirus diseases, infection is limited to macrophages and microglia, and demyelination is thought to result from cytokines released by infected cells.

Human Demyelinating Diseases of Known Viral Etiology

Postinfectious Encephalomyelitis or Acute Disseminated Encephalomyelitis (ADEM)

This is an acute perivenular demyelinating disease of the brain and spinal cord that usually follows viral infections, but on occasions follows some bacterial infections and vaccines, particularly those containing nervous system tissues. Historically, the disorder was also known as post-exanthematous encepahlomyelitis, since it was most frequent after viral diseases characterized by rashes. In the 1950s, ADEM constituted one-third of all cases of encephalitis (see Table 1-4). With the discontinuation of vaccinia virus immunization against smallpox and introduction of vaccines to prevent measles, mumps, rubella, and chickenpox,

TABLE 1-4 Postinfectious Encephalomyelitis Associated with Exanthematous Viral Infections

Disease	Case rate	Fatality rate	Sequelae rate
Vaccinia	1:63 to 1:250,000	10%	Rare
Measles	1:1,000	25%	Frequent
Varicella[a]	1:10,000	5%	10%
Rubella[a]	<1:20,000	20%	Very rare

[a]Estimates are difficult to determine because of the frequency of toxic encephalopathy or Reyes syndrome (different pathology) and acute cerebellar ataxia (unknown pathology) and the rare documentation of perivenular demyelinating disease.

ADEM constitutes less than one-tenth of the cases of acute encephalitis and now is most common after nonspecific upper respiratory infections.

The hazard of ADEM after inoculation of vaccinia virus to protect against smallpox has returned as an issue, since resumption of vaccination is being considered to counter the possible use of smallpox as a terrorist weapon. A very high rate of complications in one Dutch vaccination program was presumably due to use of a more encephalitogenic strain; the low rates during the mass vaccination in New York in 1947 probably reflects poor surveillance. In Great Britain, during the more recent outbreak of smallpox in 1962, a rate of postvaccinal encephalomyelitis of 1 per 20,000 was estimated, and CDC retrospective surveys estimated 1 per 200,000 in the United States prior to the discontinuation of vaccination. However, the risk of ADEM when starting vaccination after a hiatus of 30 years is uncertain, since neurologic complications are more frequent with primary vaccination and higher in persons over the age of 20 years.

The clinical presentation of ADEM usually follows the antecedent exanthem or respiratory or gastrointestinal symptoms by 5 to 21 days. Typically postmeasles encephalomyelitis occurs 5 to 7 days after the rash when the child is returning to normal activity. There is the abrupt recurrence of fever, depression of consciousness, and appearance of multifocal neurological findings. The spinal fluid usually contains myelin basic protein, often shows increased pressure and a mild pleocytosis (but in about one-third of cases, no increased cellularity is found). The MRI may show very dramatic changes with multiple enhancing lesions in the white matter.

The histopathology of fatal cases shows perivenular inflammation and demyelination throughout the brain and spinal cord. In most instances, virus is not found within the nervous system. For example, in measles, virus is seldom recoverable after the rash which corresponds with the humoral immune response. In measles, deaths occurring at or before the time of rash, measles virus has been found in cerebrovascular endothelial cells by in situ PCR; but no virus antigen or nucleic acid has been found in cells of the CNS in patients dying of encephalomyelitis.

The pathogenesis of ADEM is related to infection of immunocompetent cells and the alteration of immune responses. In both postmeasles and postvaricella disease activated peripheral blood lymphocytes responsive to myelin basic protein have been demonstrated. The autoimmune response against CNS myelin appears to occur without the prerequisite of infection of CNS cells. ADEM appears to be an autoimmune disease very similar to experimental autoimmune encephalomyelitis.

Progressive Multifocal Leucoencephalopathy (PML)

PML is a subacute demyelinating disease originally described as a rare complication of leukemia and Hodgkin's disease. Prior to 1982, PML was an extraordinarily rare disease. With the emergence of AIDS over the past two decades, PML has become a common opportunistic infection causing death in 3–5 percent of AIDS patients.

The clinical presentation is on a background of severe immunosuppression. Multifocal neurological symptoms and signs develop insidiously and usually follow an ingravescent course to death. With introduction of HAART therapy and recovery of T4 counts, stabilization and even improvement has been reported. There is no fever, no nuchal rigidity, and usually no pleocytosis. A very characteristic MRI pattern is seen, however, with nonenhancing multifocal lesions in the subcortical white matter.

The neuropathological changes are unique. Plaques of demyelination are seen preferentially in the grey–white junction. Histologically inflammation is slight or absent. In areas of demyelination, axons are relatively spared and oligodendrocytes are lost. Surrounding these foci, oligodendrocytes are enlarged and contain intranuclear inclusions. Astocytosis is intense, and many astrocytes contain bizarre mitotic figures and multiple nuclei resembling malignant cells.

Electron microscopic examination of the oligodendrocyte inclusions reveal profuse pseudocrystalline arrays of papovaviruses. Only occasional viral particles are seen in astrocytes but they express papovavirus T antigen. JC virus, an ubiquitous human papovavirus, has been associated with almost all cases.

The pathogenesis of demyelination in PML is the opposite of that in ADEM. JC virus causes an asymptomatic persistent infection in most persons. With intense immunosuppression the virus in some patients is transported to brain, probably in B cells. With massive replication in oligodendrocytes these cells are destroyed with secondary loss of myelin. There is no evidence of infection of neurons. Semipermissive infection of astrocytes leads to limited virus production but many astrocytic changes and proliferation resemble transformation. The tat protein of HIV may transactivate JC virus accounting for the unique frequency of PML in HIV-infected patients.

Multiple Sclerosis

A viral cause for multiple sclerosis has been postulated for over 100 years. Over the past half century this speculation has been highlighted by 3 types of studies. First, epidemiological evidence implicates childhood exposure factors (possibly viral infections) in the genesis of multiple sclerosis, and natural history studies have related "virus-like illnesses" to exacerbations of the disease. Second, studies of human and animal viral infections have documented that these infections can have incubation periods of years, cause remitting and relapsing disease and can cause myelin destruction mediated by a variety of mechanisms. Third, laboratory studies of patients with multiple sclerosis consistently show that such patients have greater antibody responses to a variety of viruses than controls and this includes intrathecal antibody synthesis. This is not to deny the clear-cut genetic susceptibility factor (a concordance of over 30 percent in monozygotic twins) or the immunologic abnormalities (which may be caused by infection or be the cause of the unusual viral immune responses in patients).

The unique geographical distribution in temperate zones may in part be explained by Nordic susceptibility genes, but because many immigration studies show that migrants after about age 13 take their risk of early homeland with them and very young migrants acquire the risk of their new land, these findings suggest a childhood exposure. Apparent outbreaks are recorded such as the increase in incidence of multiple sclerosis in the Faroe Islands following the British occupation in World War II. Little evidence is present in these studies to implicate a specific agent; but there are examples of viruses that show different ages of acquisition. For example, varicella occurs at earlier ages in temperate climates and Epstein-Barr virus infections at later ages; in addition the severity or presentation of infection may be age dependent. Early childhood Epstein-Barr virus infection is asymptomatic whereas young adult infection gives rise to infectious mononucleosis.

Specific viral infections have been suggested by serological and virus isolation studies. Over 30 studies have documented the higher levels of antibody to measles in serum and spinal fluid in multiple sclerosis patients than in controls. Although the most striking, measles is not alone as antibodies to many viruses have been found higher in multiple sclerosis patients (see Table 1-5).

Recovery of viruses from tissues or spinal fluid of patients has been repeatedly reported (see Table 1-6), but not with the consistency of serological tests.

TABLE 1-5 Higher Anti-Viral Antibodies in Multiple Sclerosis Than in Controls

Serum	CSF
Measles	Measles
Parainfluenza 3	Parainfluenza 1, 2, 3
Influenza C	Influenza A, B
Varicella	Varicella
Herpes simplex	Herpes simplex
Human herpes virus – 6	Human herpes virus – 6
Rubella	Rubella
Epstein-Barr	Epstein-Barr
	Mumps
	Respiratory syncytial
	Coronaviruses
	Adenoviruses
HTLV-I (gag)	HTLV-I (gag)
HTLV-II	Simian virus-5

SOURCE: Adapted from Johnson (1998).

TABLE 1-6 Viruses Recovered from Patients with Multiple Sclerosis

Virus	Year
Rabies virus	1946
	1964
Herpes simplex virus, type 2	1964
Scrapie agent	1965
MS-associated agent	1972
Parainfluenza virus 1	1972
Measles virus	1978
Simian virus 5	1979
Chimpanzee cytomegalovirus	1980
Coronavirus	1982
SMON-like virus (subacute myelo-optico-neuropathy)	1982
Tick-borne encephalitis flavivirus	1986
HTLV-1 (human T-cell lymphotrophic virus)	1989
LM7 (retrovirus)	1989
Herpes simplex virus, type 1	1989
Human herpesvirus 6	1994
Endogenous retroviruses	1998

Indeed most have proved to be contaminants picked up from cell cultures or laboratory animals.

Recent interest has focused on *Chlamydia pneumoniae*, herpesvirus 6, Epstein-Barr virus, and endogenous retroviruses as latent or persistent agents implicated in multiple sclerosis. While they are all normal flora of the human body, they seem to change in quantity or topography in multiple sclerosis. Again this raises the tough question of causation versus an epiphenomenon secondary to the immunological changes in the disease.

Chlamydia commonly causes chronic infection of macrophages, so its recovery from an inflammatory lesion may only reflect the ingress of macrophages. Similarly Epstein-Barr is latent in B cells, and in a disease such as multiple sclerosis, where intrathecal antibody synthesis is taking place, finding it in spinal fluid or brain by PCR is not surprising. Human herpesvirus 6 has similar latency and may be nonspecifically activated by a disease exacerbation. Endogenous retrovirus sequences are present in all our cells, but again nonspecific activation of macrophages increases the translation of these sequences.

In conclusion, patients with multiple sclerosis have abnormally active immune responses to many viruses, and these responses include intrathecal responses. Viral infections precede exacerbations of disease more often than can be explained by chance. The pathogenetic role of viruses in the cause of multiple sclerosis and the precipitation of exacerbations remain a mystery.

REFERENCES

These references are not specifically cited in text.

Buljevac D, Flach HZ, Hop WC, Hijdra D, Laman JD, Savelkoul HF, van Der Meche FG, van Doorn PA, Hintzen RQ. 2002. Prospective study on the relationship between infections and multiple sclerosis exacerbations. *Brain* 125:952–960.

Gieffers J, Pohl D, Treib J, Dittmann R, Stephan C, Klotz K, Hanefeld F, Solbach W, Haass A, Maass M. 2001. Presence of Chlamydia pneumoniae DNA in the cerebral spinal fluid is a common phenomenon in a variety of neurological diseases and not restricted to multiple sclerosis. *Annals of Neurology* 49:585–589.

Gonzalez-Scarano F and Rima B. 1999. Infectious etiology in multiple sclerosis: the database continues. *Trends in Microbiology* 7:475–477.

Johnson RT. 1994. The virology of demyelinating diseases. *Annals of Neurology* 36:S54–S60.

Johnson RT. 1998. Viral Infections of the Nervous System 2nd Ed. Philadelphia: Lippincott-Raven.

Johnston JB, Silva C, Holden J, Warren KG, Clark AW, Power C. 2001. Monocyte activation and differentiation augments human retrovirus expression: implications for inflammatory brain diseases. *Annals of Neurology* 50:434–442.

Wandinger K, Jabs W, Siekhaus A, Bubel S, Trillenberg P, Wagner H, Wessel K, Kirchner H, Hennig H. 2000. Association between clinical disease activity and Epstein-Barr virus reactivation in MS. *Neurology* 55:178–184.

Yao SY, Stratton CW, Mitchell WM, Sriram S. 2000. CSF oligoclonal bands in MS include antibodies against *Chlamydophila* antigens. *Neurology* 56:1168–1176.

COMMON INFECTIONS AND UNCOMMON DISEASE: ELUSIVE ASSOCIATIONS OF ENTEROVIRUSES AND TYPE I DIABETES MELLITUS

Mark A. Pallansch, Ph.D.; and M. Steven Oberste, Ph.D.
Respiratory and Enteric Viruses Branch,
Division of Viral and Rickettsial Diseases
National Center for Infectious Diseases,
Centers for Disease Control and Prevention, Atlanta, GA

Host genetic determinants have a major influence on an individual's risk of developing Type 1 diabetes mellitus (T1DM). At the same time, such environmental factors as foods and infectious agents are thought to play a role in the genesis of prediabetic autoimmunity or in the progression from persistent beta-cell autoimmunity to clinical diabetes (Yoon, 1990; See and Tilles, 1998). Immunity to one or more beta cell autoantigens, such as insulin, GAD65, or IA-2, may lead to destruction of beta cells and a loss of the capacity to produce insulin, ultimately resulting in clinical insulin-dependent diabetes mellitus. Postulated mechanisms by which infectious agents may trigger T1DM include:

1. direct cytolytic infection of beta cells, resulting in destruction of beta cells and loss of capacity to synthesize insulin;

2. a virus-induced immune response against infected beta cells, such as T-cell induced killing of virus-infected cells;

3. non-specific "innocent bystander" killing of beta cells through activation of non-specific immune mediators; and

4. induction of an autoimmune response to islet antigens by cross-reactivity with viral antigens (molecular mimicry) or disruption of normal immune tolerance mechanisms.

Several viruses have been proposed as infectious triggers of diabetes, but the enteroviruses (family *Picornaviridae*, genus *Enterovirus*) are the subject of the most intense scrutiny at present (Leinikki, 1998; Hyöty et al., 1998). Numerous studies have provided evidence for an association between enterovirus infection and prediabetic autoimmunity or clinical diabetes. Diabetes incidence has been epidemiologically linked to the incidence of enteroviral meningitis or enterovirus outbreaks (Karvonen et al., 1993). Serologic studies have shown that there is a correlation between enterovirus seroprevalence in patients with prediabetic autoimmunity or diabetes, compared to unaffected control individuals (Hiltunen et al., 1997; Helfand et al., 1995). Direct enterovirus detection in pancreas, blood, serum, or stool has suggested a temporal correlation between enterovirus infection and onset of diabetes (Yoon et al., 1979; Andreoletti et al., 1997; Clements et al., 1995).

Enteroviruses are among the most common of human viruses, infecting an estimated 50 million people annually in the United States and possibly a billion or more annually worldwide (Morens and Pallansch, 1995; Pallansch and Roos, 2001). Most infections are inapparent, but enteroviruses may cause a wide spectrum of acute disease, including mild upper respiratory illness (common cold), febrile rash (hand, foot, and mouth disease and herpangina), aseptic meningitis, pleurodynia, encephalitis, acute flaccid paralysis (paralytic poliomyelitis), and neonatal sepsis-like disease. Enterovirus infections result in 30,000 to 50,000 hospitalizations per year in the United States, with aseptic meningitis cases accounting for the vast majority of the hospitalizations (Pallansch and Roos, 2001). In addition to these acute illnesses, enteroviruses have also been associated with severe chronic diseases such as myocarditis (Martino et al., 1995; Kim et al., 2001), Type 1 diabetes mellitus (Leinikki, 1998; Rewers and Atkinson, 1995), and neuromuscular diseases (Dalakas, 1995). Enteroviruses are transmitted primarily by the fecal-oral route but respiratory transmission to close contacts may also be important. The incubation period between infection and onset of symptoms is usually 4–7 days. The intestinal mucosa or upper respiratory tract is the site of primary infection, with secondary spread to the central nervous system and other tissues. Viremia is usually short-lived, often waning before the onset of symptoms, except in very young children. Virus is excreted in the stool for up to 8 weeks (average 2–4 weeks) but maximal virus shedding occurs before the onset of symptoms. The maximum virus titer in stool is approximately 10^4 infectious virus particles per gram.

Of the 89 recognized enterovirus serotypes, 64 are known to infect humans (Pallansch and Roos, 2001). In addition to the human enteroviruses, human pathogenic viruses are found in four other picornavirus genera: *Rhinovirus* (human rhinoviruses), *Hepatovirus* (human hepatitis A virus), *Parechovirus* (human parechoviruses 1 and 2, formerly echoviruses 22 and 23, respectively), and *Kobuvirus* (aichivirus, an agent of gastroenteritis). Most of the human enterovirus serotypes were discovered and described between 1947 and 1963 as a result of the application of cell culture and suckling mouse inoculation to the investigation of cases of infantile paralysis (paralytic poliomyelitis) and other central nervous system diseases (Committee on Enteroviruses, 1962; Panel for Picornaviruses, 1963). The human enteroviruses were originally classified on the basis of human disease (polioviruses), replication and pathogenesis in newborn mice (coxsackie A and B viruses), and growth in cell culture without causing disease in mice (echoviruses), but they have recently been reclassified, based largely on molecular properties, into four species, A through D (King et al., 2000). Sequences in various portions of the enterovirus coding-region correlate with species, but only capsid sequence correlates with serotype.

The neutralization test, long the gold standard for enterovirus typing, is generally reliable, but it is labor-intensive and time-consuming, and may fail to identify an isolate because of aggregation of virus particles or antigenic drift (the widely used standardized typing antisera were raised against prototype strains that were isolated 40 to 50 years ago [Lim and Benyesh-Melnick, 1960]). Antisera to all serotypes are not generally available and isolates that are not of a known human enterovirus serotype (new serotypes or serotypes that normally infect animals other than humans) would obviously also present difficulties in identification by antigenic means, as the neutralization method requires the use of serotype-specific reagents. In addition, neutralization requires virus isolation, which may require the use of multiple cell lines and adds to the time required to make an identification.

The application of PCR has improved the speed and accuracy of general enterovirus detection (Rotbart and Romero, 1995; Rotbart et al., 1997), and has found wide acceptance in the clinical diagnostic laboratory. Since the enterovirus serotype is rarely relevant to clinical case management, many clinical virology laboratories are bypassing virus isolation entirely, in favor of PCR detection of viral nucleic acid directly in clinical specimens such as cerebrospinal fluid, nasopharyngeal swabs, or tissue specimens (Rotbart and Romero, 1995). This approach uses genus-specific primers targeted to the 5' non-translated region (see Figure 1-6), often coupled to probe-hybridization and detection of product in a microplate format (Rotbart and Romero, 1995). Specimens of choice for the direct detection of enteroviruses by RT-PCR are stool or rectal swab (stool is preferred because it contains a larger amount of fecal material and, hence, virus);

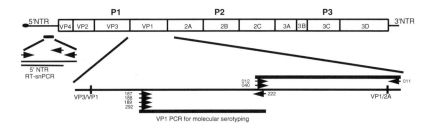

FIGURE 1-6 Schematic representation of the enterovirus genome, indicating regions that have been targeted for development of PCR diagnostics. The genome is a positive-stranded, polyadenylated RNA of ~7400 nucleotides, with a viral protein (3B/VPg) covalently linked to the 5′ end. The genome is divided into five functional regions: the 5′ non-translated region (NTR) (control of viral translation initiation and initiation of positive-strand RNA synthesis); P1 (encodes the structural proteins that comprise the virus capsid); P2 and P3 (encode the non-structural proteins involved in RNA replication, proteolytic processing of polyprotein, and host cell shut-down); and 3′ NTR (involved in initiation of negative-strand RNA synthesis).

oro- or nasopharyngeal specimens (throat swab, nasopharyngeal swab or aspirate, saliva); cerebrospinal fluid (if there is concomitant CNS disease); fresh-frozen or formalin-fixed tissue; and serum/plasma. Serum and plasma are generally only useful for RT-PCR in infants because viremia may still be present after onset of symptoms. If virus is detected only in a non-sterile site, such as stool or nasopharynx, a large number of patients are needed to establish the association between infection and disease.

Despite the advantages of enterovirus detection by RT-PCR, challenges remain. In the case of chronic diseases, the virus may act indirectly (e.g., through immune-mediated pathology). The virus may be cleared well before disease onset or virus may be present in the patient but not in the diseased tissue. Even in acute illnesses, the titer is relatively low in all specimens. As a result, a conventional single-step RT-PCR amplification may not be sensitive enough for direct detection from the original clinical specimen. Designing a prospective study and collecting multiple specimens, at multiple time points throughout the duration of the study, may overcome some of these problems; however, the only way to solve the sensitivity problem is by increasing the sensitivity of the detection method. To address this issue, we have developed an enterovirus-specific semi-nested RT-PCR assay (5′ NTR RT-snPCR) that targets the conserved regions of the 5′ NTR (see Figure 1-6). Figure 1-7 shows the sensitivity of our standard, conventional RT-PCR (Yang et al., 1992) compared with that of the 5′ NTR RT-snPCR. Ten-fold serial dilutions of a virus isolate (10^{-1} to 10^{-10}) were prepared with uninfected cell extract as diluent. RNA was extracted using the QIAamp viral RNA mini-kit (Qiagen Inc., Valencia, CA) and reverse-transcribed using the

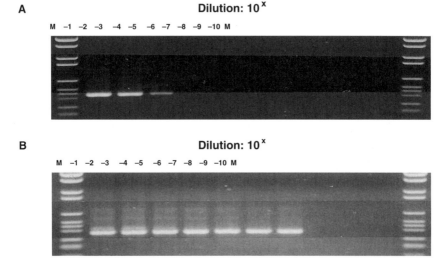

FIGURE 1-7 Sensitivity of pan-enterovirus RT-PCR methods. M-molecular weight marker. Virus dilutions are shown at the top of each panel. A. Titration of conventional two-primer RT-PCR. B. Titration of RT-semi-nested (three-primer) PCR.

antisense primer. PCR was performed using a single round of amplification (conventional PCR) or two rounds of amplification (semi-nested PCR). The second round of the semi-nested amplification used the same primers as the conventional PCR. Amplification products were visualized by polyacrylamide gel electrophoresis and staining with ethidium bromide. The RT-snPCR method (see Figure 1-7B) was approximately 10,000-fold more sensitive than the conventional RT-PCR (see Figure 1-7A). The 10^{-7} dilution corresponds to less than 20 infectious virus particles.

Enterovirus infection elicits a serotype-specific immune response directed against epitopes on the surface of the viral capsid. Mucosal immunity is most important. Antibody alone fully protects from disease, probably by limiting virus spread from the gut, but antibody does not necessarily protect from infection. The virus-specific T-cell response, directed against epitopes on both the structural and non-structural proteins, is probably involved in virus clearance but it is not needed for protection. Antigenic sites are located in each of the three enterovirus structural proteins, VP1, VP2, and VP3 (Minor, 1990; Mateu, 1995), but the epitopes responsible for serotype specificity have not been identified. Since the picornavirus VP1 protein contains a number of immunodominant neutralization domains, we hypothesized that VP1 sequence should correspond with neutralization properties (serotype) (Oberste et al., 1999b). Due to the high frequency of recombination among picornaviruses (Kopecka et al., 1995; King, 1988; Santti et al., 1999), sequence information from non-capsid regions is of little value in characterizing new serotypes within known genera.

Practical criteria must be established before molecular sequence information can be applied routinely to picornavirus identification. A partial or complete VP1 nucleotide sequence identity of at least 75 percent (minimum 85 percent amino acid sequence identity) between a clinical enterovirus isolate and serotype proto- type strain may be used to establish the serotype of the isolate (Oberste et al., 1999a,b, 2000). These criteria also appear to apply to comparisons among iso- lates of foot-and-mouth-disease virus (family *Picornaviridae*, genus *Aphthovirus*) (Vosloo et al., 1992), but a study directly comparable to the enterovirus studies has not yet been performed. A best-match nucleotide sequence identity of be- tween 70 percent and 75 percent or a second-highest score of greater than 70 percent may provide a tentative identification, pending confirmation by other means, such as neutralization with monospecific antisera (Oberste et al., 2000) or more extensive sequencing. A best-match nucleotide sequence identity below 70 percent (less than 85 percent amino acid sequence identity) may indicate that the isolate represents an unknown serotype (Oberste et al., 2000, 2001). Sequencing of the complete capsid-coding region may be useful in confirming this result, but complete capsid sequences are available for less than half of the known enterovi- rus serotypes, limiting the utility of complete capsid sequence comparisons until more sequence becomes available. More extensive characterization, possibly in- cluding complete genome sequences, may be required for viruses that appear to represent previously unknown genera (Hyypiä et al., 1992; Marvil et al., 1999; Niklasson et al., 1999; Yamashita et al., 1998).

Recognizing the technical difficulties and limitations inherent in the classic approach to enterovirus identification, we developed RT-PCR and sequencing primers that target the VP1 capsid gene and may be used to determine enterovirus serotype by sequencing of the amplicon and comparison to a database of the VP1 sequences of all enterovirus serotypes (Oberste et al., 1999a,b, 2000). These mo- lecular detection and typing methods, when coupled with well-designed prospec- tive studies, will be useful in addressing the potential causal relationship between enterovirus infection and development of prediabetic autoimmunity or progres- sion from persistent autoimmunity to clinical diabetes.

REFERENCES

Andreoletti L, Hober D, Hober-Vandenberghe C, Belaich S, Vantyghem MC, Lefebvre J, Wattre P. 1997. Detection of coxsackie B virus RNA sequences in whole blood samples from adult pa- tients at the onset of type I diabetes mellitus. *Journal of Medical Virology* 52:121–127.
Clements GB, Galbraith DN, Taylor KW. 1995. Coxsackie B virus infection and onset of childhood diabetes. *Lancet* 346:221–223.
Committee on Enteroviruses. 1962. Classification of human enteroviruses. *Virology* 16:501–504.
Dalakas MC. 1995. Enteroviruses and human neuromuscular diseases. Pp. 387–398 in Human En- terovirus Infections, HA Rotbart, ed. Washington, DC: ASM Press.

Helfand RF, Gary HE Jr, Freeman CY, Anderson LJ, Pallansch MA. 1995. Serologic evidence of an association between enteroviruses and the onset of type 1 diabetes mellitus. Pittsburgh Diabetes Research Group. *The Journal of Infectious Diseases* 172:1206–1211.

Hiltunen M, Hyoty H, Knip M, Ilonen J, Reijonen H, Vahasalo P, Roivainen M, Lonnrot M, Leinikki P, Hovi T, Akerblom HK. 1997. Islet cell antibody seroconversion in children is temporally associated with enterovirus infections. Childhood Diabetes in Finland (DiMe) Study Group. *The Journal of Infectious Diseases* 175:554–560.

Hyöty H, Hiltunen M, Lonnrot M. 1998. Enterovirus infections and insulin dependent diabetes mellitus—evidence for causality. *Clinical and Diagnostic Virology* 9:77–84.

Hyypiä T, Horsnell C, Maaronen M, Khan M, Kalkkinen N, Auvinen P, Kinnunen L, Stanway G. 1992. A distinct picornavirus group identified by sequence analysis. *Proceedings of the National Academy of Sciences* 89:8847–8851.

Karvonen M, Tuomilehto J, Libman I, LaPorte R. 1993. A review of the recent epidemiological data on the worldwide incidence of type 1 (insulin-dependent) diabetes mellitus. World Health Organisation DIAMOND Project Group. *Diabetologia* 36:883–892.

Kim KS, Hufnagel G, Chapman NM, Tracy S. 2001. The group B coxsackieviruses and myocarditis. *Reviews in Medical Virology* 11:355–368.

King AMQ. 1988. Genetic recombination in positive strand RNA viruses. Pp. 149–165 in RNA Genetics, E Domingo, JJ Holland, and P Ahlquist, eds. Boca Raton, FL: CRC Press, Inc.

King AMQ et al. 2000. Picornaviridae. Pp. 657–678 in Virus Taxonomy: Seventh Report of the International Committee on Taxonomy of Viruses, MH Van Regenmortel et al., eds. San Diego: Academic Press.

Kopecka H, Brown B, Pallansch M. 1995. Genotypic variation in coxsackievirus B5 isolates from three different outbreaks in the United States. *Virus Research* 38:125–136.

Leinikki P. 1998. Viruses and type 1 diabetes: elusive problems and elusive answers. *Clinical and Diagnostic Virology* 9:65–66.

Lim KA and Benyesh-Melnick M. 1960. Typing of viruses by combinations of antiserum pools. Application to typing of enteroviruses (coxsackie and ECHO). *Journal of Immunology* 84:309–317.

Martino TA et al. 1995. Enteroviral myocarditis and cardiomyopathy: a review of clinical and experimental studies. Pp. 291–351 in Human Enterovirus Infections, HA Rotbart, ed. Washington, DC: ASM Press.

Marvil P, Knowles NJ, Mockett AP, Britton P, Brown TD, Cavanagh D. 1999. Avian encephalomyelitis virus is a picornavirus and is most closely related to hepatitis A virus. *Journal of General Virology* 80:653–662.

Mateu MG. 1995. Antibody recognition of picornaviruses and escape from neutralization. *Virus Research* 38:1–24.

Minor PD. 1990. Antigenic structure of picornaviruses. *Current Topics in Microbiology and Immunology* 161:121–154.

Morens DM and Pallansch MA. 1995. Epidemiology. Pp. 3–23 in Human Enterovirus Infections, HA Rotbart, ed. Washington, DC: ASM Press.

Niklasson B, Kinnunen L, Hornfeldt B, Horling J, Benemar C, Hedlund KO, Matskova L, Hyypia T, Winberg G. 1999. A new picornavirus isolated from bank voles (Clethrionomys glareolus). *Virology* 255:86–93.

Oberste MS, Maher K, Kilpatrick DR, Flemister MR, Brown BA, Pallansch MA. 1999a. Typing of human enteroviruses by partial sequencing of VP1. *Journal of Clinical Microbiology* 37:1288–1293.

Oberste MS, Maher K, Kilpatrick DR, Pallansch MA. 1999b. Molecular evolution of the human enteroviruses: correlation of serotype with VP1 sequence and application to picornavirus classification. *Journal of Virology* 73:1941–1948.

Oberste MS, Maher K, Flemister MR, Marchetti G, Kilpatrick DR, Pallansch MA. 2000. Comparison of classic and molecular approaches for the identification of "untypable" enteroviruses. *Journal of Clinical Microbiology* 38:1170–1174.

Oberste MS, Schnurr D, Maher K, al-Busaidy S, Pallansch M. 2001. Molecular identification of new picornaviruses and characterization of a proposed enterovirus 73 serotype. *Journal of General Virology* 82:409–416.

Pallansch MA and Roos RP. 2001. Enteroviruses: polioviruses, coxsackieviruses, echoviruses, and newer enteroviruses. Pp. 723–775 in Fields Virology, DM Knipe and PM Howley, eds. Philadelphia: Lippincott Williams and Wilkins.

Panel for Picornaviruses. 1963. Picornaviruses: classification of nine new types. *Science* 141:153–154.

Rewers M and Atkinson M. 1995. The possible role of enteroviruses in diabetes mellitus. Pp. 353–385 in Human Enterovirus Infections, HA Rotbart, ed. Washington, DC:ASM Press.

Rotbart HA and Romero JR. 1995. Laboratory diagnosis of enteroviral infections. Pp. 401–418 in Human Enterovirus Infections, HA Rotbart, ed. Washington, DC: ASM Press.

Rotbart HA, Ahmed A, Hickey S, Dagan R, McCracken GH Jr, Whitley RJ, Modlin JF, Cascino M, O'Connell JF, Menegus MA, Blum D. 1997. Diagnosis of enterovirus infection by polymerase chain reaction of multiple specimen types. *The Pediatric Infectious Disease Journal* 16:409–411.

Santti J, Hyypia T, Kinnunen L, Salminen M. 1999. Evidence of recombination among enteroviruses. *Journal of Virology* 73:8741–8749.

See DM and Tilles JG. 1998. The pathogenesis of viral-induced diabetes. *Clinical and Diagnostic Virology* 9:85–88.

Vosloo W, Knowles NJ, Thomson GR. 1992. Genetic relationships between southern African SAT-2 isolates of foot-and-mouth-disease virus. *Epidemiology and Infection* 109:547–558.

Yamashita T, Sakae K, Tsuzuki H, Suzuki Y, Ishikawa N, Takeda N, Miyamura T, Yamazaki S. 1998. Complete nucleotide sequence and genetic organization of Aichi virus, a distinct member of the Picornaviridae associated with acute gastroenteritis in humans. *Journal of Virology* 72:8408–8412.

Yang CF, De L, Yang SJ, Ruiz Gomez J, Cruz JR, Holloway BP, Pallansch MA, Kew OM. 1992. Genotype-specific in vitro amplification of sequences of the wild type 3 polioviruses from Mexico and Guatemala. *Virus Research* 24:277–296.

Yoon JW. 1990. The role of viruses and environmental factors in the induction of diabetes. *Current Topics in Microbiology and Immunology* 164:95–123.

Yoon JW, Austin M, Onodera T, Notkins AL. 1979. Isolation of a virus from the pancreas of a child with diabetic ketoacidosis. *New England Journal of Medicine* 300:1173–1179.

INFECTIOUS AGENTS AND SCHIZOPHRENIA[*]

Robert H. Yolken
Johns Hopkins School of Medicine, Baltimore, MD
E. Fuller Torrey
Stanley Medical Research Institute, Bethesda, MD

Schizophrenia is a pervasive neuropsychiatric disorder of worldwide importance. This disease and related serious psychiatric diseases exact an enormous cost in terms of medical resources, lost productivity, and social ills such as crime and homelessness (see Box 1-2). Despite more than 100 years of extensive research, the causes of schizophrenia remain obscure. Much of the recent research

---

[*]The research described in this presentation was supported by the Stanley Medical Research Institute.

Box 1-2
Clinical and Epidemiological Features of Schizophrenia

Positive symptoms:

- Hallucinations
- Delusions
- Disordered thinking

Negative symptoms:

- Withdrawal
- Amotivation
- Retricted expressiveness

Impairment in cognitive and social functioning
Structural and functional brain abnormalities
Lifetime prevalence = ~1 percent
Peak onset of symptoms in young adulthood
Significant societal consequences worldwide

Characteristics of available medicines:

- Symptomatic improvement
- High rate of side effects
- Do not affect overall disease process

---

in schizophrenia has focused on possible genetic etiologies. The rationale for this approach is based on numerous studies indicating a strong risk associated with having a biological parent with this disease. Extensive genetic analyses of families with schizophrenia have led to the identification of a number of broad genomic regions which appear to be inherited in a non-random fashion by individuals with schizophrenia. However, despite intensive searches, no genes of major, or even minor effect, have been consistently linked to the schizophrenia phenotype (see Box 1-3).

Due to the limited success of genetic investigations, there has been renewed interest in the role of environmental factors in the etiopathogenesis of schizophrenia. This approach derives its rationale from a number of epidemiological studies which indicate that environmental factors may contribute to the risk of schizophrenia in some individuals. Many of these studies identify environmental events occurring during fetal development and early infancy as risk factors for the development of schizophrenia in adult life. Risk factors which have been identified

Box 1-3
Genetics of Schizophrenia

Increased incidence in biological first-degree relatives:

- General Population ~1 percent
- First Degree Relatives ~7–9 percent
- Monozygotic Twins ~30 percent

Most individuals with schizophrenia lack a first degree relative with the disease.
Genetic factors have a large relative risk but a small risk (5 percent) in the overall population.

Intensive search for genes using molecular methods:

- Multiple chromosomal regions of linkage
- Genetic polymorphisms of minor effect (OR-2)
- No genes of major effect in different populations

include infections, nutritional deprivation, and animal exposures in pregnancy (Yolken and Torrey, 1995; Torrey et al., 2000). Additional studies have documented an association between risk of schizophrenia with place and season of birth (Torrey et al., 1997; Torrey and Yolken, 1998). While the relative risks associated with these factors are relatively modest, the common nature of these exposures indicates that they may have a large effect on a population basis (Mortensen et al., 1999).

Based on this background, we have devised the working hypothesis that most cases of schizophrenia are caused by infections and other environmental events occurring in genetically susceptible individuals (Torrey and Yolken, 2000). It is of note that infections relating to schizophrenia occurring in this context would not be expected to follow satisfy Koch's postulates since they would not lead to disease in individuals who did not have the appropriate genetic susceptibility. It is also likely that different microbial agents could lead to a similar disease process in individuals who share common genetic predispositions. It will thus be necessary to move beyond Koch's postulates in order to analyze the interaction between genetic and environmental factors as causative agents of schizophrenia and other serious psychiatric diseases.

We have applied a number of laboratory techniques to the examination of these hypotheses (Johnston-Wilson et al., 2001). These techniques have been used to analyze brain tissues obtained postmortem from individuals with psychiatric diseases and control conditions. These brains were obtained by the Stanley Foundation from a consortium of neuropathologists located in several different regions of the United States and are available to researchers with an interest in the studies of these disorders.

One of the most informative techniques which we have applied to these samples has been that of differential display. This method has indicated that there are several differences in RNA transcription in the brains of individuals with schizophrenia as compared to unaffected controls (Yee and Yolken, 1997). Sequence analysis of differentially expressed transcripts has indicated that many have a high degree of homology with a range of endogenous retroviruses. These elements are components of the human genome which arose from retrotransposition of infectious retroviruses in our evolutionary past. Endogenous retroviruses are integrated into the human genome. Upon activation, they can modulate the transcription of genes located upstream or downstream from the site of chromosomal integration (see Figure 1-8). Since they share properties of both genes and infectious agents, they are a potential link between genetic and environmental causes of human disease (Yolken et al., 2000).

Further studies were performed on cerebrospinal fluids (CSFs) obtained from living individuals with early symptoms of schizophrenia. Amplification of RNA extracted from these fluids indicated an increased rate of transcription of an endogenous retrovirus called HERV-W. This endogenous retrovirus was found in the CSFs of approximately 30 percent of individuals with recent-onset schizophrenia and 5 percent of individuals with chronic forms of the disease (see Figure 1-9). HERV-W transcription was not detected in the CSF of individuals without psychiatric disorders (Karlsson et al., 2001). HERV-W is of interest since its

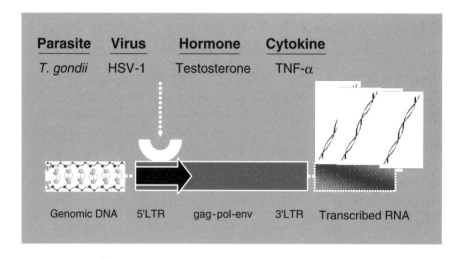

FIGURE 1-8 Integration and transcription of endogenous retroviruses.

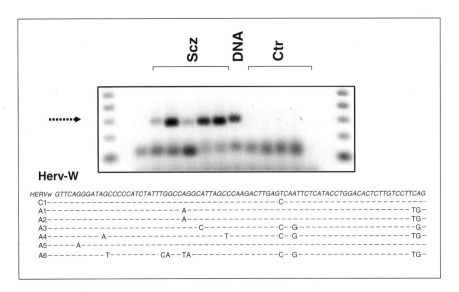

FIGURE 1-9 Endogenous retrovirus was found in the CSFs of approximately 30 percent of individuals with recent-onset schizophrenia and 5 percent of individuals with chronic forms of the disease.
SOURCE: Karlsson et al. (2001).

transcription has also been found to be increased in the CSFs of individuals with multiple sclerosis (Perron et al., 1997). It has also been demonstrated to be active during human fetal development and to encode a protein with syncytium forming activity in the human placenta (Mi et al., 2000). Furthermore , the envelope protein of HERV-W is capable of causing polyclonal T-lymphocyte activation (Perron et al., 2001). HERV-W may thus also provide a link between environmental events active both during fetal development and adult life.

The transcription of endogenous retroviruses can be activated by a number of infectious agents and other environmental factors. We have examined the prevalence of potential activating infections in different stages of schizophrenia. We have found an increased level of antibodies to *Toxoplasma gondii* in individuals with the recent onset of schizophrenia (see Figure 1-10) (Yolken et al., 2001). This finding is consistent with epidemiological studies documenting an increased rate in schizophrenia in individuals who were exposed to cats in early life (Torrey et al., 2000). We have also found that serological evidence of infection with Herpes Simplex Virus Type 1 and *Toxoplasma gondii* are associated with increased levels of cognitive and memory impairments in individuals with established forms of schizophrenia (Dickerson et al., 2003b). We also examined the possible association between infections in pregnancy in the occurrence of schizophrenia in

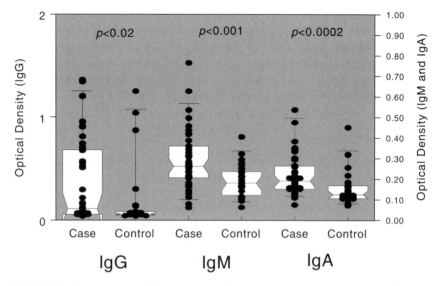

FIGURE 1-10 An increased level of antibodies to *Toxoplasma gondii* is found in individuals with recent onset of schizophrenia.
SOURCE: Yolken et al. (2001).

later life. These analyses were accomplished by the testing of sera which had been obtained from healthy pregnant women as part of the National Collaborative Perinatal Study performed in the United States during the 1950s and 1960s. Initial analyses of this cohort indicates that the offspring of mothers who had evidence of infection, as indicated by increased levels of IgG, IgM, and of IgG antibodies to Herpes Simplex Virus type 2, have higher rates of schizophrenia in adult life (see Figure 1-11) (Buka et al., 2001). There was also a risk of schizophrenia associated with IgM antibodies to *Toxoplasma gondii*, although the antigenic source of these antibodies is still under investigation.

These studies indicate that infectious agents play a role in the generation of schizophrenia in some individuals. The activation of endogenous retroviruses within the central nervous system is likely to be one of several mechanisms by means of which infections can lead to disease. If this is the case, it is possible that the treatment of infectious agents which activate retroviral transcription may be capable of modulating the course of disease at different times in the lifelong course of disease. For example, the treatment of active infection with herpes simplex virus might prevent endogenous retrovirus activation due to this organism. It is of note in this regard that several of the medications which are commonly used for the treatment of schizophrenia also have the ability to inhibit the replication of infectious agents (Jones-Brando et al., 1997). Preliminary analysis of a clinical

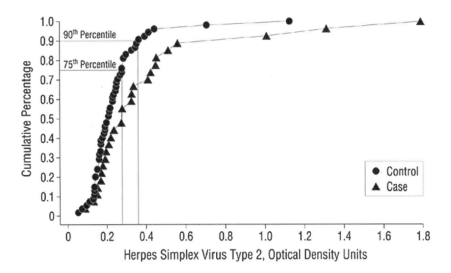

FIGURE 1-11 Association between HSV infections in pregnant women and the occurrence of schizophrenia in their adult offspring. The adult offspring of mothers whose sera showed evidence of HSV infection during pregnancy have higher rates of schizophrenia than the adult offspring of mothers whose sera did not show such evidence during pregnancy. SOURCE: Reprinted from Buka et al. (2001).

trial of the anti-herpesvirus medication valacyclovir indicates that it is effective in reducing the symptoms of some individuals with schizophrenia (Dickerson et al., 2003a). Ongoing studies are directed at the further evaluation of the role of anti-viral and anti-parasitic agents in the treatment of schizophrenia. The definitive establishment of the role of infectious agents in the etiopathogenesis of schizophrenia may lead to new methods for the diagnosis, prevention, and treatment of this devastating disease.

REFERENCES

Buka SL, Tsuang MT, Torrey EF, Klebanoff MA, Bernstein D, Yolken RH. 2001. Maternal infections and subsequent psychosis among offspring. *Archives of General Psychiatry* 58:1032–1037.

Dickerson F, Boronow JJ, Stallings C, Origoni A, Yolken R. 2003a. Valacyclovir reduces symptoms in individuals with schizophrenia who are seropositive for cytomegalovirus. Paper presented at the International Congress on Schizophrenia Research, Colorado Springs, March 2003.

Dickerson FB, Boronow JJ, Stallings C, Origoni AE, Ruslanova I, Yolken RH. 2003b. Association of serum antibodies to herpes simplex virus 1 with cognitive deficits in individuals with schizophrenia. *Archives of General Psychiatry* 60:466–472.

Johnston-Wilson NL, Bouton CM, Pevsner J, Breen JJ, Torrey EF, Yolken RH. 2001. Emerging technologies for large-scale screening of human tissues and fluids in the study of severe psychiatric disease. *The International Journal of Neuropsychopharmacology* 4:83–92.

Jones-Brando LV, Buthod JL, Holland LE, Yolken RH, Torrey EF. 1997. Metabolites of the antipsycotic agent clozapine inhibit the replication of human immunodeficiency virus type 1. *Schizophrenia Research* 25:63–70.

Karlsson H, Bachmann S, Schroder J, McArthur J, Torrey EF, Yolken RH. 2001. Retroviral RNA identified in the cerebrospinal fluids and brains of individuals with schizophrenia. *Proceedings of the National Academy of Sciences* 98:4634–4639.

Mi S, Lee X, Li X, Veldman GM, Finnerty H, Racie L, LaVallie E, Tang XY, Edouard P, Howes S, Keith JC Jr, McCoy JM. 2000. Syncytin is a captive retroviral envelope protein involved in human placental morphogenesis. *Nature* 403:785–789.

Mortensen PB, Pederson CB, Westergaard T, Wohlfahrt J, Ewald H, Mors O, Andersen PK, Melbye M. 1999. Effects of family history and place and season of birth on the risk of schizophrenia. *New England Journal of Medicine* 340:603–608.

Perron H, Garson JA, Beden F, Beseme F, Paranhos-Baccala G, Komurian-Pradel F, Mallet F, Tuke PW, Voisset C, Blond JL, Lalande B, Seigneurin JM, Mandrand B. 1997. Molecular identification of a novel retrovirus repeatedly isolated from patients with multiple sclerosis. The Collaborative Research Group on Multiple Sclerosis. *Proceedings of the National Academy of Sciences* 94:7583–7588.

Perron H, Jouvin-Marche E, Michael M, Quanonian-Paroz A, Camelo S, Dumon A, Jolivet-Reynaud C, Marcel F, Souillet Y, Barel E, Gebeihrer L, Santoro L, Marcel S, Seigreurin JM, Marche PN, Lafon M. 2001. Multiple sclerosis retrovirus particles and recombinant envelope trigger on abnormal immune response in vitro, by inducing polyclonal Vbetal 6 T-lymphocyte activation. *Virology* 287:321–332.

Torrey EF and Yolken RH. 1998. At issue: is household crowding a factor for schizophrenia and bipolar disorder. *Schizophrenia Bulletin* 24:321–324.

Torrey EF and Yolken RH. 2000. Familial and genetic mechanisms in schizophrenia. *Brain Research Reviews* 31:113–117.

Torrey EF, Miller J, Rawlings R, Yolken RH. 1997. Seasonality of births in schizophrenia and bipolar disorder: a review of the literature. *Schizophrenia Research* 28:1–38.

Torrey EF, Rawlings R, Yolken RH. 2000. The antecedents of psychoses: a case-control study of selected risk factors. *Schizophrenia Research* 46:17–23.

Yee F and Yolken RH. 1997. Identification of differentially expressed RNA transcripts in neuropsychiatric disorders. *Biological Psychiatry* 41:759–761.

Yolken RH and Torrey EF. 1995. Viruses, schizophrenia and bipolar disorder. *Clinical Microbiology Reviews* 8:131–145.

Yolken RH, Karlsson H, Yee F, Johnston-Wilson NL, Torrey EF. 2000. Endogenous retroviruses and schizophrenia. *Brain Research Reviews* 31:193–199.

Yolken RH, Bachmann S, Rouslanova I, Lillehoj E, Ford G, Torrey EF, Schroeder J. 2001. Antibodies to Toxoplasma gondii in individuals with first-episode schizophrenia. *Clinical Infectious Diseases* 32:842–844.

OVINE PULMONARY ADENOCARCINOMA: IDENTIFYING THE CAUSATIVE AGENT FOR A NEOPLASTIC DISEASE AND IMPLICATIONS FOR HUMAN LUNG CANCER

Hung Fan, Ph.D.
Department of Molecular Biology and Biochemistry
Cancer Research Institute, University of California, Irvine, CA

Cancer is a collection of diseases that result from uncontrolled cell growth. Progression from a normal cell to a fully malignant one is a multi-step process, and numerous factors can contribute. Over the years, it has been shown that environmental factors (e.g., radiation and heavy metals) and lifestyle habits (e.g., tobacco smoking) can increase the rates of particular cancers. In some cases, infectious agents have been identified as causative to certain cancers. In animal model systems, several classes of viruses have been shown to cause cancers, including retroviruses (e.g., avian sarcoma/leukemia viruses and murine leukemia viruses) and small DNA viruses (e.g., polyoma and SV40). Viruses associated with human cancers include retroviruses (human T-cell leukemia virus—adult T-cell leukemia), human papillomavirus (cervical cancer), hepatitis virus types B and C (hepatocellular carcinoma) and gamma herpes viruses (EBV—lymphomas and nasopharyngeal carcinoma; HHV8—Kaposi's sarcoma). In addition, the bacterium *Helicobacter pylori* has been associated with stomach cancer. Proving the involvement of viruses and bacteria in human cancers has typically taken many years. Steps involved include appreciating an epidemiological pattern of the particular cancer suggesting an infectious agent, identification of an infectious agent whose distribution fits the epidemiological pattern, and ultimately demonstrating in an animal model or in vitro culture system that the putative infectious agent is carcinogenic.

Lung cancer is one of the most common human neoplasms. While a substantial portion of lung cancer can be attributed to tobacco smoking, other factors may also contribute to development of disease. Moreover, in some cases tobacco smoking is not involved in causation of the tumor. Human adenocarcinoma of the lung represents neoplasms of secretory epithelia cells. In the distal airways (alveoli and bronchioles), the targets of transformation are Type II pneumocytes and Clara cells. Bronchiolo alveolar carcinoma (BAC) is a sub-classification of lung adenocarcinoma in which the tumor cells line the alveoli or bronchioles and spread in a sideways (lepidic) fashion (Mornex et al., 2003). BAC does not appear to be tightly associated with tobacco smoking, and the incidence of this cancer may be rising. Thus the possibility that an infectious agent may be involved in BAC or human lung adenocarcinoma in general has been suggested by a number of investigators (Jackson et al., 2000; Koyi et al., 2001; Laurila et al., 1997).

A very interesting animal model for human lung adenocarcinoma exists: ovine pulmonary adenocarcinoma (OPA), a contagious lung cancer of sheep (Fan, 2003). The disease was first described in the late 1800s in South Africa, and was named jaagsiekte—"driving sickness" in Afrikaans (York and Querat, 2003). The disease is prevalent worldwide, and is particularly well-documented in Europe and Africa. It is estimated that the lifetime risk of developing OPA in high incidence flocks is approximately 25 percent (Sharp and DeMartini, 2003). The spread of OPA may result from inhalation of aerosols. A noteworthy feature of the disease is production of excess surfactant by the tumor cells—the normal function of Type II pneumocytes and Clara cells is to produce lung surfactant and other molecules important for lung physiology. As a result, animals with end-stage OPA exhibit respiratory distress; "tipping" of OPA animals results in lung fluid (excess surfactant) draining from the nose. In the mid-1970s, researchers in the United Kingdom showed that filtered OPA lung fluid could transfer the disease to unaffected animals, indicating a viral etiology of OPA (York and Querat, 2003). In the 1960s and 1970s, further evidence was obtained that supported this notion. In particular, OPA lung fluid was shown to contain reverse transcriptase activity (characteristic of retroviruses), and OPA lung fluid was shown to contain antigens that cross-react with two retroviruses—Mason Pfizer monkey virus (MPMV) and murine mammary tumor virus (MMTV) (Sharp and Herring, 1983). MPMV and MMTV are relatively closely related viruses, belonging to the betaretrovirus class. However, the experiments were complicated by the presence of another retrovirus, an ovine lentivirus, that was also present in many of the animals with OPA. This confounded experiments to isolate and purify the causative agent of OPA. Moreover, attempts to propagate the OPA-inducing virus from lung fluid in tissue culture were unsuccessful. A major advance was made in 1990, when York et al. deduced the presence and sequence of a novel retrovirus in OPA lung fluid (York et al., 1991, 1992). This was accomplished by first developing a technique that partially removed the contaminating ovine lentivirus from the OPA lung fluid (treatment with a fluorocarbon). The treated lung fluid was then banded to equilibrium in a sucrose density gradient, and RNA was extracted from the peak of reverse transcriptase activity. This RNA was then reverse transcribed in vitro using purified reverse transcriptase and an oligodT primer, and a series of overlapping partial cDNA clones was obtained. Sequencing of the cDNA clones and overlapping the resulting sequences revealed a novel complete retroviral sequence; this retrovirus was designated jaagsiekte sheep retrovirus or JSRV. Consistent with the previous serology, sequence homology analyses indicated that JSRV is also a beta retrovirus, with sequence similarities to both MPMV and MMTV. A diagram of the JSRV sequence is shown in Figure 1-12. Disappointingly, attempts to isolate a replication-competent retrovirus from assembled cDNA clones were unsuccessful.

The availability of the JSRV sequence allowed generation of important molecular reagents for detection of the putative virus. Initial Southern blot experiments indicated that, as for many other retroviruses, endogenous JSRV-related proviruses are present in the germ line of all sheep and goats (DeMartini et al., 2003; Hecht et al., 1996; York et al., 1991). There are 15–20 endogenous JSRV-related proviruses in most sheep. On an evolutionary scale, these endogenous viruses entered the sheep germ line relatively recently—1–5 million years ago (Palmarini et al., 2000a). The existence of endogenous proviruses complicated experiments, in that it was necessary to distinguish the endogenous proviruses from the exogenous JSRV present in lung fluid. PCR-based assays were developed that allowed distinguishing exogenous from endogenous JSRV's (Palmarini et al., 1996). This allowed demonstration that tumor samples from OPA animals consistently contain exogenous JSRV DNA above and beyond the endogenous JSRV-related sequences. The JSRV cDNA clones were also used for production

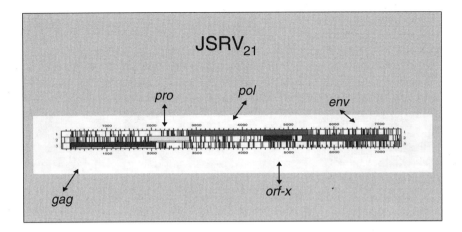

FIGURE 1-12 Genetic organization of the genome of jaagsiekte sheep retrovirus. NOTE: The acronyms and abbreviations in the diagram stand for genes that code for the following: gag = viral packaging protein; pro = promoter; pol = polymerase; orf = open reading frame; env = viral envelope protein.

of bacterial expression plasmids, for development of anti-JSRV antisera. A rabbit polyclonal antibody to JSRV capsid (CA) has been particularly useful. Immunohistochemistry with this antiserum indicated that in OPA animals, the tumor cells consistently show the presence of JSRV CA antigens, while normal cells of the lung do not. In addition, lung cells from uninfected animals do not show JSRV CA protein. These results further strengthened the likelihood that JSRV is the causative agent of OPA.

A major goal was isolation of an infectious and oncogenic molecular clone of JSRV. We undertook such experiments (Palmarini et al., 1999), taking advantage of the prior work. Most notably, the availability of the complete JSRV sequence, and the PCR-based diagnosis for exogenous JSRV were important. A lambda phage genomic library was prepared from a naturally occurring OPA tumor from the United Kingdom. The library was screened by a combination of sib-selection and PCR diagnosis for exogenous JSRV recombinants, followed by standard filter hybridizations with JSRV-specific probes. One lambda phage recombinant was obtained that contained a complete JSRV provirus integrated into adjacent cellular sequences, $JSRV_{21}$. Sequencing of this clone revealed a genome with very high (~95 percent) homology to the previously deduced South African JSRV sequence. All of the open reading frames in the initial sequence deduced by York et al. were present, and there were no other additional frames. Thus the failure of previous attempts to obtain infectious virus from the assembled cDNA clones did not reflect the absence of sequences in the partial cDNA clones. To test whether the $JSRV_{21}$ genome was infectious, we carried out in vivo DNA transfections in newborn lambs. In vivo transfection of retroviral DNA was first demonstrated for bovine leukemia virus (Willems et al., 1993). In vivo transfection of JSRV DNA was accomplished by incorporating a plasmid form of $JSRV_{21}$, pJS21, into liposomes containing a lipid that favors DNA transfer into lung epithelial cells. The pJS21 liposomes were injected intratracheally into newborn lambs, and PBMCs were tested for the presence of JSRV DNA at different times post-transfection. Nested PCR amplifications revealed the presence of exogenous JSRV DNA in PBMCs from the transfected animals at various times up to nine months, when the animals were sacrificed. These results indicated that the $JSRV_{21}$ was an infectious provirus. However, at necropsy (9 months), no tumors were observed, so this experiment did not indicate if $JSRV_{21}$ was an oncogenic clone.

The failure to observe tumors in the pJS21-transfected animals might have been due to the relative inefficiency of in vivo DNA transfection. Therefore, a method for generating genuine JSRV virus from the pJS21 clone was developed. Ultimately, we were able to prepare significant amounts of JSRV virus from a version of the pJS21 plasmid in which the human cytomegalovirus immediate early promoter drives expression of the JSRV sequences. Transient transfection of pJS21 into human 293T cells resulted in the production of JSRV particles. When concentrated JSRV stocks prepared in this way were inoculated intratracheally into four newborn lambs, two lambs developed classic OPA within four months. The resulting tumors were positive for viral CA antigen and DNA (Palmarini et al., 1999). This proved that JSRV is the causative agent of OPA. The availability of an infectious and oncogenic molecular clone of JSRV has opened up several avenues of research that are being pursued.

Two features of JSRV molecular biology are particularly noteworthy. First, JSRV is unusual among retroviruses in that its expression is highly restricted in vivo. In infected animals, JSRV DNA sequences can be detected in various cells, including different lineages of hematopoietic cells in the PBMCs (Holland et al., 1999). The level infection is low—detection requires a nested PCR—and this infection is apparently not productive, since CA antigen-positive cells cannot be detected in PBMCs. Even in lungs of animals with end-stage OPA, CA antigen is only detected in the tumor cells. In particular, other lung cells (even normal lung epithelial cells) do not typically express the CA antigen (Sharp and DeMartini, 2003). Thus, lung epithelial cells may be the only cell types in which JSRV infection is productive. The basis for the expression specificity is the enhancer sequences in the JSRV long terminal repeat (LTR). Retroviral LTRs containing enhancer sequences in the U3 region that are responsible for driving transcription of the provirus. We showed that the JSRV LTR is quite specific for lung epithelial cells in transient transfection assays using a JSRV LTR-driven luciferase reporter gene in mouse cell lines of different differentiation lineages (Palmarini et al., 2000b). Deletional analysis indicated that the JSRV enhancers function in lung epithelial-derived cell lines, while they are inactive in most other cell types.

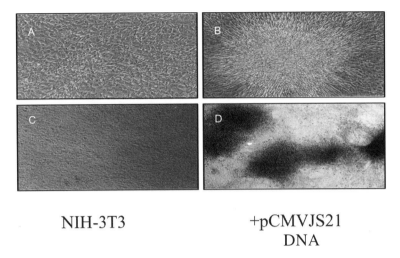

NIH-3T3   +pCMVJS21
DNA

FIGURE 1-13 Foci of transformation induced by the transfection of clone JSRV DNA into mouse NIH 3T3 cells. Such transfection is a standard assay for detecting viral and cellular oncogenes. Panels (a) and (c) show untransfected NIH3T3 cells. Panel (b) shows a focus of transformed cells resulting from transfection with CMV-driven plasmid DNA (pCMV2JS21). Panel (d) shows a pCMV2JS21 transfected culture that had been passaged several times prior to plating under focus-forming conditions.

Detailed analysis of the factors responsible for the lung epithelial-specific expression is in progress.

The second interesting feature of JSRV biology is that the viral genome appears to contain a transforming gene. In fact, JSRV is an extremely potent carcinogen in the laboratory setting. Experimentally inoculated newborn animals develop end-stage OPA with a mean time of six weeks, and in some cases tumors have been observed as early as 10 to 14 days. The rapid oncogenesis, coupled with the multi-focal pattern of the tumors is consistent with a direct transforming function (oncogene) in the virus. We showed that transfection of clone JSRV DNA into mouse NIH 3T3 cells could induce foci of transformation, a standard assay for detection of viral and cellular oncogenes (see Figure 1-13) (Maeda et al., 2001). Further studies indicated that the envelope gene of JSRV is responsible for the transformation. Transformation appears to occur through the cytoplasmic tail of the envelope transmembrane (TM) protein (Palmarini et al., 2001a). The cytoplasmic tail contains a docking site for PI 3 kinase, an important cellular kinase involved in signal transduction and oncogenic transformation. Mutation of the critical tyrosine for methionine residues in the PI3K docking site led to loss of transformation. It is noteworthy that all exogenous JSRV envelopes sequenced so far contain the PI3K binding domain, while endogenous JSRV-related envelope genes do not.

The finding that the JSRV envelope gene contains oncogenic potential is unusual for replication-competent retroviruses. Most other replication-competent retroviruses do not normally cause tumors by a direct mechanism (i.e., oncogenes). More typically, oncogenesis is a byproduct of the replication cycle (e.g., insertional activation of cellular proto-oncogenes). However, the fact that all exogenous JSRVs have a transforming envelope suggests that this property is important for replication of the virus. We have proposed a hypothesis to explain this. In studies of the endogenous JSRV-related proviruses, we found that the endogenous JSRV LTRs do not show transcriptional specificity for lung epithelial cells (Palmarini et al., 2000a). The endogenous viruses provide a view into the primordial progenitor of JSRV, since they reflect the JSRV progenitor from 1 million to 5 million years ago. (Mutation rates of retroviral DNAs decrease markedly when they are transmitted in the proviral [DNA] form.) Thus the progenitor to exogenous JSRV likely replicated through different cells in the animals than lung epithelial cells. Indeed, the endogenous JSRV proviruses in current day sheep are not expressed in lung epithelial cells, but they are expressed in cells of the female reproductive tract (Palmarini et al., 2001b). During evolution of exogenous JSRV, presumably alterations in the enhancer sequences in the LTR arose that conferred transcriptional specificity for lung epithelial cells. However, in the normal adult lung there is relatively little division and growth of Type II pneumocytes and close cells. Most retroviruses require cell division for efficient infection and production. Thus during evolution of exogenous JSRV, the mutation in the cytoplasmic tail of the envelope TM protein would allow for more efficient infection and expression in lung epithelial cells, to which JSRV is transcriptionally restricted.

As mentioned above, JSRV-induced OPA is histologically very similar to human adenocarcinoma and BAC. In light of the lack of association of human BAC with tobacco smoking and its increasing incidence, the possibility of a viral involvement in human lung adenocarcinoma has also been raised. Several investigators have specifically explored whether a human virus related to JSRV might be associated with human lung cancer. In particular, De las Heras and colleagues recently reported a study in which they screened a series of human lung cancers and other tumors for immunological staining with a polyclonal antibody to JSRV CA protein (De las Heras et al., 2000). They found that approximately 30 percent of human BACs and nearly 25 percent of human lung adenocarcinomas showed immunohistochemical staining with the JSRV CA antibody. In contrast, little or no reactivity was detected in squamous cell carcinomas of the lung and other tumors. Thus the reactivity appears to be rather specific for human lung adenocarcinomas and BACs. Another laboratory has been able to replicate these immunohistochemistry findings (J. DeMartini, personal communication). On the other hand, several investigators have attempted to clone a JSRV-related retrovirus from these human tumors by using PCR amplification with degenerative oligonucleotide primers. So far no one has succeeded.

The antigenic cross-reactivity to JSRV observed in some human lung adenocarcinomas might result from two possibilities. First, it could reflect infection with an exogenous human retrovirus with some relationship to JSRV. Alternatively, it could reflect expression of a human endogenous retrovirus (HERV) with antigenic cross-reactivity to JSRV. The human genome contains many copies of HERVs, divided into several classes. It has been shown that different HERVs are expressed in normal versus malignant tissues. It has been noted that the JSRV sequence has some similarity to the HERV-K class, so it is possible that these tumors are expressing a HERV-K (J. DeMartini, personal communication). A third possibility is that the antigenic cross-reactivity could reflect a human cellular protein unrelated to a retrovirus. Identification of the nucleic acid encoding the JSRV antigenic cross-reactivity in the human lung adenocarcinomas and BACs is a goal of primary importance, and several laboratories are actively pursuing this. Once the genetic material encoding the cross-reactivity is identified, if it corresponds to an exogenous or endogenous human retrovirus, the next important issue will be to ascertain whether it has a causal role in lung carcinogenesis. For such experiments, the JSRV OPA system and sheep will provide a valuable framework for designing experiments to address this question.

REFERENCES

De las Heras M, Barsky SH, Hasleton P, Wagner M, Larson E, Egan J, Ortin A, Gimenez-Mas JA, Palmarini M, Sharp JM. 2000. Evidence for a protein related immunologically to the jaagsiekte sheep retrovirus in some human lung tumors. *The European Respiratory Journal* 15:330–332.

DeMartini J, Carlson J, Leroux C, Spencer T, Palmarini M. 2003. Endogenous retroviruses related to jaagsiekte sheep retrovirus. Pp. 117–137 in Jaagsiekte Sheep Retrovirus and Lung Cancer, H Fan, ed. Berlin: Springer-Verlag.

Fan H, ed. 2003. Jaagsiekte Sheep Retrovirus and Lung Cancer, Vol. 275. Berlin: Springer-Verlag.

Hecht SJ, Stedman KE, Carlson JO, DeMartini JC. 1996. Distribution of endogenous type B and type D sheep retrovirus sequences in ungulates and other mammals. *Proceedings of the National Academy of Sciences* 93:3297–3302.

Holland MJ, Palmarini M, Garcia-Goti M, Gonzalez L, de las Heras M, McKendrick I, Sharp JM. 1999. Jaagsiekte retrovirus is widely distributed both in T and B lymphocytes and in mononuclear phagocytes of sheep with naturally and experimentally acquired pulmonary adenomatosis. *Journal of Virology* 73:4004–4008.

Jackson LA, Wang SP, Nazar-Stewart V, Grayston JT, Vaughan TL. 2000. Association of *Chlamydia pneumoniae* immunoglobulin A seropositivity and risk of lung cancer. *Cancer Epidemiology Biomarkers and Prevention* 9:1263–1266.

Koyi H, Branden E, Gnarpe J, Gnarpe H, Steen B. 2001. An association between chronic infection with *Chlamydia pneumoniae* and lung cancer. A prospective 2-year study. *APMIS* 109:572–580.

Laurila AL, Anttila T, Laara E, Bloigu A, Virtamo J, Albanes D, Leinonen M, Saikku P. 1997. Serological evidence of an association between *Chlamydia pneumoniae* infection and lung cancer. *International Journal of Cancer* 74:31–34.

Maeda N, Palmarini M, Murgia C, Fan H. 2001. Direct transformation of rodent fibroblasts by jaasiekte sheep retrovirus DNA. *Proceedings of the National Academy of Sciences* 98:4449–4454.

Mornex JF, Thivolet F, de las Heras M, Leroux C. 2003. Pathology of human bronchioloalveolar carcinoma and its relationship to the ovine disease. Pp. 225–248. In Fan H, editor. *Jaagsiekte Sheep Retrovirus and Lung Cancer.* Berlin: Springer-Verlag.

Palmarini M, Cousens C, Dalziel RG, Bai J, Stedman K, DeMartini JC, Sharp JM. 1996. The exogenous form of Jaagsiekte retrovirus is specifically associated with a contagious lung cancer of sheep. *Journal of Virology* 70:1618–1623.

Palmarini M, Sharp JM, de las Heras M, Fan H. 1999. Jaagsiekte sheep retrovirus is necessary and sufficient to induce a contagious lung cancer in sheep. *Journal of Virology* 73:6964–6972.

Palmarini M, Hallwirth C, York D, Murgia C, de Oliveira T, Spencer T, Fan H. 2000a. Molecular cloning and functional analysis of three type D endogenous retroviruses of sheep reveal a different cell tropism from that of the highly related exogenous jaagsiekte sheep retrovirus. *Journal of Virology* 74:8065–8076.

Palmarini M, Datta S, Omid R, Murgia C, Fan H. 2000b. The long terminal repeat of Jaagsiekte sheep retrovirus is preferentially active in differentiated epithelial cells of the lungs. *Journal of Virology* 74:5776–5787.

Palmarini M, Maeda N, Murgia C, De-Fraja C, Hofacre A, Fan H. 2001a. A phosphatidylinositol 3-kinase docking site in the cytoplasmic tail of the jaagsiekte sheep retrovirus transmembrane protein is essential for envelope-induced transformation of NIH 3T3 cells. *Journal of Virology* 75:11002–11009.

Palmarini M, Gray CA, Carpenter K, Fan H, Bazer FW, Spencer TE. 2001b. Expression of endogenous betaretroviruses in the ovine uterus: effects of neonatal age, estrous cycle, pregnancy and progersterone. *Journal of Virology* 75:11319–11327.

Sharp J and DeMartini J. 2003. Natural history of JSRV in sheep. Pp. 55–79. In Fan H, editor. *Jaagsiekte Sheep Retrovirus and Lung Cancer.* Berlin: Springer-Verlag.

Sharp JM and Herring AJ. 1983. Sheep pulmonary adenomatosis: demonstration of a protein which cross-reacts with the major core proteins of Mason-Pfizer monkey virus and mouse mammary tumour virus. *The Journal of General Virology* 64:2323–2327.

Willems L, Kettmann R, Dequiedt F, Portetelle D, Voneche V, Cornil I, Kerkhofs P, Burny A, Mammerickx M. 1993. In vivo infection of sheep by bovine leukemia virus mutants. *Journal of Virology* 67:4078–4085.

York D and Querat G. 2003. A history of ovine pulmonary adenocarcinoma (Jaagsiekte) and experiments leading to the deduction of the JSRV nucleotide sequence. Pp. 1–23. In Fan H, editor. *Jaagsiekte Sheep Retrovirus and Lung Cancer.* Berlin: Springer-Verlag.

York DF, Vigne R, Verwoerd DW, Querat G. 1991. Isolation, identification, and partial cDNA cloning of genomic RNA of jaagsiekte retrovirus, the etiological agent of sheep pulmonary adenomatosis. *Journal of Virology* 65:5061–5067.

York DF, Vigne R, Verwoerd DW, Querat G. 1992. Nucleotide sequence of the jaagsiekte retrovirus, an exogenous and endogenous type D and B retrovirus of sheep and goats. *Journal of Virology* 66:4930–4939.

PROPIONIBACTERIUM ACNES AND CHRONIC DISEASES

Ajay Bhatia, Ph.D.; Jean-Francoise Maisonneuve, Ph.D.; and David H. Persing, M.D., Ph.D.

Corixa Corporation, Seattle, WA

Propionibacterium acnes is a gram-positive human skin commensal that prefers anaerobic growth conditions and is involved in the pathogenesis of acne (Kirschbaum and Kligman, 1963). Acne is one of the most common skin diseases, affecting more than 45 million individuals in the United States. It is estimated that nearly 20 percent of all visits to dermatologists are related to the treatment of acne. Acne often debuts during changes in hormonal levels in pre-teens; however, it is also very common as an adult-onset condition, often associated with hormonal fluctuation during the menstrual cycle and pregnancy. While not life-threatening, acne can persist for years and is known to have serious psychosocial effects such as decreased self-esteem, depression, frustration, and social withdrawal. In addition to dermatological pathology, *P. acnes* is also suspected to be discreetly involved in post-operative infections, prostheses failure, and more recently, in inflammation of lumbar nerve roots leading to sciatica.

P. acnes, previously known by the name *Corynebacterium parvum*, has been studied extensively by immunologists for its ability to stimulate the reticuloendothelial system (Adlam and Scott, 1973). Not too long ago, an important cytokine, interleukin (IL)-18 was cloned from the liver of mice primed with *P. acnes* followed by challenge with LPS (Okamura et al., 1995). In the early eighties, certain bacteria, including BCG and *P. acnes,* were commonly used to stimulate the innate immune response against cancer in mice and human cells (Cantrell and Wheat, 1979; Davies, 1982). One of the great ironies of this organism is that it is a powerful nonspecific immune stimulant that resides naturally in the skin; its role as an immunostimulant in humans is appreciated when cases of severe acne also develop adjuvant-type arthritis.

Some investigators have gone so far as to suggest that severe acne, by virtue of the nonspecific immunostimulatory effects of *P. acnes*, might have played a role in natural protection against life-threatening diseases such as malaria and plague. In contrast, the acquired immune response to *P. acnes* has received little attention in humans.

Pathogenesis of Acne

Chronic inflammatory acne cannot be defined as an infectious disease, since the bacteria are normally present on the skin of a vast majority of individuals, irrespective of the presence of acne lesions. *P. acnes* apparently only triggers the disease when it meets favorable dermatophysiological terrain; *P. acnes* colonization of the skin is therefore necessary but not sufficient for the establishment of the pathology. The 4 major recognized pathophysiological features of acne include androgen stimulated seborrhea, hyperkeratinization and obstruction of the follicular epithelium, proliferation of *P. acnes,* and then inflammation.

Comedogenesis, the transformation of the pilosebaceous follicle into the primary acne lesion, the comedone, is the product of abnormal follicular keratinization related to excessive sebum secretion. During this process, *P. acnes* often gets trapped in layers of corneocytes and sebum and rapidly colonizes the comedonal kernel, resulting in a microcomedone, a structure invisible to the naked eye (Plewig and Kligman, 2000). A microcomedone can develop into larger structures, called comedones. Comedones can be a closed structure (whitehead) that appears like a colored bump on the skin or an open structure (blackhead). Unlike open comedones, closed comedones cannot evacuate the thread-looking conglomerate of cell debris, sebum, *P. acnes* and its products to the skin surface, and this makes them more prone to inflammation and rupture. In inflammatory acne, comedones rupture and the follicular material becomes dispersed in the dermis rather than on the skin surface. Depending on the extent of the damage to the comedone wall, various types of inflammatory lesions are produced and these are classified as papules, pustules, or nodules. Nodules are the most severe types of acne lesions and scarring may be associated with any form of severe inflammatory acne.

A break in the lining of the comedone was initially attributed to free fatty acids generated by *P. acnes*-mediated triglyceride hydrolysis, but for several reasons, it is now thought that substances produced by *P. acnes* are directly involved in the rupture the comedone epithelial lining (Holland et al., 1981). The bacteria secrete many polypeptides, among which are numerous extracellular enzymes such as proteases, hyaluronidases, neuraminidases, and others that could be involved in epithelium permeabilization and inflammatory infiltration (Noble, 1984). *P. acnes* is also known to produce chemotactic factors (Puhvel and Sakamoto, 1977), proinflammatory cytokine inducing-factors (Vowels et al., 1995), and to activate both the direct and indirect complement pathways (Webster et al., 1978). The infiltrate of an early inflamed lesion consists of polymorphonuclear cells that certainly contribute to the lining breakage, but eventually, as time goes by and infection becomes chronic, these cells attract and are replaced by mononuclear cells, predominantly T-cells of the CD4 phenotype (Norris and Cunliffe, 1988; Layton et al., 1994). As the inflammation propagates to the lining of adjacent sebaceous follicules, it can start a chain reaction that results in multiple lesions connected together and called a sinus. Studies by Hoffler et al. (1985) have revealed differences in the production of various enzymes by *Propionibacterium* isolates of acne lesions versus bacteria isolated from healthy controls. These studies are important for differentiating bacterial antigens that lead healthy controls to generate a protective immune response and those that might be involved in pathogenesis.

Antibody against *P. acnes* antigenic determinants are found in the blood of most adults, whether they have had acne or not (Ingham et al., 1987); amounts may vary between the two populations, and possibly the nature of the determinants the antibodies recognize (Holland et al., 1993). Recent investigations by our group suggest that differential recognition might involve surface molecules with physiological functions. *P. acnes* specific IgG and IgA are also found at the level of the follicular infudibulum (Knop et al., 1983); these antibodies might be of great importance in limiting or preventing *P. acnes* proliferation, and maybe more importantly, in preventing comedonal lining destruction by *P. acnes*-derived soluble factors. Our preliminary data suggests that a robust *P. acnes* specific T-cell response is also common in adult donors, but its specificity at the antigen level is currently under investigation. We like to think that there possibly exists a *P. acnes*-specific protective immunity against acne. This hypothesis is supported by the fact that some people never get acne, as well as by the observation that acne is mostly a disease of young people, (although there are numerous exceptions), and that even in countries where people are unable to afford sophisticated medications, chronic disease of adolescents eventually resolves with age. Finally, there have been successful human trials of therapeutic vaccination against *P. acnes*, and although the rate of success has not been high, some individuals refractory to conventional approaches experienced remission (Goldman et al., 1979; Vymola et al., 1970).

Role of *P. acnes* in Chronic Inflammation and Systemic Infections

The chronic inflammatory condition of the pilosebaceous follicle caused by *P. acnes* is generally considered non-pathogenic. However, there is a growing body of evidence that point to the bacterium as being low virulence pathogen in several types of postoperative infections and other chronic conditions. *P. acnes* have been associated with endocarditis of prosthetic (Lazar and Schulman, 1992) and native aortic valves (Mohsen et al., 2001), corneal infections (Underdahl et al., 2000) and postoperative endophthalmitis (Clark et al., 1999). It has also been recognized as a source of infection in focal intracranial infections (Chu et al., 2001) and various cerebrospinal fluid shunt infections (Thompson and Albright, 1998).

A recent study from Japan (Ishige et al., 1999) has shown that *P. acnes* DNA can be detected in lymph nodes of Japanese individuals with sarcoidosis. Sarcoidosis is a granulomatous disease that results in the inflammation of lymph nodes, lungs, eyes, liver, and other tissues. *P. acnes* have also been implicated in sciatica, a chronic inflammatory condition of the lower back. Stirling et al. (2001) have isolated *P. acnes* from intervertebral disc material of patients with severe sciatica and they hypothesize that low virulent organisms such as *P. acnes* can gain access to the injured spinal disc and initiate chronic inflammation. However, until confirmatory data is available, the proposed role of *P. acnes* in sarcoidosis and sciatica should be considered intriguing but preliminary.

It also appears to be significant that *P. acnes* have been isolated from several orthopedic infections, silicone breast prosthesis, and prosthetic joint infections (Yu et al., 1997; Tunney et al., 1999). The infected prostheses have been shown to contain bacterial biofilms of *P. acnes* and/or *Staphylococcus epidermidis*. The adhesion of *P. acnes* to the surface of the prostheses has been postulated to be a result of binding of propionibacterial cell surface proteins or adhesion molecules to host plasma or connective tissue proteins such as fibronectin (Yu et al., 1997). Evidence for this hypothesis comes from the studies of Herrmann et al. (1988), who show that fibronectin, fibrinogen, and laminin are mediators of adherence of staphylococcal isolates to polymer surfaces in intravenous device infection.

Corixa Acne Vaccine Program

The gamut of acne treatments range from topical and systemic antibiotics to oral and topical isotretinoins, chemicals like benzoyl peroxide, oral contraceptives and corticosteroids. Antibiotics have been in use for several decades as one of the most common treatments for acne. Antibiotics, both topical and systemic, take a relatively long time to reduce the numbers of *P. acnes* bacteria in the skin and do not address other causative factors of acne. More recently, vitamin A derivatives called retinoids have been used effectively for acne treatment since these drugs help unclog pores, reduce sebum production and help normalize skin shedding and growth. However, oral isotretinoins are also known to cause severe side effects including elevated serum triglyceride levels, acute pancreatitis, hepatotoxicity, clinical depression, and birth defects in pregnant women.

To help identify components of *P. acnes* involved in pathogenesis or a protective immune response and develop a therapeutic vaccine for acne, we recently sequenced the genome of *P. acnes*. The genome is approximately 2.6 Mb and organized into 100 contigs. It shares similarity with the genomes of other bacteria, including *Streptomyces coelicor*, *Mycobacterium tuberculosis*, and other gram-positive cocci. Numerous homologues to virulence factors of other gram-positive pathogens have been found in the *P. acnes* genome, including homologues of known vaccine targets.

Whole genome sequencing of microbial pathogens has been used successfully to predict vaccine candidates in *Streptococcus pneumoniae* and *Haemophilus influenzae* (Adamou et al., 2001; Wizemann et al., 2001; Chakravarti et al., 2000). We are using a multifaceted approach that combines traditional immunological and biochemical antigen discovery strategies along with a genomics approach to identify antigens for use as vaccine targets. This approach includes serological expression cloning, proteomics, and CD4 T-cell expression cloning. We are further enhancing antigen discovery methods by using in-silico approaches to predict targets for antibody-based vaccines and antimicrobial agents. The products of these various research strategies provide attractive antigen candidates, i.e., a polypeptide that is detected by serum from adult individuals who never suffered acne, and predicted to be extracellular and involved in *P. acnes* metabolism, or an immunogenic extracellular enzyme potentially involved in epithelial destruction. Such antigens may prove to be valuable vaccine candidates for the other chronic diseases associated with *P. acnes* as well.

Knowing the physiological function of our targets allows us to tailor in-vitro and in-vivo assays to evaluate the potential of specific immune components to limit or abolish the events that lead to inflammatory acne. Since the antigens of choice will be delivered under a recombinant protein format, they will require a strong adjuvant that induces an adequate immune response at the correct site. Recent data indicates that Corixa's proprietary adjuvants, MPL® and AGPs (aminoalkyl glucosaminide phosphates), induce strong mucosal and systemic immunity when administered mucosally. Adjuvants such as these would be useful to prime a local immune system against *P. acnes* at the pilosebaceous level.

Lastly, the molecules discovered by immunological methods could be used in immunodiagnostic assays. For example, we might be able to develop serological markers to predict in early adolescence the likelihood of future acne flares. In addition, since many of the studies of the involvement of *P. acnes* outside of the skin have so far relied on culture-based and molecular techniques that are prone to false positive results, future studies of disease associations of *P. acnes* might be facilitated by the availability of a specific immunoassay comprising recombinant *P. acnes* proteins.

REFERENCES

Adamou JE, Heinrichs JH, Erwin AL, Walsh W, Gayle T, Dormitzer M, Dagan R, Brewah YA, Barren P, Lathigra R, Langermann S, Koenig S, Johnson S. 2001. Identification and characterization of a novel family of pneumococcal proteins that are protective against sepsis. *Infection and Immunity* 69:949–958.

Adlam C and Scott MT. 1973. Lympho-reticular stimulatory properties of Corynebacterium parvum and related bacteria. *Journal of Medical Microbiology* 6:261–274.

Cantrell JL and Wheat RW. 1979. Antitumor activity and lymphoreticular stimulation properties of fractions isolated from Corynebacterium parvum. *Cancer Research* 39:3554–3563.

Chakravarti DN, Fiske MJ, Fletcher LD, Zagursky RJ. 2000. Application of genomics and proteomics for identification of bacterial gene products as potential vaccine candidates. *Vaccine* 19:601–612.

Chu RM, Tummala RP, Hall WA. 2001. Focal intracranial infections due to Propionibacterium acnes: report of three cases. *Neurosurgery* 49:717–720.

Clark WL, Kaiser PK, Flynn HW Jr, Belfort A, Miller D, Meisler DM. 1999. Treatment strategies and visual acuity outcomes in chronic postoperative Propionibacterium acnes endophthalmitis. *Ophthalmology* 106:1665–1670.

Davies M. 1982. Bacterial cells as anti-tumour agents in man. *Reviews on Environmental Health* 4:31–56.

Goldman L, Michael JG, Riebel S. 1979. The immunobiology of acne. A polyvalent proprionibacteria vaccine. *Cutis* 23:181–184.

Herrmann M, Vaudaux PE, Pittet D, Auckenthaler R, Lew PD, Schumacher-Perdreau F, Peters G, Waldvogel FA. 1988. Fibronectin, fibrinogen, and laminin act as mediators of adherence of clinical staphylococcal isolates to foreign material. *The Journal of Infectious Diseases* 158:693–701.

Hoffler U, Gehse M, Gloor M, Pulverer G. 1985. Enzyme production of propionibacteria from patients with acne vulgaris and healthy persons. *Acta Dermato-Venereologica* 65:428–432.

Holland KT, Ingham E, Cunliffe WJ. 1981. A review, the microbiology of acne. *The Journal of Applied Bacteriology* 51:195–215.

Holland KT, Holland DB, Cunliffe WJ, Cutcliffe AG. 1993. Detection of Propionibacterium acnes polypeptides which have stimulated an immune response in acne patients but not in normal individuals. *Experimental Dermatology* 2:12–16.

Ingham E, Gowland G, Ward RM, Holland KT, Cunliffe WJ. 1987. Antibodies to P. acnes and P. acnes exocellular enzymes in the normal population at various ages and in patients with acne vulgaris. *The British Journal of Dermatology* 116:805–812.

Ishige I, Usui Y, Takemura T, Eishi Y. 1999. Quantitative PCR of mycobacterial and propionibacterial DNA in lymph nodes of Japanese patients with sarcoidosis. *Lancet* 354:120–123.

Kirschbaum JO and Kligman AM. 1963. The pathogenic role of Corynebacterium acnes in acne vulgaris. *Archives of Dermatology* 88:832–833.

Knop J, Ollefs K, Frosch PJ. 1983. Anti-P. acnes antibody in comedonal extracts. *The Journal of Investigative Dermatology* 80:9–12.

Layton AM, Henderson CA, Cunliffe WJ. 1994. A clinical evaluation of acne scarring and its incidence. *Clinical and Experimental Dermatology* 19:303–308.

Lazar JM and Schulman DS. 1992. Propionibacterium acnes prosthetic valve endocarditis: a case of severe aortic insufficiency. *Clinical Cardiology* 15:299–300.

Mohsen AH, Price A, Ridgway E, West JN, Green S, McKendrick MW. 2001. Propionibacterium acnes endocarditis in a native valve complicated by intraventricular abscess: a case report and review. *Scandinavian Journal of Infectious Diseases* 33:379–380.

Noble WC. 1984. Skin microbiology: coming of age. *Journal of Medical Microbiology* 17:1–12

Norris JF and Cunliffe WJ. 1988. A histological and immunocytochemical study of early acne lesions. The British Journal of Dermatology 118:651–659.

Okamura H, Nagata K, Komatsu T, Tanimoto T, Nukata Y, Tanabe F, Akita K, Torigoe K, Okura T, Fukuda S. 1995. A novel costimulatory factor for gamma interferon induction found in the livers of mice causes endotoxic shock. *Infection and Immunity* 63:3966–3972.

Plewig G and Kligman AM, eds. 2000. Acne and Rosacea, 3rd ed., 744 pages. New York: Springer-Verlag.

Puhvel SM and Sakamoto M. 1977. Chemoattractant properties of Corynebacterium parvum and pyran copolymer for human monocytes and neutrophils. *Journal of the National Cancer Institute* 58:781–783.

Stirling A, Worthington T, Rafiq M, Lambert PA, Elliott TS. 2001. Association between sciatica and Propionibacterium acnes. *Lancet* 357:2024–2025.

Thompson TP and Albright AL. 1998. Propionibacterium [correction of Proprionibacterium] acnes infections of cerebrospinal fluid shunts. *Childs Nervous System* 14:378–380.

Tunney MM, Patrick S, Curran MD, Ramage G, Hanna D, Nixon JR, Gorman SP, Davis RI, Anderson N. 1999. Detection of prosthetic hip infection at revision arthroplasty by immunofluorescence microscopy and PCR amplification of the bacterial 16S rRNA gene. *Journal of Clinical Microbiology* 37:3281–3290.

Underdahl JP, Florakis GJ, Braunstein RE, Johnson DA, Cheung P, Briggs J, Meisler DM. 2000. Propionibacterium acnes as a cause of visually significant corneal ulcers. *Cornea* 19:451–454.

Vymola F, Buda J, Lochmann O, Pillich J. 1970. Successful treatment of acne by immunotherapy. *Journal of Hygiene, Epidemiology, Microbiology, and Immunology* 14:135–138.

Vowels BR, Yang S, Leyden JJ. 1995. Induction of proinflammatory cytokines by a soluble factor of Propionibacterium acnes: implications for chronic inflammatory acne. *Infection and Immunity* 63:3158–3165.

Webster GF, Leyden JJ, Norman ME, Nilsson UR. 1978. Complement activation in acne vulgaris: in vitro studies with Propionibacterium acnes and Propionibacterium granulosum. *Infection and Immunity* 22:523–529.

Wizemann TM, Heinrichs JH, Adamou JE, Erwin AL, Kunsch C, Choi GH, Barash SC, Rosen CA, Masure HR, Tuomanen E, Gayle A, Brewah YA, Walsh W, Barren P, Lathigra R, Hanson M, Langermann S, Johnson S, Koenig S. 2001. Use of a whole genome approach to identify vaccine molecules affording protection against Streptococcus pneumoniae infection. *Infection and Immunity* 69:1593–1598.

Yu JL, Mansson R, Flock JI, Ljungh A. 1997. Fibronectin binding by Propionibacterium acnes. *FEMS Immunology and Medical Microbiology* 19:247–253.

2

Endemic Infectious Diseases Linked to Chronic Diseases: Implications for Developing Countries

OVERVIEW

Successful disease control efforts in some economically developing countries have increased life expectancy and resulted in changes in demographics from predominantly youthful populations to older and aging ones. Consequently, during the next 20 years, chronic diseases are expected to become increasingly important in economically developing regions and to encompass chronic conditions currently attributed to industrialized nations. Not only will changing economics, demographic shifts with lower childhood mortality, and changing lifestyles affect this trend, but migration from rural to urban areas and into previously uninhabited ecosystems may expose populations to new infectious agents that underlie chronic disease. Both newly identified and well-recognized infectious etiologies of chronic disease, including infections known to enter a chronic state, such as tuberculosis and malaria, will acquire increasing importance to domestic and global health. As such, countries with limited research capacities and health care services will face increasing burdens from both infectious and chronic disease.

Richard Guerrant illustrated the wide-ranging nature of the threats from chronic diseases caused by infections, using as an example the long-term consequences of early childhood enteric and parasitic infections. The chronic impact of repeated malnourishing diarrheal illnesses is greater than that of acute deaths from enteric illness, which claims more than 6,000 children each day. Early diarrheal illnesses have significant long-term effects not only on physical fitness, but on growth, cognition, and school performance. Diarrhea appears to be a cofactor with malnutrition in that it reduces nutritional absorption.

Josemir Sander detailed the relationship between epilepsy, the most common serious neurological condition worldwide, and a number of parasites. Epilepsy is a symptom complex, so diagnosis relies on clinical history rather than a specific test. Incidence is higher in developing countries than in the industrialized world, and appears to be higher in rural areas than in urban areas. Furthermore, endemic infections may be responsible for the increased incidence in low-income countries.

Maureen Durkin discussed ostensibly preventable or controllable infections that are important causes of childhood cognitive disability, paralysis, epilepsy, blindness, and deafness in developing countries. These infections include congenital disorders, such as syphilis, rubella, and cytomegalovirus, as well as infections occurring during infancy and childhood, such as malaria, meningitis, Japanese viral encephalitis, measles, poliomyelitis, and trachoma.

Eduardo Gotuzzo described clinical experience with HTLV-1, a retrovirus that causes adult T-cell leukemia and is endemic in much of Latin America.The virus produces 3 different clinical patterns: cancer, autoimmune disease, and immunosuppression disease. In developing countries, 80 percent of lymphomas are non-Hodgkins lymphoma, and 10 pecent of the non-Hodgkins lymphomas seen by the Peruvian national cancer center are associated with HTLV-1. A second clinical presentation is tropical dysplastic paraparesia (TSP). The third clinical pattern associated with the infection is immunosuppression.

Sanaa Kamal described chronic hepatitis C infection with and without schistosomiasis. Patients typically present in their thirties or forties with gastrointestinal bleeding, usually massive, and compromised liver function and status. These patients progress rapidly to end stage disease, usually dying in their forties. Coinfected individuals have significantly higher fibrosis levels and are unable to achieve spontaneous viral clearance.

Altaf Lal described interactions between the human immunodeficiency virus (HIV) and malaria to illustrate how different pathogens interact with each other and how they modulate the disease process. Infant mortality is higher in babies born to mothers who are infected with placental malaria and HIV-1, and these infants have lower levels of acquired passive immunity. Concurrent infections also promote pathogen diversity. The interactions, however, are extremely complex. For example, acute measles suppresses HIV replication significantly.

POTENTIAL LONG-TERM CONSEQUENCES OF EARLY CHILDHOOD ENTERIC AND PARASITIC INFECTIONS*

Richard L. Guerrant, M.D.; Aldo A.M. Lima, M.D., Ph.D.; Sean R. Moore, M.S.; Breyette Lorntz, M.S.; and Peter Patrick, Ph.D.
Center for Global Health, University of Virginia School of Medicine; and Federal University of Ceara, Fortaleza, Brazil

The assessment of the global burden of diseases is increasingly important in recognizing and analyzing their importance as well as the priority of economic investments in their amelioration. In this perspective we recognize the quality of life or years lived with varying degrees of disability in addition to the quantity of life lost to premature mortality, as important outcomes or consequences of all diseases or conditions. Recognizing disability or quality of life is especially important, as mortality from a growing list of acute diseases is reduced, and chronic diseases or long-term consequences of diseases or conditions are now being appreciated. Only such a global view can begin to capture the full human and economic costs of diseases, injuries, or other conditions. Only as these true costs are appreciated, can we affect the necessary investments in their alleviation (Guerrant, 2001; Guerrant and Blackwood, 1999).

Importance of Measuring Morbidity as well as Mortality

Major advances have been made in understanding the quality and quantity elements of health outcomes and the global burdens of disease. Two of these "quality of life" measures are Quality-Adjusted Life Years (QALYs) and Disability-Adjusted Life Years (DALYs). QALYs have been devised by economists to capture both quality and quantity elements of a health care outcome in a single measure, and have been used primarily in assessing the effectiveness of specific interventions to improve health. However, QALYs suffer problems of subjective value assignments that vary considerably with who makes the choices, and they do not capture wider benefits (externalities) that may accrue to society, family, or friends.

DALYs involve not only calculating age-specific mortality (as years of potential life lost [YPLL] to fatal conditions) but also taking into account the quality of life affected by disabilities (by formulating years lost to disability [YLD] with nonfatal conditions, injuries, and diseases) (Murray et al., 1994; Murray and Lopez, 1997). In calculating DALYs, perfect health is weighted as 0 disability with disability weights progressing to 1, the equivalent of death. DALYs have the

---

*Parts of this paper have been published in a perspective article (Guerrant et al, 2002a) and in a review (Guerrant et al., 2002b).

advantages that they can also help assess effectiveness of interventions as well as the burden of disease and are standardized to permit age weighting and comparability across studies.

All conditions affecting health as well as interventions that prevent or reverse the adverse effects of these conditions are measured in economic as well as human terms. These include, in addition to the causes of death and the YPLL due to premature mortality, the *morbidity* costs or YLD from conditions that impair the ability of individuals to reach their full human and economic potential or productivity. As causes of premature mortality are brought under control worldwide, the morbidity costs are becoming increasingly recognized and their quantitation is increasingly important. Thus, in addition to diseases or conditions like meningitis, AIDS, or automobile accidents that are often fatal at young ages and are thus responsible for disproportionately greater years of life lost, we must also weigh the burden of chronic diseases, like arthritis or depression, that often disable much more than they kill. Both YPLL and YLD are included in the DALYs that are being used to assess the burdens of all diseases or conditions that threaten healthy life worldwide, as well as the "cost-effectiveness" of interventions designed for their amelioration. Both mortality (YPLL) and morbidity (YLD) pose profound economic costs, whether a young, productive working parent dies with AIDS or violence, or whether a child with repeated bouts of diarrhea, parasitic infection, or malnutrition fails to develop normally to meet his or her full human and economic potential.

It is just such an analysis that has brought appropriate attention to conditions like neuropsychiatric diseases or depression that kill few but disable many. Likewise, from placebo-controlled prospective studies of albendazole treatment of helminthic infections in Kenyan and Jamaican schoolchildren, intestinal helminths have been found to impair growth, fitness, and even cognitive function (Adams et al., 1994; Nokes et al., 1992a,b; Nokes and Bundy, 1992; Stephenson et al., 1993). Such studies have enabled Chan and Bundy to suggest potential recalculation of the long-term impact of childhood helminthic infections on DALYs to essentially double their previous values (Chan et al., 1994; Guerrant and Blackwood, 1999).

Indeed, the disability component of the DALY calculations for malnutrition and the "tropical cluster" (trypanosomiasis, Chagas' disease, schistosomiasis, and leishmaniasis), like neuropsychiatric conditions, chronic obstructive lung disease, and rheumatoid arthritis, outweigh their mortality components (Guerrant and Blackwood, 1999; Murray and Lopez, 1997). However, the initially calculated DALY for diarrheal diseases, from a 1997 assessment (Murray and Lopez, 1997), initially comprised 95 percent mortality (YPLL) and only 5 percent disability (YLD, from the transient 10 percent incapacitation during just the overt diarrheal illness [i.e., liquid stools] itself). No long-term disability from repeated dehydrating and malnourishing diarrheal illnesses in the critical formative developmental first 2 years of life is considered, largely because there had been no data to suggest such long-term effects (Guerrant and Blackwood, 1999).

Potential Long-Term Morbidity from Diarrheal Disease

The challenge is to obtain data implicating specific diseases or conditions with long-term impaired outcomes. Best studied perhaps are nutritional effects that may even involve genetic "imprinting" from the regulation of critical developmental genes at pivotal times by DNA methylation, that might further extend the developmental impact of early childhood illnesses perhaps even beyond 2–3 generations (Golden, 1994). In addition, iron deficiency has a well recognized impact on cognitive development (Basta et al., 1979; Soewondo et al., 1989). Nevertheless, despite the lack of a specific single drug (like albendazole for intestinal helminths) to control diarrheal diseases, long-term cohort studies are now enabling associations to be made of heavy early childhood disease burdens with later functional as well as nutritional outcomes. The growing evidence for lasting disability consequences of early childhood diarrhea and specific parasitic infections (including cryptosporidiosis and intestinal helminthic infections in the first 6–24 months of life) is presented in Table 2-1.

Perhaps one of the greatest of all overlooked costs of the diseases of poverty, such as diarrhea and intestinal parasitic infections, are the increasingly recognized, long-term developmental impact of early childhood illnesses, so common in developing areas. For example, we are now learning that the 4–8 dehydrating, malnourishing diarrheal illnesses that often occur each year in the critically formative first two years of life may have profound, lasting consequences for impaired fitness, growth, cognitive development, and school performance several years later. Initial studies in Northeast Brazil show reduced fitness 4 to 6 years later associated with early childhood diarrhea, and specifically with cryptosporidial infections in the first 2 years of life, *independent* of respiratory illnesses, anthropometry, anemia, and intestinal helminths (Guerrant and Blackwood, 1999). The fitness deficits alone that associate with the median diarrhea burdens in the first 2 years of life in these studies in Northeast Brazil are comparable to that associated with a 17 percent decrement in work productivity in Zimbabwe sugarcane workers (Guerrant et al., 1999; Ndamba et al., 1993).

Furthermore, these early childhood diarrheal illnesses and intestinal helminthic infections in the first 2 years of life independently and additively associate with substantial long-term linear growth shortfalls that continue beyond six years of age (totaling an average of 8.2 cm [3 $1/_4$ inches] growth shortfall at 7 years old, 3.6 cm with diarrhea alone after controlling for early childhood intestinal helminthic infections) (Moore et al., 2001). In addition, longitudinal studies in Peru (Checkley et al., 1997, 1998) have also shown that cryptosporidial infections (even without overt diarrhea) in young or stunted children predispose to an average 1 cm growth shortfall 1 year after infection.

TABLE 2-1 Evidence for Lasting Disability Effects from Early Childhood Diarrhea

Disease	Outcome	References
Growth shortfalls		
Cryptosporidial infections and persistent diarrhea	Increased diarrhea morbidity and nutritional shortfalls for up to 18 months	Agnew et al., 1998 Lima et al., 2000 Newman et al., 1999
Cryptosporidial infections at < 6 months of age and in stunted children	0.95–1.05 cm growth deficits at 1 year later	Checkley et al., 1998
Early childhood diarrhea (0–2 y.o.)	Lasting growth shortfalls, persisting at 3.6 cm at 7 y.o. (additive to 8.2 cm with intestinal helminths at 0–2 y.o.)	Moore et al., 2001
Fitness impairment		
Early childhood diarrhea (0–2 y.o.)	Impaired fitness scores (assessed by the Harvard Step Test, HST) 4–7 years later (by 4–8.2 percent for median and high diarrhea burdens, respectively; for comparison, fitness scores improved 6.9 percent 4 months after albendazole treatment of schoolboys in Kenya and a 4.3 percent increase in HST scores correlated with a 16.6 percent increase in work productivity in sugarcane cutters in Zimbabwe	Stephenson et al., 1993 Guerrant et al., 1999 Ndamba et al., 1993
Cognitive impairment Early childhood diarrhea (0–2 y.o.)	Impaired cognitive function at 6–9 y.o. by McCarthy Draw-A-Design ($p = 0.017$ when controlling for early childhood helminthic infections), and WISC coding and reverse digit span testing ($p = 0.045$)	Guerrant et al., 1999

We also find significant associations of early childhood diarrhea with long-term cognitive deficits (by standard "Test of Nonverbal Intelligence" [TONI]) even when controlling for maternal education, breast feeding duration, and early helminthic infections (Niehaus et al., 2002). Furthermore, WISC (Wechsler Intelligence Scale for Children; The Psychological Corp, San Antonio, TX) coding and digit span scores were lower in children with persistent diarrheal illnesses in their first 2 years of life, even when controlling for helminths and maternal education (Niehaus et al., 2002). And these effects are seen in a "best case" scenario in which we have documented substantial improvements in disease rates and in nutritional status over the several years in which we have conducted close, long-term surveillance of this population (Moore et al., 2000), effects that we have subsequently *not* found in other nearby shantytown communities that had not

TABLE 2-1 Continued

Disease	Outcome	References
Early childhood diarrhea (0–2 y.o.)	Impaired Test of Nonverbal Intelligence (TONI-III) scores at 6–10 y.o., when controlling for maternal education, breast feeding duration, and early helminthic infections; and WISC coding and digit span scores were lower in children who had one or more persistent diarrheal illnesses in their first 2 years of life.	Niehaus et al., 2002
School performance (increased age at starting school and age-for-grade)		
Early childhood diarrhea	Delayed age at starting school and older age-for-grade, independent of maternal education, socioeconomic status, other illnesses and of also significant effects (of ECD) on height for age Z scores (i.e., stunting) at 0, 2, or 7 years of age ($p < 0.02$, N = 77). Late starters also are 2-fold more likely to have experienced cryptosporidial infections in their first 2 years of life.	Lorntz et al., 2000

been under such intensive surveillance (Lima, Guerrant et al., unpublished observations).

We are now finding that these correlations of early childhood diarrhea are also extending to school performance, with significant associations of diarrhea in the first 2 years of life with delayed age at starting school and age for grade that remain even after controlling for maternal education and (also affected) stature. Late starters are also two-fold more likely to have experienced cryptosporidial infections (Lorntz et al., 2000).

A recent report describes the significant associations of stunting in the first 2 years of life and multiple episodes of *Giardia* infection with impaired intelligence quotients on the WISC-R test among children in Peru (Berkman et al., 2002). This is the setting in which diarrhea is also associated with reduced WISC-R scores albeit not independently of its association with stunting. This is also the setting in which cryptosporidial infections are associated with persistent stunting as well (Checkley et al., 1997, 1998).

Most recently we have launched studies of sensitive measures of higher order frontal lobe development and critical "executive" functioning that predict functional recovery from brain injury in children. We conducted semantic and phonetic fluency testing among 74 children who have now reached 6–12 years old from our prospective surveillance population (with their diarrheal illnesses recorded from birth). Early childhood diarrhea, whether measured by total numbers of episodes or as days of diarrhea in the first 2 years of life was a highly significant predictor of total fluency scores at 6–12 years of age (i.e., 4–10 years later). Impressively, early childhood diarrhea remained a significant predictor of fluency even when controlling for maternal education and for household income ($p = 0.02$; beta = –0.31)[1] or when controlling for birth size ($p = 0.007$; beta = –0.325) or height-for-age Z score (HAZ) at 6.5 years old. Since early childhood diarrhea has such profound effects on TONI III scores and on HAZ at age 2 years old, its association with fluency was not significantly independent of TONI III or HAZ at 2 years old. The persistence of strong associations of early diarrhea with fluency to 6–12 years old and its independence of HAZ at birth and at 6.5 years old (despite persistent associations of diarrhea with HAZ to 6–7 years old) suggests that despite the growth effects recovering in part, the lasting impact of early childhood diarrhea does not recover and is even greater on functional verbal fluency than on growth. We conclude that the higher frontal lobe executive functioning impairment seen at 6–12 years old associated with diarrhea in the first 2 years of life, especially with impaired schooling, growth and cognition, suggest that early childhood diarrhea results in critical neurodevelopmental impairment that greatly magnifies the importance of ameliorating these diarrheal illnesses and their long-term consequences.

These potential consequences of early childhood malnourishing and dehydrating diarrheal illnesses should not be a great surprise when one considers the importance of early childhood years in human brain development (Dobbing, 1985; 1990; Dobbing and Sands, 1985; Niehaus et al., 2002). Unlike other species such as monkeys, sheep or opossums, which have most of their brain development in utero, it is during the first 2 years of life in humans that the major brain growth and synapse formation occurs. Furthermore, if impaired at this formative stage, it is apparently difficult if not impossible to compensate or build these synapses later in life. Add to this the recognized potential for genetic imprinting noted above, and the duration of impact of early childhood illnesses may well be life-long and even extend even to the next generation(s).

Thus the disability impact and ultimate societal costs of these early child-

---

[1]The statistical symbol p stands for the probability that the observed difference could have been obtained by chance alone, given random variation and a single test of the null hypothesis.

hood diarrheal illnesses of poverty is potentially far greater and more critical a global investment than is generally appreciated, i.e., a global "tax" that is paid for the impaired work productivity in the global economy because these largely preventable illnesses continue unabated. Thus, beyond their obvious human toll, the diseases of poverty may well require an economic investment (as they are readily prevented) that we cannot afford *not* to make.

Persistent High Diarrhea Morbidity Despite Improving Mortality

The importance of an accurate assessment of the YLD, years lost to disability from early childhood illnesses like diarrheal diseases is further accentuated by the striking relative shift from mortality to morbidity seen over recent decades. Despite clear reductions in diarrhea mortality (from 4.2 to 3.3 to 2.5 million) from 1955 to the present (Bern et al., 1992; Kosek et al., 2003; Snyder and Merson, 1982), the morbidity *rates* from a third 10-year update review (Kosek et al., 2003) have not decreased; instead, with the fastest growing populations occurring in the poorest areas with the highest disease rates, the total global morbidity from diarrhea has actually substantially *increased*. The potential impact of these still common early childhood diarrheal illnesses on long-term development or disability only further adds to their morbidity costs.

Refining DALYs for Diarrheal Disease

As shown in the first row of Table 2-2, following the standard formulas with age-weighting and discounting at 3 percent, and all disability falling into the lowest class (weight of 0.096), the DALY calculations for diarrheal diseases are presented.

The morbidity in 0–4 year olds is presented in 5 different scenarios as follows:

• Scenario 1 applies the original assumptions by Murray and Lopez of 2.27 million attacks of 1 week duration, in which the 1.3 million DALYs from morbidity in 0–4 year olds represents 1 percent of the total of 100.9 million global diarrhea DALYs.

• Scenario 2 assumes that 17 percent of 0–4 year olds (or 33 percent at half the 9.6 percent disability weight) are at risk of at least 1 diarrheal attack (or a diarrhea burden) which could have life-long disability (with a life expectancy of 81.25 years as used by Murray and Lopez).

• Scenario 3 assumes that 25 percent of 0–4 year olds (or 50 percent at half the 9.6 percent disability weight) are at life-long risk.

• Scenario 4 assumes that 10 percent of 0–4 year olds (or 50 percent at 20 percent of the 9.6 percent disability weight, i.e., half experience a 2 percent life-long disability).

TABLE 2-2 Revised Calculations of Disability-Adjusted Life Years (DALYs) for Diarrheal Diseases

Scenario	Attack rate/year	Proportion disabled	Duration of disability	DALYS for morbidity in 0–4 year olds (millions) [percentage of total]		Total DALYs (millions)
1	3.6	1	0.02	1.3	[1]	100.9
2	1	0.17	81.25	351.7	[78]	451.3
3	1	0.25	81.25	517.2	[84]	616.8
4	1	0.10	81.25	215.2	[68]	314.8
5	1	0.05	81.25	107.6	[52]	207.2

• Scenario 5 assumes that only 5 percent of 0–4 year olds (or half experience a 1 percent life-long disability).

Thus, a 1 to 4.8 percent disability affecting one-third to one-half of 0–4-year-old children would increase the total global diarrhea DALYs to 2 to 6-fold the current estimates. Considered differently, for every 5 percent of children affected lifelong, DALYs increase by about 100 million; 25 percent of children affected would increase current DALY estimates by over six-fold; only 5 percent affected lifelong (or 10 percent affected for only 25 years) would more than double the total global diarrhea DALYs (Guerrant et al., 2002a).

Add to this the concept that even subclinical enteric infections that may alter critical absorptive function without necessarily producing overt symptoms of liquid stools, like those with *Cryptosporidium* or enteroaggregative *E. coli* may impair growth (Checkley et al., 1997, 1998; Steiner et al., 1998), or impede the absorption of (and potentially thus enhance resistance to) key anti-HIV or anti-tuberculosis drugs (Lima et al., 1997; Brantley et al., 2003), and the potential cost of these diseases of poverty, inadequate water, and inadequate sanitation become increasingly unacceptable.

Conclusions

Critical to understanding and making this case for investing adequate resources in the presentation or amelioration of the diseases of poverty like diarrhea is obtaining solid information about the potential long-term correlates with illness rates and even subclinical infections, controlling to the extent possible the numerous confounding variables, and careful studies of potential interventions that could alter these adverse outcomes. Only improved data and careful, accurate analyses will direct adequate attention to alleviation of these diseases of poverty that are so potentially costly to human and societal development for us all.

REFERENCES

Adams EJ, Stephenson LS, Latham MC, Kinoti SN. 1994. Physical activity and growth of Kenyan school children with hookworm, *Trichuris trichiura* and *Ascaris lumbricoides* infections are improved after treatment with albendazole. *Journal of Nutrition* 124:1199–1206.

Agnew DG, Lima AA, Newman RD, Wuhib T, Moore RD, Guerrant RL, Sears CL. 1998. Cryptosporidiosis in northeastern Brazilian children: association with increased diarrhea morbidity. *Journal of Infectious Diseases* 177:754–760.

Basta SS, Soerkirman, D Karyadi, NS Scrimshaw. 1979. Iron deficiency anaemia and the productivity of males in Indonesia. *The American Journal of Clinical Nutrition* 32: 916–925.

Berkman DS, Lescano AG, Gilman RH, Lopez SL, Black MM. 2002. Effects of stunting, diarrhoeal disease, and parasitic infection during infancy on cognition in late childhood: a follow-up study. *Lancet* 359:564–571.

Bern C, Martines J, de Zoysa I, Glass RI. 1992. The magnitude of the global problem of diarrhoeal disease: a ten-year update. *Bulletin of the World Health Organization* 70:705–714.

Brantley RK, Williams KR, Silva TM, Sistrom M, Thielman NM, Ward H, Lima AA, Guerrant RL. 2003. AIDS-associated diarrhea and wasting in Northeast Brazil is associated with subtherapeutic plasma levels of antiretroviral medications and with both bovine and human subtypes of *Cryptosporidium parvum*. *Brazilian Journal of Infectious Diseases* 7:16–22.

Chan MS, Medley GF, Jamison D, Bundy DA. 1994. The evaluation of potential global morbidity attributable to intestinal nematode infections. *Parasitology* 109:373–387.

Checkley W, Gilman RH, Epstein LD, Suarez M, Diaz JF, Cabrera L, Black RE, Sterling CR. 1997. Asymptomatic and symptomatic cryptosporidiosis: their acute effect on weight gain in Peruvian children. *American Journal of Epidemiology* 145:156–163.

Checkley W, Epstein LD, Gilman RH, Black RE, Cabrera L, Sterling CR. 1998. Effects of *Cryptosporidium parvum* infection in Peruvian children: growth faltering and subsequent catch-up growth. *American Journal of Epidemiology* 148:497–506.

Dobbing J. 1985. Infant nutrition and later achievement. *The American Journal of Clinical Nutrition* 41:477–484.

Dobbing J. 1990. Boyd Orr memorial lecture. Early nutrition and later achievement. *Proceedings of the Nutrition Society* 49:103–118.

Dobbing J and Sands J. 1985. Cell size and cell number in tissue growth and development. An old hypothesis reconsidered. *Archives Francaises de Pediatrie* 42:199–203.

Golden MH. 1994. Is complete catch-up possible for stunted malnourished children? *European Journal of Clinical Nutrition* 48:S58–S70.

Guerrant DI, Moore SR, Lima AA, Patrick PD, Schorling JB, Guerrant RL. 1999. Association of early childhood diarrhea and cryptosporidiosis with impaired physical fitness and cognitive function four-seven years later in a poor urban community in northeast Brazil. *The American Journal of Tropical Medicine and Hygiene* 61:707–713.

Guerrant RL. 2001. The unacceptable costs of the diseases of poverty. *Current Infectious Disease Reports* 3:1–3.

Guerrant RL and Blackwood BL. 1999. Threats to global health and survival: the growing crises of tropical infectious diseases—our "unfinished agenda." *Clinical Infectious Diseases* 28:966–986.

Guerrant RL, Kosek M, Lima AA, Lorntz B, Guyatt HL. 2002a. Updating the DALYs for diarrhoeal disease. *Trends in Parasitology* 18:191–193.

Guerrant RL, Kosek M, Moore S, Lorntz B, Brantley R, Lima AA. 2002b. Magnitude and impact of diarrheal diseases. *Archives of Medical Research* 33:351–355.

Kosek M, Bern C, Guerrant RL. 2003. The global burden of diarrhoeal disease, as estimated from studies published between 1992 and 2000. *Bulletin of the World Health Organization* 81:197–204.

Lima AA, Silva TM, Gifoni AM, Barrett LJ, McAuliffe IT, Bao Y, Fox JW, Fedorko DP, Guerrant RL. 1997. Mucosal injury and disruption of intestinal barrier function in HIV-infected individuals with and without diarrhea and cryptosporidiosis in northeast Brazil. *American Journal of Gastroenterology* 92:1861–1866.

Lima AA, Moore SR, Barboza MS, Soares AM, Schleupner MA, Newman RD, Sears CL, Nataro JP, Fedorko DP, Wuhib T, Schorling JB, Guerrant RL. 2000. Persistent diarrhea signals a critical period of increased diarrhea burdens and nutritional shortfalls: A prospective cohort study among children in northeastern Brazil. *Journal of Infectious Diseases* 181:1643–1651.

Lorntz et al. 2000. Presentation at the ASTMH.

Moore SR, Lima AA, Schorling JB, Barboza MS Jr., Soares AM, Guerrant RL. 2000. Changes over time in the epidemiology of diarrhea and malnutrition among children in an urban Brazilian shantytown, 1989 to 1996. *International Journal of Infectious Diseases* 4:179–186.

Moore SR, Lima AA, Conaway MR, Schorling JB, Soares AM, Guerrant RL. 2001. Early childhood diarrhoea and helminthiases associate with long-term linear growth faltering. *International Journal of Epidemiology* 30:1457–1464.

Murray CJ and Lopez AD, eds. 1997. The Global Burden of Disease: A Comprehensive Assessment of Mortality and Disability from Diseases, Injuries, and Risk Factors in 1900 and Projected to 2020. Cambridge, MA: Harvard University Press.

Murray CJ, Lopez AD, Jamison DT. 1994. The global burden of disease in 1990: summary results, sensitivity analysis and future directions. *Bulletin of the World Health Organization* 72:495–509.

Ndamba J, Makaza N, Munjoma M, Gomo E, Kaondera KC. 1993. The physical fitness and work performance of agricultural workers infected with *Schistosoma mansoni* in Zimbabwe. *Annals of Tropical Medicine & Parasitology* 87:553–561.

Newman RD, Sears CL, Moore SR, Nataro JP, Wuhib T, Agnew DA, Guerrant RL, Lima AA. 1999. Longitudinal study of *Cryptosporidium* infection in children in northeastern Brazil. *Journal of Infectious Diseases* 180:167–175.

Niehaus MD, Moore SR, Patrick PD, Derr LL, Lorntz B, Lima AA, Guerrant RL. 2002. Early childhood diarrhea is associated with diminished cognitive function 4 to 7 years later in children in a northeast Brazilian shantytown. *The American Journal of Tropical Medicine and Hygiene* 66:590–593.

Nokes C and Bundy DA. 1992. *Trichuris trichiura* infection and mental development in children. *Lancet* 339:500.

Nokes C, Grantham-McGregor SM, Sawyer AW, Cooper ES, Bundy DA. 1992a. Parasitic helminth infection and cognitive function in school children. *Proceedings of the Royal Society of London. Series B Biological Sciences* 247:77–81.

Nokes C, Grantham-McGregor SM, Sawyer AW, Cooper ES, Robinson BA, Bundy DA. 1992b. Moderate to heavy infections of *Trichuris trichiura* affect cognitive function in Jamaican school children. *Parasitology* 104:539–547.

Snyder JD and Merson MH. 1982. The magnitude of the global problem of acute diarrhoeal disease: a review of active surveillance data. *Bulletin of the World Health Organization* 60:605–613.

Soewondo S, Husaini M, Pollitt E. 1989. Effects of iron deficiency on attention and learning processes in preschool children: Bandung, Indonesia. *The American Journal of Clinical Nutrition* 50:667–673.

Steiner TS, Lima AA, Nataro JP, Guerrant RL. 1998. Enteroaggregative *Escherichia coli* produce intestinal inflammation and growth impairment and cause interleukin-8 release from intestinal epithelial cells. *Journal of Infectious Diseases* 177:88–96.

Stephenson LS, Latham MC, Adams EJ, Kinoti SN, Pertet A. 1993. Physical fitness, growth and appetite of Kenyan school boys with hookworm, *Trichuris trichiura* and *Ascaris lumbricoides* infections are improved four months after a single dose of albendazole. *Journal of Nutrition* 123:1036–1046.

INFECTIOUS AGENTS AND EPILEPSY

Josemir W. Sander, M.D., Ph.D., M.R.C.P.
Department of Clinical and Experimental Epilepsy
University College London Institute of Neurology, and
WHO Collaborative Centre for Research and Training in Neurosciences
London, United Kingdom

Epilepsy is the tendency to have unprovoked epileptic seizures. Anything causing structural or functional derangement of the cortical physiology may lead to seizures and different conditions may express themselves solely by recurrent seizures and thus be labelled "epilepsy." The semiology of seizures and the consequences for the sufferers are, however, similar and therefore epilepsy could be better described as a symptom complex or a condition rather than a disease on its own right (Sander, 2003).

Throughout the world, epilepsy is the most common serious neurological condition (Bergen, 1998). In high-income economies its incidence is around 50 per 100,000/year (range 40 to 70 per 100,000/year) and socioeconomically deprived people are at higher risk (Heaney et al., 2002). In low income countries incidence is generally quoted as between 100 and 190 cases per 100,000/year (Sander, 2003). Most large-scale studies have reported prevalence rates for active epilepsy between 4 and 10/1,000; many of these studies, particularly in low-income countries, have reported different rates for urban and rural areas, usually with higher rates in the latter (Sander and Shorvon, 1996). No clear explanation has been advanced for these differences. It is estimated that worldwide there are at least 50 million sufferers from epilepsy, the great majority of whom are in low-income countries (Scott et al., 2001). The overall prognosis for seizure control is quite good if epilepsy is treated. Epilepsy does, however, carry an increased mortality, particularly if untreated (Cockerell et al., 1994; Sander, 2003).

The range of risk factors for the development of epilepsy varies with age and geographic location (Sander, 2003). Congenital, developmental and genetic conditions are mostly associated with the development of epilepsy in childhood, adolescence and early adulthood. Head trauma, infections of the central nervous system and tumours may occur at any age and may lead to the development of epilepsy. Infections of the central nervous system have one of the highest risks for causing epilepsy (Hauser and Annegers, 1991; Annegers et al., 1996; Bittencourt et al., 1999). For instance, over three-quarters of the survivors of cerebral abscess develop severe epilepsy and survivors of viral encephalitis have an odds ratio of 16.2 for the development of epilepsy (Annegers et al., 1996). In the elderly, cerebrovascular disease is the commonest risk factor and accounts for over half the cases of epilepsy in this age group (Sander, 2003). The presence of a family history of epilepsy seems to enhance other risk factors and this suggests that the aetiology of epilepsy is multifactorial, with genetic predisposition playing a role (Johnson and Sander, 2001). It might be difficult, however, to say whether individuals share predisposition or are exposed to the same environmental sources. In epilepsy due to infections, it could also be argued that the interaction between infective agents and social, genetic, and environmental factors determines the extent of the risk (Bittencourt et al., 1999).

Endemic infections such as malaria, neurocysticercosis and paragonomiasis are associated with epilepsy in certain environments particularly in low-income countries (Sander, 2003). Neurocysticercosis, for instance, is the commonest cause of newly diagnosed epilepsy in large areas of the tropical belt, and malaria is the commonest cause of fever in febrile convulsions in endemic areas (Medina et al., 1990; Waruiru et al., 1996; Carpio, 2002). These infections are probably responsible for the higher incidence of epilepsy in low-income economies and this makes epilepsy one of the world's most preventable non-communicable conditions (Commission on Tropical Diseases of the International League Against Epilepsy, 1994; Bittencourt et al., 1999; Bergen and Silberberg, 2002). This paper briefly reviews central nervous infections and infestations that may lead to chronic epilepsy. The contribution of social and geographic factors and the putative pathophysiology are discussed in general terms and the natural history of the commonest infections is reviewed. Seizures that occur during the acute phase of an infection are termed acute symptomatic seizures and do not constitute epilepsy even if repeated, and are not covered here.

Social and Geographical Factors

The fact that the incidence of epilepsy seems to be higher in low-income countries is often attributed to social problems in these countries (Commission on Tropical Diseases of the International League Against Epilepsy, 1994; Sander and Shorvon, 1996; Bittencourt et al., 1999). Indeed, poor sanitation and malnutrition are risk factors for infections and these are common in low-income countries. In the past, malaria, schistosomiasis and neurocysticercosis were problems in parts of the high-income countries but improvements in social conditions and basic sanitation have resolved this. In most low-income countries there are inadequate health delivery systems, which results in late or no diagnosis and treatment for infective conditions that would carry a low risk if prompt action were instituted. As a result, neurological disabilities, including seizures, may be higher in survivors of CNS infection in low-income countries than in more developed economies (Bittencourt et al., 1999).

The tropics provide the ideal environment for a number of organisms that may occasionally invade the CNS; most of them would not thrive in colder or temperate climates. Other factors may also play a role: malaria, highly prevalent in endemic coastal areas and lowlands, is non-existent at higher altitudes. Some fungi are restricted to small ecological niches. Other agents exhibit seasonal variation in their infectability. The interaction between infective organism and social, geographic and environmental factors determine the extent of infection (Bittencourt et al., 1999). There is, however, no objective information on the relative distribution of risk factors or attributable risk for the epilepsies in the community in most of the world and this is an area that requires urgent research (Sander and Shorvon, 1996).

Pathophysiology

Seizures in the aftermath of CNS infectious diseases are usually partial or focal in nature, i.e., they start in the epileptic focus, a localised area of (usually damaged) cortex (Bittencourt et al., 1999). The route of entry of infective agents to the CNS may be arterial—(through the blood-brain barrier or the choroid plexus), by passive venous transport through the spinal plexuses, by direct invasion through trauma or from cranial sinuses. Viruses may enter the CNS by the haematogenous route or via neuronal routes (Eeg-Olofsson, 2003). The infectious agent needs to reach and damage the cerebral cortex for seizures to develop, and this may be achieved through various mechanisms (Bittencourt et al., 1999). Fungal infections are often dependent on the immunological status of the person, and are therefore more prevalent in immunocompromised subjects. Cortical damage will not invariably lead to epilepsy but is a major risk factor affected by the location, severity and individual predisposition, which is likely to be genetically determined (Sander and Shorvon, 1996). There may be months, or even years, between the insult and the onset of epilepsy and the reasons for this are not well understood. The existence of critical modulators, which can turn damaged cortical tissue into an epileptic focus, has been postulated (Walker et al., 2002).

Arteritis, ischaemia and infarction are the main pathological outcome of severe viral or bacterial CNS disease and if this affects the cortical ribbon it may be the substrate for an epileptic focus (Bittencourt et al., 1999). Cerebral malaria may lead to capillary thrombosis, which is probably caused by intravascular aggregates of parasitised erythrocytes in cerebral tissues, particularly in white matter (Molyneux, 2000). Astroglial reaction results in the formation of granulomata and infarcts affecting the cortical ribbon and leading to seizures. Most other protozoan and helminthic infestations of the CNS lead to formation of granulomata, which, if located in cortical tissues, may lead to partial seizures (Bittencourt et al., 1999).

Viral Infections

Among the many viruses that have been associated with the development of encephalitis are arboviruses, coxsackie, rubella, measles, herpes simplex, flavivirus (Japanese encephalitis), and cytomegalovirus. Patients may present with seizures during the acute encephalitic process but more often develop neurological disability, including epilepsy, as a long-term complication (Eeg-Olofsson, 2003).

Herpes simplex virus is the commonest and most severe viral encephalitis in immunocompetent subjects and epilepsy as its aftermath is particularly devastating (Marks et al., 1992).

HIV infections may be complicated by a subacute cortical and subcortical encephalopathy with progressive dementia, myoclunus and tonic-clonic seizures (Modi et al., 2000). Partial seizures in patients with HIV are usually the result of secondary infections with cytomegalovirus, cryptococcus or toxoplasmosis.

Bacterial Infections

Bacterial infections of the CNS usually involve the meninges or cerebral parenchyma and present as either meningitis or cerebral abscess. Acute bacterial meningitis is usually caused by *H. influenzae, N. meningitidis, S. pneumoniae* or streptococcus infections. Although it may occur in any age group, children are the group more likely to contract bacterial meningitis. Five to ten percent of survivors of acute bacterial meningitis will develop chronic epilepsy and this is usually associated with learning deficits and other neurological disabilities (Marks et al., 1992; Bittencourt et al., 1999; Oostenbrink et al., 2002).

Cerebral abscesses and intracranial empyemas are usually associated with a clear port of entry like sinusitis, otitis media, dental abscess or cardiac valvopathies (Bittencourt et al., 1999). In the majority of cases anaerobic organisms are involved. Epilepsy in the aftermath of a cortical abscess is the rule, and it is usually highly refractory to treatment and often associated with other neurological disabilities. Tuberculosis of the central nervous system may involve the meninges and cerebral parenchyma and is associated with neurological disabilities in a large number of survivors (Bittencourt et al., 1999). Many of these will have partial epilepsy that is often refractory to treatment.

Fungal Infections

Fungal infections of the CNS are rare in immunocompetent subjects, particularly in high-income economies. The fungi are acquired by inhalation of spores that lodge initially in the lungs or paranasal sinuses and may seed to any organ, although with certain topographic preferences depending on the organism (Bittencourt et al., 1999). *C. neoformans, C. immitis, H. capsulatum, C. albicans, A. fumigatus* and *A. flavus,* and *Mucoraceae sp.* are the fungal species most likely to be involved and all of them may eventually provoke seizures.

Protozoal Infections

Plasmodium falciparum and *Toxoplasma gondii* are associated with epilepsy, although the former is by far the bigger culprit. Cerebral malaria may develop abruptly or subacutely, during systemic uncomplicated, as well as during severe, falciparum malaria and may have severe consequences. Survivors are at high risk of neurological disabilities including epilepsy (Waruiru et al., 1996; Molyneux, 2000; Versteeg et al., 2003). It is likely that this is responsible for the higher prevalence of epilepsy in endemic area. Intrauterine *T. gondii* infections are associated with a severe congenital encephalopathy with epilepsy as one of the symptoms. It may also cause seizures in immunocompromised patients. Recently, a suggestion has been made that it may be responsible for many cases of cryptogenic partial epilepsy but this has not been fully elucidated (Stommel et al., 2001).

Helminthic Infestations

A number of helminthic infestations can occasionally reach the CNS and lead to seizures. *Taenia solium* is probably the commonest of these helminthic infestations but *Paragonomiasis westermani, Echinoccocus granulosis, Spargonomiasis mansonoides* and *Schistosoma japonicum* and *S. mansoni* have also been implicated (Pal et al., 2000; Bittencourt et al., 1999). Recently, suggestions have been made that *Toxocara canis* could be a major culprit for the higher prevalence of epilepsy in low-income economies (Nicoletti et al., 2002).

Taeniasis and cysticercosis are caused by *Taenia solium* (Carpio, 2002). They are closely related to poor sanitation, and the coexistence of humans and pigs is a major factor. Humans are the final host for *Taenia solium* while hogs are the intermediate host. Eating uncooked pork contaminated with taenia cysts will lead to intestinal taeniasis. When humans, instead of pigs, ingest taenia eggs they may become the intermediate host and this may lead to neurocysticercosis. In pigs the cysts tend to lodge in subcutaneous and muscle tissues but in humans there is an attraction for the brain, particularly well irrigated areas like the cortex and the choroidal plexus, Here infestation may lead to epilepsy and other neurological symptoms. Indeed, neurological problems resulting from neurocysticercosis are very common in vast areas of South America, West Africa and Asia (Medina et al., 1990; Bergen, 1998; Sander, 2003). Neurocysticercosis is probably the most preventable form of epilepsy worldwide.

Cerebral hydatidosis is caused by *Echinococcus granulosus* and occurs in sheep-raising areas. It is acquired mainly by eating food contaminated with dog feces. Epilepsy is a rare complication of this condition (Bittencourt et al., 1999).

Paragonimiasis is a parasitic disease caused by *Paragonimiasis westermanii* and is common in some endemic areas in the Far East. Like neurocysticercosis, it may be associated with epilepsy when humans become the intermediate host (usually a fish). It is acquired by eating undercooked or raw crab or crayfish (Bittencourt et al., 1999).

A recent report has suggested the possibility of *Toxocara canis* being the culprit for partial epilepsy in low-income countries (Nicoletti et al., 2002). An odds ratio of 18.2 for the development of late onset epilepsy has been reported in association with positive serology for *Toxocara canis*. This same study in Bolivia found an odds ratio for positive serology for *Taenia solium* of 3.6. This is interesting as, over 30 years ago, Woodruff claimed that dog ownership was a major risk factor for epilepsy, but this was never taken forward (Woodruff et al., 1966). Further studies are urgently needed to clarify this issue.

Conclusion

Much of the existing evidence indicates that epilepsy resulting from infections is a major cause of neurological disability in low-income countries. Indeed, it is probably responsible for the higher incidence of epilepsy in these areas and is the commonest preventable cause of epilepsy worldwide. Improvement in basic sanitation is likely to be crucial to decrease the global burden of epilepsy. Much remains to be done in this area. Studies are urgently needed to elucidate the whole spectrum of attributable risk factors for epilepsy. More research is also needed to understand the molecular basis of all epilepsies particularly the ones caused by infectious agents.

REFERENCES

Annegers JF, Rocca WA, Hauser WA. 1996. Causes of epilepsy: contributions of the Rochester epidemiology project. *Mayo Clinic Proceedings* 71:570–575.

Bergen DC. 1998. Preventable neurological diseases worldwide. *Neuroepidemiology* 17:67–73.

Bergen DC and Silberberg D. 2002. Nervous system disorders: a global epidemic. *Archives of Neurology* 59:1194–1196.

Bittencourt PR, Sander JW, Mazer S. 1999. Viral, bacterial, fungal and parasitic infections associated with seizure disorders. Pp. 145–174 in Handbook of Clinical Neurology, Vol. 72: The Epilepsies, H.Meinardi, ed. Amsterdam: Elsevier Sciences.

Carpio A. 2002. Neurocysticercosis: an update. *Lancet Infectious Diseases* 2:751–762.

Cockerell OC, Johnson AL, Sander JW, Hart YM, Goodridge DM, Shorvon SD. 1994. Mortality from epilepsy: results from a prospective population-based study. *Lancet* 344:918–921.

Commission on Tropical Diseases of the International League Against Epilepsy. 1994. Relationship between epilepsy and tropical diseases. *Epilepsia* 35:89–93.

Eeg-Olofsson O. 2003. Virological and immunological aspects of seizure disorders. *Brain and Development* 25:9–13.

Hauser WA and Annegers JF. 1991. Risk factors for epilepsy. *Epilepsy Research Supplement* 4:45–52.

Heaney DC, MacDonald BK, Everitt A, Stevenson S, Leonardi GS, Wilkinson P, Sander JW. 2002. Socioeconomic variation in incidence of epilepsy: prospective community based study in south east England. *British Medical Journal* 325:1013–1016.

Johnson MR and Sander JW. 2001. The clinical impact of epilepsy genetics. *Journal of Neurology, Neurosurgery, and Psychiatry* 70:428–430.

Marks DA, Kim J, Spencer DD, Spencer SS. 1992. Characteristics of intractable seizures following meningitis and encephalitis. *Neurology* 42:1513–1518.

Medina MT, Rosas E, Rubio-Donnadieu F, Sotelo J. 1990. Neurocysticercosis as the main cause of late-onset epilepsy in Mexico. *Archives of Internal Medicine* 150:325–327.

Modi G, Modi M, Martinus I, Saffer D. 2000. New-onset seizures associated with HIV infection. *Neurology* 55:1558–1561.

Molyneux ME. 2000. Impact of malaria on the brain and its prevention. *Lancet* 355:671–672.

Nicoletti A, Bartoloni A, Reggio A, Bartalesi F, Roselli M, Sofia V, Rosado Chavez J, Gamboa Barahona H, Paradisi F, Cancrini G, Tsang VC, Hall AJ. 2002. Epilepsy, cysticercosis, and toxocariasis: a population-based case-control study in rural Bolivia. *Neurology* 58:1256–1261.

Oostenbrink R, Moons KG, Derksen-Lubsen G, Grobbee DE, Moll HA. 2002. Early prediction of neurological sequelae or death after bacterial meningitis. *Acta Paediatrica* 91:391–398.

Pal DK, Carpio A, Sander JW. 2000. Neurocysticercosis and epilepsy in developing countries. *Journal of Neurology, Neurosurgery, and Psychiatry* 68:137–143.

Sander JW. 2003. The epidemiology of epilepsy revisited. *Current Opinion in Neurology* 16:165–170.

Sander JW and Shorvon SD. 1996. Epidemiology of the epilepsies. *Journal of Neurology, Neurosurgery, and Psychiatry* 61:433–443.

Scott RA, Lhatoo SD, Sander JW. 2001. The treatment of epilepsy in developing countries: where do we go from here? *Bulletin of the World Health Organization* 79:344–351.

Stommel EW, Seguin R, Thadani VM, Schwartzman JD, Gilbert K, Ryan KA, Tosteson TD, Kasper LH. 2001. Cryptogenic epilepsy: an infectious etiology? *Epilepsia* 42:436–438.

Versteeg AC, Carter JA, Dzombo J, Neville BG, Newton CR. 2003. Seizure disorders among relatives of Kenyan children with severe falciparum malaria. *Tropical Medicine and International Health* 8:12–16.

Walker MC, White HS, Sander JW. 2002. Disease modification in partial epilepsy. *Brain* 125:1937–1950.

Waruiru CM, Newton CR, Forster D, New L, Winstanley P, Mwangi I, Marsh V, Winstanley M, Snow RW, Marsh K. 1996. Epileptic seizures and malaria in Kenyan children. *Transactions of the Royal Society of Tropical Medicine and Hygiene* 90:152–155.

Woodruff AW, Bisseru B, Bowe JC. 1966. Infection with animal helminths as a factor in causing poliomyelitis and epilepsy. *British Medical Journal* 5503:1576–1579.

CONTROL OF INFECTIOUS CAUSES OF CHILDHOOD DISABILITY IN DEVELOPING COUNTRIES

Maureen Durkin, Ph.D., Dr.P.H.
Department of Population Health Sciences and Waisman Center
University of Wisconsin-Madison, Madison, WI

Too often, infectious diseases have been distinguished from chronic diseases, as though these are mutually exclusive categories competing for recognition as a leading public health priority. Nowhere is this view less sustainable than in the field of childhood disability, particularly in developing countries. Worldwide, infections are among the leading causes of chronic, developmental disabilities in children, along with and sometimes interacting with genetic and nutritional causes (Institute of Medicine, 2001). In developing countries today, infections that are ostensibly preventable or controllable continue to be important causes of damage to the developing nervous system resulting in early and long-term cognitive, motor, seizure, hearing, vision, and behavioral disabilities. Infectious causes of developmental disabilities thus take a major and potentially unavoidable toll on the population health and economies of low-income countries today. This paper reviews some of the major infectious causes of developmental disabilities in low-income countries and discusses strategies and inputs needed for their prevention.

Congenital Infections

Numerous prenatal infections can damage the developing nervous system or senses, causing long-term disabilities in children (Levine et al., 2001). The occurrence, nature, and severity of effects vary not only with the type of organism but also often with the timing of the exposure. For example, first or second trimester exposure to toxoplasmosis, cytomegalovirus, and varicella infections may result in a range of impairments recognizable at birth, including microcephaly, hydrocephaly, growth retardation, blindness, seizures, and skin disorders (Remington et al., 1995; Dunn et al., 1999), whereas exposure late in pregnancy or during delivery may result in unapparent infection at birth and onset of developmental delay during infancy or childhood (Koppe et al., 1986).

Congenital Syphilis

The first congenital disability to be linked to an infectious cause (the spirochete *Treponema pallidum*), congenital syphilis is preventable through routine antenatal screening and treatment with penicillin. As a result, it is now a relatively rare occurrence in developed countries, but in some low-resource settings where routine antenatal care is lacking or where cost barriers prevent access to treatment, recent studies have reported that 4 to 11 percent of births occur to women with positive syphilis tests at delivery (Southwick et al., 2001; Frank and Duke, 2000; Walker and Walker, 2002). The outcomes of congenital syphilis range from fetal and infant death to premature birth, and survival with or without neurological manifestations, which can include deafness, interstitial keratitis, and mental retardation. The most severe outcomes generally result when conception occurs during the early stages of maternal syphilis infection. Outcomes are less severe when conception occurs during the latent state of maternal infection, and clinical manifestations of congenital syphilis are thought to be least severe when onset of maternal infection occurs during the third trimester of pregnancy (Wicher and Wicher, 2001). Animal studies suggest that outcomes may also be modulated by the genetic background of the conceptus (Wicher et al., 1994). Prevention of congenital syphilis requires interventions to reduce the risk of sexual transmission to women of childbearing age, and expansion of antenatal screening and access to treatment. Although the effectiveness and cost-effectiveness of these interventions have been established in developed countries, a recent study in South Africa identified logistical difficulties that prevent timely diagnostic results and access to treatment even when antenatal screening can be accomplished (Beksinska et al., 2002). These difficulties include late presentation for antenatal care, transportation delays that delay access to accurate laboratory results, and lack of record keeping, tracking mechanisms, and counseling services. Considerations such as these have led some to recommend antibiotic treatment of all pregnant women in selected high risk populations (Walker and Walker, 2002).

Congenital Toxoplasmosis

Congenital toxoplasmosis results from transplacental transmission of infection with the protozoan parasite *Toxoplasma gondii* following an acute episode of maternal infection during pregnancy. The clinical manifestations can include chorioretinitis, intracranial calcification, necrotizing encephalopathy, microcephaly, cranial nerve palsies, spastic hemi- or quadriparesis, seizures, cognitive disability, and death. Clinical signs may be absent at birth, but infants with congenital toxoplasmosis may develop cognitive and vision disabilities by late childhood. While the risk of transplacental transmission has been found to increase with increasing gestational age, approaching 90 percent during the third trimester, the severity of clinical manifestations appears to decrease with increasing gestational age (Jones et al., 2001). Those previously uninfected are susceptible to acute toxoplasmosis infection through ingestion of raw or inadequately cooked infected meat, contaminated unwashed fruits and vegetables, or oocytes from the feces of infected cats. Although little is known about the frequency of congenital toxoplasmosis in low- and middle-income countries generally, a recent study from Brazil reported a prevalence of 1 per 3,000 live births (Neto et al., 2000), more than three times the rate reported in developed countries (Jara et al., 2001). Evidence of the cost-effectiveness and safety of early detection (via prenatal or newborn screening) and treatment of acute infection with antiparasitics is not consistent or conclusive at this time (Jones et al., 2001; Roizen et al., 1995). Thus, prevention of congenital toxoplasmosis in low-income countries requires further research and perhaps more emphasis on educational programs regarding the risks and specific hygienic precautions that can prevent acute infections during pregnancy.

Congenital Rubella

Congenial rubella leads to a range of adverse pregnancy outcomes or birth defects but only when maternal rubella virus infection occurs within the first 18 weeks of pregnancy. Outcomes include fetal death, spontaneous abortion, stillbirth, premature birth and, among surviving infants, sensorineural deafness, cataracts and other visual impairments, mental retardation, autistic features, cardiac defects, and increased susceptibility to juvenile diabetes and other chronic conditions (Peckham and Newell, 2001). The earlier in gestation that the fetus becomes infected, the greater the likelihood of multiple defects. Although congenital rubella has been nearly eliminated in successfully vaccinated populations and with a very high benefit-to-cost ratio (Plotkin et al., 1999), epidemics continue to occur in many developing countries (Lawn et al., 2000). Cutts and Vynnycky have concluded from an extensive review of evidence that "Congenital rubella syndrome is an under-recognized public health problem in many developing countries. There is an urgent need for collection of appropriate data to estimate the cost-effectiveness of a potential global rubella control program" (Cutts and Vynnycky, 1999). A difficulty facing developing countries is that vaccination can prevent congenital rubella only if high coverage is maintained. Incomplete vaccine coverage may actually increase the risk of congenital rubella infection by reducing opportunities for natural immunity and increasing the mean age of infection, thus increasing the susceptibility to infection of women of childbearing age (Panagiotopoulos et al., 1999). The availability of a combined measles and rubella vaccine may increase the feasibility of achieving adequate rubella vaccination and improve opportunities to prevent congenital rubella throughout the world (Banatvala, 1998).

Mother-to-Child Transmission of HIV and Herpes Viruses

This is an emerging cause of developmental disabilities in populations where high HIV prevalence among childbearing women is combined with lack of access to antenatal antiretroviral therapy and cesarean delivery, which in combination are highly effective in preventing vertical transmission of HIV (European Mode of Delivery Collaboration, 1999; International Perinatal HIV Group, 1999). The neurodevelopmental effects of pediatric AIDS include microcephaly and significant delays in cognitive and motor development (Belman, 1990; Macmillan et al., 2001). These effects may be greater when transmission of the virus from mother to child occurs in utero or early in gestation versus during parturition (Smith et al., 2000). In developed countries, improvements in postnatal treatment and survival of children with HIV may be associated with a reduction in adverse neurodevelopmental outcomes. One study of HIV-infected children in the US found no detriment in verbal or performance IQ when compared to controls matched on ethnicity and prenatal drug exposure (Fishkin et al., 2000). Estimates are not available of the prevalence of pediatric HIV-associated neurodevelopmental disorders from low-income countries where few infected children have access to antiretroviral therapy. In addition to direct effects of AIDS on the developing nervous system, the AIDS epidemic may increase children's exposure to social, emotional, and economic deprivation during critical periods of development. Cost-effective and accessible methods of prevention and treatment of HIV in developing countries are needed.

Perinatal transmission of herpes viruses, including cytomegalovirus and *Herpes simplex* can also result in severe neurodevelopmental disorders (Levine et al., 2001; Peckham et al., 1983), but little is known about their occurrence in developing countries.

Infections Contributing to Perinatal Complications

In addition to infections known to directly damage the developing nervous system or senses, other prenatal and perinatal infections associated with perinatal complications may contribute to developmental disabilities either directly or indirectly (Breslau et al., 1994). Perinatal complications that occur more frequently in the presence of maternal and fetal infections include premature birth, low birth weight, intrauterine growth restriction and asphyxia. For example, maternal malaria infection may result in placental parasitemia and intrauterine growth restriction, as well as maternal anemia and death. Infants born with perinatal complications are often at increased risk for brain and sensory abnormalities and disabilities. For example, retinopathy of prematurity is a leading cause of childhood blindness worldwide (WHO, 2000a), and prematurity is an important risk factor for cerebral palsy and cognitive disabilities in childhood. Yet the role and timing of infections in these disorders are not fully understood (Donders et al., 1993; O'Shea and Dammann, 2000). Many factors may contribute to the elevated frequency of perinatal complications in low-income countries, including the scarcity of resources for obstetrical care and management of complications of labor and delivery, nutritional deficiencies, and increased risk of maternal infections. Research is urgently needed on the role of maternal infections in the etiology of adverse perinatal outcomes; on the causal role of infections in developmental disabilities; and on the impact of infection treatment and control on the prevalence of neurodevelopmental disabilities in low-income countries.

Infections During Infancy and Childhood

Infections acquired during infancy and childhood that continue to cause developmental disabilities among children in low-income countries, where access to prophylaxis and treatment is often limited and delayed, include neonatal infections (Wolf et al., 1999; Durkin et al., 2000) as well as bacterial meningitis, viral encephalitis, measles, poliomyelitis, trachoma, and parasitic conditions such as malaria, neurocysticercosis, and other helminth conditions (Institute of Medicine, 2001).

Malaria and Helminthic Diseases

Malaria is a public health problem in many countries and is estimated to cause hundreds of millions of cases and approximately one million deaths in children each year (WHO, 1998). Repeated episodes of malaria are responsible for poor school attendance and childhood anemia. Cerebral malaria occurs in a percentage of affected children, with major clinical manifestations, including convulsions and coma. Measures to prevent malaria infection include use of protective clothing, insect repellents, insecticide-treated bednets, and environmental management to control mosquito vectors. Once infection has occurred, chemo-prophylaxis is effective against the development of disease. The cost-effectiveness of malaria prophylaxis and treatment programs is well established in populations where malaria is endemic, even without accounting for the potential for long-term neurological deficits in children who survive cerebral malaria. Other parasitic diseases, such as intestinal helminthic diseases, also affect a large proportion of the world's child population and may adversely affect school performance and cognitive development (Dickson et al., 2000).

Meningitis

Meningitis from major bacterial agents probably occurs more commonly in the developing than in developed countries, though specific data are lacking. Children under age 5 and the elderly are at highest risk. In developing countries, pneumonia is the most common presentation of *Haemophilus influenzae* Type b meningitis; it has been estimated that this cause of meningitis in developing countries has a case fatality rate of 30 percent and results in permanent nervous system impairment in 20 percent of survivors (WHO, 2001a). Meningococcal meningitis occurs sporadically in developed countries, but major epidemics of the disease occur every several years in sub-Saharan Africa and South America. Case fatality exceeds 50 percent in the absence of early and adequate treatment, and it is estimated that 15 to 20 percent of survivors are left with deafness, seizures, and mental retardation (Levine et al., 1998). Primary prevention of *Haemophilus influenzae* Type b meningitis can be achieved by means of vaccination of all infants or by chemoprophylaxis following close contact with an affected child. Vaccination is the only practical method of preventing infection on a population level. In developed countries where immunization against this disease during infancy is routine, the incidence of *Haemophilus influenzae* Type b meningitis has dropped dramatically (Levine et al., 1998). It has been argued that vaccination against *Haemophilus influenzae* Type b infection is cost-effective in developing countries as well (Levine et al., 1998), but information on the frequency of the disease and its sequelae in developing countries is needed to guide the implementation of control strategies. Epidemics of meningococcal meningitis can be controlled effectively by means of mass immunization campaigns resulting in over 80 percent coverage, while infection in endemic situations can be prevented by chemoprophylaxis administered to close contacts of patients (Levine et al., 1998). Information on the cost-effectiveness of these interventions in developing countries is needed.

Japanese Viral Encephalitis

Japanese viral encephalitis is the leading cause of viral encephalitis in Asia, where it is responsible for at least 50,000 cases of clinical disease each year, primarily among children (Siraprapasiri et al., 1997). Case fatality is as high as 20 percent, and the frequency of neuropsychiatric sequelae among survivors is thought to be high, though specific data are lacking. Following an infectious mosquito bite, the virus replicates in the lymph nodes, spreads to the central nervous system and propagates in the brain, leading to seizures, cognitive and motor disabilities, and progressive coma (Siraprapasiri et al., 1997). Effective vaccines have been developed against the viral agent causing Japanese encephalitis. One is a mouse-brain derived vaccine that has been incorporated effectively into the national childhood vaccination program of Thailand (Siraprapasiri et al., 1997). The high cost of this vaccine and the potential for serious neurological sequelae, however, are barriers to its widespread use in endemic and epidemic situations (Siraprapasiri et al., 1997).

Measles

Measles is an acute viral disease that is still a leading cause of death worldwide, largely because of its occurrence among children under age 5 in developing countries. Rarely (about 1/1,000 cases), measles infection causes encephalitis, which can result in long-term nervous system sequelae among survivors. While Vitamin A deficiency has been shown to increase the severity of measles infection, it is thought the infection can, in turn, exacerbate Vitamin A deficiency and lead to blindness (Strebel, 1998). Vaccination using live, attenuated measles virus produces long-lasting immunity. Eradication of measles is theoretically feasible, given the effectiveness of available vaccines and the likelihood that humans are the only reservoir capable of sustaining transmission of the measles virus. Widespread vaccination has successfully prevented the spread of measles in a number of developing countries, and is considered one of the most cost-effective public health interventions ever undertaken (Strebel, 1998). However, measles continues to be a major contributor to childhood death and disease worldwide. Global eradication of this cause of developmental disability will require sustained efforts.

Poliomyelitis

Polio was eradicated from the Western Hemisphere, the Western Pacific region, and Eastern Europe following a concerted international initiative (WHO, 2000b). This enteroviral disease, however, continues to threaten children in tropical Africa and to a lesser extent in South and Southeast Asia. Once established in the intestines, poliovirus can enter the blood stream and invade the central nervous system. As it multiplies, the virus destroys motor neurons and leads to irreversible paralysis. Immunization programs have effectively eradicated poliomyelitis from much of the world, but the disease remains endemic in much of sub-Saharan Africa and parts of South and Southeast Asia. Reported immunization coverage with the oral polio vaccine is still low in most African countries (WHO, 2001b). Although worldwide eradication of polio as a cause of childhood paralysis can be achieved by vaccination during infancy, meeting this goal will require major commitments that may be difficult to sustain in the face of the decline of the disease in much of the world (WHO, 2001b).

Trachoma and Leprosy

Trachoma is a bacterial disease of the conjunctiva caused by *Chlamydia trachomatis* (Cook, 1998). Repeated infections, which often begin in childhood, result in blindness in adulthood. Trachoma is endemic in many impoverished areas of the world where access to clean water is compromised. An estimated 5.9 million people worldwide have become blind or are at immediate risk for blindness as a result of trachoma infection (Cook, 1998). Improvements in hygiene, including access to clean water and education to promote frequent face washing, are highly cost-effective in the prevention of blindness due to trachoma (Helen Keller International, 2001). Leprosy is another neglected disease with neurological effects that continues to affect large numbers of children throughout the developing world (Jain et al., 2002).

Conclusions

Children in developed countries have benefited for decades from interventions such as maternal vaccination to prevent congenital rubella, pediatric vaccinations to prevent potentially brain-damaging childhood infections such as *Haemophilus influenza* Type b, and early detection and effective management of bacterial infections that can lead to meningitis or hearing loss. In addition, antiretroviral therapies have become available in developed countries to prevent pediatric HIV transmission. Unfortunately, cost and attitudinal and logistical barriers prevent these interventions from reaching children at greatest risk in the developing world. Extension of such interventions to low-income countries is a necessary step toward the reduction of international inequalities in child health.

To effectively respond to the impacts of infectious causes of developmental disabilities worldwide, proven methods of prevention must be implemented and expanded within primary health care systems in low-income countries. Specific interventions should be tailored to local epidemiology and resources and needs, and should include vaccination programs with high coverage to prevent conditions such as congenital rubella, bacterial meningitis and poliomyelitis, development of laboratory facilities and networks to facilitate accurate diagnoses, and commitment of resources to prevent other infectious diseases, such as pediatric AIDS, malaria, neurocysticercosis, leprosy, viral encephalitis, and trachoma. Additional recommendations articulated in the Institute of Medicine report on

Neurological, Psychiatric and Developmental Disorders: Meeting the Challenge in the Developing World (Institute of Medicine, 2001) are as follows:

1. Increase training and expertise at all levels of health care, as well as in the educational and research sectors, in the intersection between infectious disease control and child development.

2. Develop and maintain Internet cababilities to facilitate international communication among those involved in the implementation of primary prevention and rehabilitation programs for children with developmental disabilities in low-income countries.

3. In the context of the successes of current primary health care child survival initiatives in low-income countries, it is essential that increased emphasis be placed in low-income countries on prevention and early identification of developmental disabilities within the primary and maternal and child health care systems. Those systems must in turn be linked to and supported by secondary and tertiary medical services, as well as rehabilitation programs.

4. Develop increased capacity for evidence-based research by establishing regional coordinating centers in low-income countries to enable the conduct of clinical and community trials of the effectiveness of interventions to prevent infectious causes of developmental disabilities.

5. Support research on factors that are crucial to understanding how to prevent developmental disabilities in low-income countries, such as the etiology and prevention of adverse perinatal outcomes and the impact of maternal education and alleviation of poverty on the prevention of infections resulting in developmental disabilities.

6. Develop practical methods for surveillance of infections leading to childhood disabilities.

7. Document nervous system sequelae of cerebral malaria and their prevention.

8. Determine the cost-effectiveness of methods for the prevention of prevalent infections that result in developmental disabilities.

REFERENCES

Banatvala JE. 1998. Rubella—could do better. *Lancet* 351:849–850.

Beksinska ME, Mullick S, Kunene B, Rees H, Deperthes B. 2002. A case study of antenatal syphilis screening in South Africa: successes and challenges. *Sexually Transmitted Diseases* 29:32–37.

Belman AL. 1990. AIDS and pediatric neurology. *Neurologic Clinics* 8:571–603.

Breslau N, DelDotto JE, Brown GG, Kumar S, Ezhuthachan S, Hufnagle KG, Peterson EL. 1994. A gradient relationship between low birth weight and IQ at age 6 years. *Archives of Pediatric and Adolescent Medicine* 148:377–383.

Cook JA. 1998. Trachoma. *Bulletin of the World Health Organization* 76(Suppl 2):139–140.

Cutts FT and Vynnycky E. 1999. Modelling the incidence of congenital rubella syndrome in developing countries. *International Journal of Epidemiology* 28:1176–1184.

Dickson R, Awasthi S, Williamson P, Demellweek C, Garner P. 2000. Effects of treatment for intestinal helminth infection on growth and cognitive performance in children: systematic review of randomized trials. *British Medical Journal* 320:1697–1701.

Donders GG, Desmyter J, De Wet DH, Van Assche FA. 1993. The association of gonorrhoea and syphilis with premature birth and low birthweight. *Genitourinary Medicine* 69:98–101.

Dunn D, Wallon M, Peyron F, Petersen E, Peckham C, Gilbert R. 1999. Mother-to-child transmission of toxoplasmosis: risk estimates for clinical counselling. *Lancet* 353:1829–1833.

Durkin MS, Khan NZ, Davidson LL, Huq S, Munir S, Rasul E, Zaman SS. 2000. Prenatal and postnatal risk factors for mental retardation among children in Bangladesh. *American Journal of Epidemiology* 152:1024–1033.

European Mode of Delivery Collaboration. 1999. Elective caesarean-section versus vaginal delivery in prevention of vertical HIV-1 transmission: a randomized clinical trial. *Lancet* 353:1035–1039.

Fishkin PE, Armstrong FD, Routh DK, Harris L, Thompson W, Miloslavich K, Levy JD, Johnson A, Morrow C, Bandstra ES, Mason CA, Scott G. 2000. Brief report: relationship between HIV infection and WPPSI-R performance in preschool-age children. *Journal of Pediatric Psychology* 25:347–351.

Frank D and Duke T. 2000. Congenital syphilis at Goroka Base Hospital: incidence, clinical features and risk factors for mortality. *Papua New Guinea Medical Journal* 43:121–126.

Helen Keller International. 2001. Trachoma. Available at: http://www.hki.org/programs/trachoma.html.

Institute of Medicine. 2001. Neurological, Psychiatric, and Developmental Disorders: Meeting the Challenge in the Developing World. Washington, DC: National Academy Press.

International Perinatal HIV Group. 1999. The mode of delivery and the risk of vertical transmission of human immunodeficiency virus type 1: a meta-analysis of 15 prospective cohort studies. *New England Journal of Medicine* 340:977–987.

Jain S, Reddy RG, Osmani SN, Lockwood DN, Suneetha S. 2002. Childhood leprosy in an urban clinic, Hyderabad, India: clinical presentation and the role of household contacts. *Leprosy Review* 73:248–253.

Jara M, Hsu HW, Eaton RB, Demaria A Jr. 2001. Epidemiology of congenital toxoplasmosis identified by population-based newborn screening in Massachusetts. *Pediatric Infectious Disease Journal* 20:1132–1135.

Jones JL, Lopez A, Wilson M, Schulkin J, Gibbs R. 2001. Congenital toxoplasmosis: a review. *Obstetrical and Gynecological Survey* 56:296–305.

Koppe JG, Loewer-Sieger DH, de Roever-Bonnet H. 1986. Results of 20-year follow-up of congenital toxoplasmosis. *Lancet* 1:254–256.

Lawn JE, Reef S, Baffoe-Bonnie B, Adadevoh S, Caul EO, Griffin GE. 2000. Unseen blindness, unheard deafness, and unrecorded death and disability: congenital rubella in Kumasi, Ghana. *American Journal of Public Health* 90:1555–1561.

Levine MI, Chervenak FA, Whittle M, eds. 2001. Fetal and Neonatal Neurology and Neurosurgery. London: Churchill Livingston.

Levine OS, Schwartz B, Pierce N, Kane M. 1998. Development, evaluation and implementation of *Haemophilus influenzae* type b vaccines for young children in developing countries: current status and priority actions. *Pediatric Infectious Disease Journal* 17 (9 Suppl):S95–113.

Macmillan C, Magder LS, Brouwers P, Chase C, Hittelman J, Lasky T, Malee K, Mellins CA, Velez-Borras J. 2001. Head growth and neurodevelopment of infants born to HIV-1 infected drug-using women. *Neurology* 57:1402–1411.

Neto EC, Anele E, Rubim R, Brites A, Schulte J, Becker D, Tuuminen T. 2000. High prevalence of congenital toxoplasmosis in Brazil estimated in a 3-year prospective neonatal screening study. *International Journal of Epidemiology* 29:941–947.

O'Shea TM and Dammann O. 2000. Antecedents of cerebral palsy in very low birthweight infants. *Clinics in Perinatology* 27:285–302.

Panagiotopoulos T, Antoniadou I, Valassi-Adam E. 1999. Increase in congenital rubella occurrence after immunization in Greece: retrospective survey and systematic review. *British Medical Journal* 319:1462–1467.

Peckham CS and Newell ML. 2001. Viral infections. Pp. 553–572 in Fetal and Neonatal Neurology and Neurosurgery, MI Levine, FA Chervenak, M Whittle, eds. London: Churchill Livingston.

Peckam CS, Chin KS, Coleman JC, Henderson K, Hurley R, Preece PM. 1983. Cytomegalovirus infection in pregnancy: preliminary findings from a prospective study. *Lancet* 1:1352–1355.

Plotkin SA, Katz M, Cordero JF. 1999. The eradication of rubella. *Journal of the American Medical Association* 281:561–562.

Remington JS, McLeod R, Desmonts G. 1995. Toxoplasmosis. Pp. 140–267 in Infectious Diseases of the Fetus and Newborn Infant, JS Remington and JO Klein, eds. Philadelphia: WB Saunders.

Roizen N, Swisher CN, Stein MA, Hopkins J, Boyer KM, Holfels E, Mets MB, Stein L, Patel D, Meier P, et al. 1995. Neurologic and developmental outcome in treated congenital toxoplasmosis. *Pediatrics* 95:11–20.

Siraprapasiri T, Sawaddiwudhipong W, Rojanasuphot S. 1997. Cost benefit analysis of Japanese encephalitis vaccination program in Thailand. *Southeast Asian Journal of Tropical Medicine and Public Health* 28:143–148.

Smith R, Malee K, Charurat M, Magder L, Mellins C, Macmillan C, Hittleman J, Lasky T, Llorente A, Moye J. 2000. Timing of perinatal human immunodeficiency virus type 1 infection and rate of neurodevelopment. The Women and Infant Transmission Study Group. *Pediatric Infectious Disease Journal* 19:862–871.

Southwick KL, Blanco S, Santander A, Estenssoro M, Torrico F, Seoane G, Brady W, Fears M, Lewis J, Pope V, Guarner J, Levine WC. 2001. Maternal and congenital syphilis in Bolivia, 1996: prevalence and risk factors. *Bulletin of the World Health Organization* 79:33–42.

Strebel PM. 1998. Measles. *Bulletin of the World Health Organization* 76 (Suppl. 2):154–155.

Walker DG and Walker GJ. 2002. Forgotten but not gone: the continuing scourge of congenital syphilis. *Lancet Infectious Diseases* 2:432–436.

Wicher V and Wicher K. 2001. Pathogenesis of maternal-fetal syphilis revisited. *Clinical Infectious Diseases* 33:354–363.

Wicher V, Baughn RE, Wicher K. 1994. Congenital and neonatal syphilis in guinea pigs show a different pattern of immune response. *Immunology* 82:404–409.

Wolf MJ, Wolf B, Beunen G, Casaer P. 1999. Neurodevelopmental outcome at 1 year in Zimbabwean neonates with extreme hyperbilirubinaemia. *European Journal of Pediatrics* 158:111–114.

World Health Organization. 1998. Malaria: Fact Sheet Number 94. Available at: http://www.who.int/inf-fs/en/fact094.html.

World Health Organization. 2000a. Control of Major Blinding Diseases and Disorders: Fact Sheet Number 214. Available at: http://www.who.int/inf-fs/en/fact214.html.

World Health Organization. 2000b. Global Polio Eradication Initiative. Available at: http://www.polioeradication.org/vaccines/polioeradication/all/partners/default.asp.

World Health Organization. 2001a. Haemophilus Influenzae Type b Disease. [Online] Available at: http://www.who.int/vaccines-diseases/diseases/hib.shtml.

World Health Organization. 2001b. Polio Eradication: Final 1% Poses Greatest Challenge. Available at: http://www.who.int/inf-pr-2001/en/pr2001-17.html.

HTLV-1: CLINICAL IMPACT OF A CHRONIC INFECTION

Eduardo Gotuzzo
Instituto de Medicina Tropical Alexander von Humboldt, Universidad Peruana
Cayetano Heredia
Lima, Peru
and
Kristien Verdonck
Prince Leopold Institute of Tropical Medicine, Antwerp, Belgium

Human T-cell lymphotropic virus type 1 (HTLV-1) was the first human retrovirus to be described. It was discovered simultaneously in the United States and in Japan in 1980 (Poiesz et al., 1980; Hinuma et al., 1981). As documented for all retroviruses, HTLV-1 produces a permanent cell infection. Therefore, all carriers are potential sources of transmission of the infection.

Epidemiology

Geographical Distribution

HTLV-1 has an ubiquitous distribution, with well-described endemic areas. An area is called endemic for HTLV-1 if 2–10 percent of the healthy adult population is infected. The islands of Kyushu and Okinawa, in southwestern Japan, are hyperendemic areas for HTLV-1, 15 percent of the healthy adult population carry the virus (Blattner, 1990). Moderate rates of infection have been reported in West Africa, Australia, and the Caribbean (Caribbean Epidemiology Center, 1990; Delaporte et al., 1989; Nerurkar et al., 1993). In South America, Brazil, Colombia, and Peru are HTLV-1 endemic areas (Zurita et al., 1997; Gabbai et al., 1993; Zaninovic et al., 1994); the virus is also present in Ecuador (Guderian et al., 1994), Paraguay (de Cabral et al., 1995), Chile (Cartier and Cartier, 1996) and Argentina (Bouzas et al., 1994). In Peru, the virus is highly prevalent in some population and ethnic groups. Sixteen percent of immigrants from Japan—particularly from Okinawa—are seropositive. However, in the first generation of these immigrants born in Peru, the virus is prevalent in 4 percent of the population, and is not present in the second generation (Gotuzzo et al., 1996). Similar trends were reported in Hawaii (Blattner et al., 1986) and Bolivia (Tsugane et al., 1988). A study of HTLV-1 infection in asymptomatic women in Peru found prevalence rates of 3.8 percent among Afro-American women in Chincha, a coastal town south of Lima, 1.3 percent among the Quechua population of the central highlands (Ayacucho) and 3.8 percent in the population of northern Lima (Sanchez-Palacios, 2003). In other regions in South America, in which there is a strong presence of African Americans, such as Tumaco (Colombia) and Bahia (Brazil), the prevalence of HTLV-1 ranges from 2–5 percent in the healthy adult population.

Transmission

HTLV-1 is transmitted through modes similar to those described for HIV, but there are also important differences that are explained by the requirement of infected lymphocytes for the transmission of HTLV-1.

Vertical Transmission

Intrauterine transmission of HTLV-1 is very rare, and prolonged breastfeeding seems to be the main risk factor associated with this type of transmission. In Peru, breastfeeding is the most common route of transmission of HTLV-1. In a study of 120 HTLV-1-infected Peruvian women and their offspring, infection was not detected in children who were not breastfed, but was documented in 14 percent of those who received maternal milk for less than 6 months and in 31 percent of those breastfed for more than 6 months (E. Gotuzzo, unpublished data). Moreover, in a hyperendemic area in southwestern Japan, screening pregnant women and abstaining from breastfeeding has been documented to dramatically decrease the prevalence of HTLV-1 (Katamine, 1999). HTLV-1-related disease in mothers may also be associated with the increased risk of transmission of the virus to their children, as suggested by a recent study which found that HTLV-1 is present in 43 percent of children born from mothers with strongyloidiasis, and 20 percent of children born from mothers with tropical spastic paraparesis ($p < 0.01$). Gender also seemed to be a factor, as HTLV-1 is transmitted to 17 percent of males and to 32 percent of females ($p < 0.01$) (E. Gotuzzo, submitted for publication).

Parenteral Transmission

HTLV-1 is transmitted less efficiently than HIV in whole blood transfusions. Fresh frozen plasma, which can transmit HIV, has not been associated with the transmission of HTLV-1. In addition, the efficacy of HTLV-1 transmission decreases when blood is stored for more than one week (Okochi et al., 1984). These observations point to the need for viable lymphocytes to establish infection with HTLV-1. Transmission through transfusion of whole blood has been estimated to infect between 50 and 60 percent of recipients (Larson and Taswell, 1988). A national survey in Peru indicated that 1.2 percent of 142,500 blood donors were HTLV-1 seropositive. Epidemiologic studies of the general population in Caribbean countries have consistently shown that the prevalence of HTLV-1 significantly increases with age, is higher in women, specifically in low socioeconomic strata, and correlates with a history of blood transfusion (Murphy et al., 1996). The efficacy of HTLV-1 transmission through needle sharing by intravenous drug users is very low (Gradilone et al., 1986).

HTLV-1 as a Sexually Transmitted Disease (STD)

There are several arguments indicating that HTLV-1 is an STD in Latin America. The virus has been found in semen and cervical secretions of infected people and sexual intercourse is an important factor for HTLV-1 transmission (Tajima et al., 1982). Male-female sexual transmission is more efficient than female-male transmission. Seropositivity is more prevalent in sexual risk groups such as female commercial sex workers (CSW) (Khabbaz et al., 1990) and promiscuous men engaged in homosexual activities (Bartholomew et al., 1987). In such cases, the seropositivity rate is associated with the number of sexual partners, time in prostitution activities, and presence of other STDs. Sexual transmission of HTLV-1 can be significantly reduced by the consistent use of condoms. Surveys among female CSW in Peru have shown rates of infection ranging between 7 and 25 percent (Wignall et al., 1992).

Diseases Associated with HTLV-1

Although HTLV-1 is a life-long retroviral infection, symptoms occur only in a minority of infected subjects. Classical complications include lymphoproliferative disorders, such as Adult T-cell Leukemia/Lymphoma (ATLL) and autoimmune disorders (Tropical Spastic Paraparesis). Both syndromes may occur in 1–5 percent of HTLV-1-infected subjects (Murphy et al., 1989). Several reports have suggested immune-suppression in HTLV-1-positive patients.

Adult T-Cell Leukemia/Lymphoma (ATLL)

In the 1970s, an epidemic of ATLL was described in Japan (Takatsuki et al., 1977)—the striking observation being that this phenomenon occurred in Okinawa and Kyushu and not in northern Japan. In 1980, two groups determined the relationship between HTLV-1 and ATLL; the HTLV-1 provirus is integrated into the neoplastic cell DNA and the virus can be isolated from malignant cells (Seiki et al., 1983). The clinical presentation of ATLL involves fever, lymphadenopathy, hepatosplenomegaly, bone lesions with hypercalcemia, skin lesions, and a fatal course with poor response to chemotherapy. Chronic and smoldering types of leukemia, with more lymphoma-like characteristics, slower courses, and more extensive skin involvement have also been described. Males aged 50–60 years are the group most frequently affected. Studies conducted in the HTLV-1 hyperendemic areas of Japan have estimated a lifetime risk for ATLL of 2–4 percent (Tajima and Hinuma, 1992). In Jamaica, Murphy reported the lifetime risk of ATLL to be 4 percent for those infected with HTLV-1 before 20 years of age (Murphy et al., 1996). In South America, the association between HTLV-1 and ATLL has been recognized in Brazil, Colombia, and in Argentina. Three hundred new cases of non-Hodgkin's lymphoma are detected at the National Institute of

Cancer in Lima, Peru, each year, and 10 percent (30) of these cases are associated with HTLV-1.

Tropical Spastic Paraparesis

The general term "tropical spastic paraparesis" (TSP) was introduced by Mani et al. in 1969 for a chronic progressive paraparesis of unknown cause observed in tropical areas; however, it was not until 1985 that the association between this syndrome and HTLV-1 infection was recognized (Gessain et al., 1985). The designation HTLV-1-associated myelopathy/tropical spastic paraparesis (HAM/TSP) was proposed in 1989.

It has been reported that TSP occurs in 1–4 percent of people infected with HTLV-1 (Kaplan et al., 1990). TSP predominantly affects adult females, an observation that is also confirmed in WHO's guidelines for diagnosis of TSP. The risk of TSP appears to be higher in Latin America than in Japan and associations have been reported between TSP and certain HLA alleles (Jeffrey et al., 1999). Furthermore, the association between HTLV-1 and TSP varies between geographical regions; in Colombia, 87 percent of TSP cases were HTLV-1-seropositive and in Peru, 55–65 percent of TSP patients were carriers of HTLV-1. On the other hand, in a study in Mexico, less than 1 percent of TSP cases were found to carry HTLV-1 (unpublished data, J. Sotelo, Inst Nal Neurol, Mexico City). These observations suggest that genetic background can influence susceptibility to TSP, and that HTLV-1 and other cofactors, that remain unknown, are involved in the pathogenesis of this disease.

An autoimmune mechanism has been proposed to explain the pathogenesis of TSP. According to this hypothesis, cytokines, such as tumor necrosis factor-α, are released against viral proteins in the surface of infected lymphocytes thereby causing chronic inflammation and tissue damage within the thoracic middle portion of the spinal cord.

The clinical symptoms of TSP consist of a gradually appearing symmetrical paraparesis with signs of pyramidal tract involvement that usually progresses slowly and relentlessly. However, some patients present rapid progression of the neurological symptoms; in these patients, higher antibody titers to HTLV-1 have been found (Nakagawa et al., 1995). In a recent retrospective study in Peru, 22 percent of TSP patients presented rapid progression, defined as less than 2 years between onset of symptoms and confinement to a wheelchair. Some patients presented more rapid progression, with the time between onset of symptoms and the inability to walk unaided as short as 6 months. As noted in a previous report (Nakagawa et al., 1995), there was an association between age of onset and rapid progression of TSP; 67 percent of patients with rapid progression were at least 50 years of age at disease onset, compared with 38 percent among slow progressors, $p < 0.01$. With the exception of unintentional tremor, no differences were found in clinical symptoms (38 percent of patients with rapid progression reported tremor versus 9 percent among slow progressors, $p < 0.001$) (E. Gotuzzo, unpublished data).

Urinary symptoms are a frequent complaint of TSP patients. Initially, patients report difficulties to initiate voiding. Not uncommonly, patients mention the need to put external pressure on their lower abdomen in order to urinate. In severe cases, patients cannot maintain voiding without compressing the abdomen, sometimes leading to urinary retention. Recurrent urinary infections are common, probably reflecting disorders in bladder emptying. Dysfunction of the detrusor muscle has been implicated in the urinary tract involvement in TSP.

Manifestations of immune hyperactivity other than TSP—such as Sjögren's syndrome, uveitis, arthritis, Behçet's disease and thyroiditis—have been repeatedly observed among patients with TSP.

Currently, there is neither specific nor standardized treatment for HTLV-1 and TSP. Prolonged periods of systemic steroids appear to improve clinical symptoms of TSP and recently, antiretroviral drugs effective in treating HIV, such as lamivudine and zidovudine, have been used with relative success in treating patients with TSP (Sheremata et al., 1993). A combination of corticosteroids, antiretroviral drugs, and rehabilitation might considerably improve the quality of life of TSP patients—particularly if treatment is started early in the course of the disease in those cases with rapid progression (Araujo et al., 1995).

Association of HTLV-1 with Strongyloidiasis

Strongyloides stercoralis is a soil-transmitted intestinal nematode that has been estimated to infect at least 60 million people worldwide. Infection is often asymptomatic, but can cause nonspecific abdominal symptoms and mild diarrhea. While strongyloidiasis is generally a self-limited disease in immunocompetent hosts, *S. stercoralis* behaves as an opportunistic pathogen, producing disseminated and life-threatening infections (Neva, 1986) in immunocompromised hosts who are incapable of mounting an appropriate immune response. An association of disseminated *S. stercoralis* infection with malignant tumors, severe malnutrition, acquired immunodeficiency syndrome (AIDS), corticosteroid therapy, and renal transplantation has been well documented. Studies in Japan and Jamaica have shown a significant association between the presence of *S. stercoralis* infection and HTLV-1 (Nakada et al., 1984). In Sao Paulo, 12 percent of HTLV-1-positive blood donors carried strongyloidiasis, compared to 1.6 percent of the control group (Nakada et al., 1984). In our institute in Lima, Peru, 10 percent of strongyloidiasis patients are HTLV-1-positive. Another study conducted in Lima, Peru reveals a strong association between the phenomenon of hyperinfection with *S. stercoralis* and HTLV-1. Eighty-six percent (18 out of 21) of patients with *S. stercoralis* hyperinfection were infected with HTLV-1, but were not infected with other immunosuppressive diseases such as AIDS or cancer. The difference with the HTLV-1 prevalence in a carefully matched control group (5 percent, 1 out of 21) and in a group with intestinal strongyloidiasis (10 percent, 6 of 62) was statistically significant ($p < 0.001$) (Gotuzzo et al., 1999). A report of decreased therapeutic efficacy of thiabendazole exists among patients with concomitant *S. stercoralis*-HTLV-1 infection in Okinawa (Sato et al., 1994). Terashima showed that the failure of the standard treatment against intestinal strongyloidiasis with thiabendazole or ivermectin was an important marker for suspecting HTLV-1 infection. Some reports suggest that there is a relation between strongyloidiasis and ATLL in HTLV-1-positive patients. It is not clear whether *Strongyloides* acts as a trigger, shortening the incubation time of leukemia, or a marker of high proviral load.

Association of HTLV-1 with Crusted Scabies

Crusted scabies, a severe form of scabies with generalized itching and massive numbers of mites, has been described among patients undergoing chemotherapy and with various immunosuppressive conditions, such as Down's syndrome, cancer, and AIDS (Paterson et al., 1973). Several reports on the association between HTLV-1 and severe scabies have been published. In a study in 6 hospitals in Lima, Peru, 23 patients were diagnosed with Norwegian scabies over 19 months. Seventy percent of patients were serologically confirmed to have HTLV-1 infection; 9 percent were on long-term oral corticosteroid treatment; 1 patient had Down's syndrome; 2 patients were chronically malnourished; and 2 patients had no known risk factors for crusted scabies. A study conducted in Bahia, Brazil, found a similar association between HTLV-1 and severe scabies but also identified dual infection (HIV/HTLV-1) as a risk factor for even more severe forms of scabies. The crusted form of the disease was highly predictive of double retroviral infection and seemed to be associated with severe immunodeficiency, because HIV/HTLV-1 coinfected patients were more likely to die during the study period. These data suggest that coinfection by HIV-HTLV-1 is associated with a deeper degree of immunodeficiency, which increases the risk of developing severe forms of scabies (Brites et al., 2002).

Coinfection of HTLV-1 with HIV

In spite of the similarities between HTLV-1 and HIV with respect to transmission, both epidemics are still largely separated in Peru. Nevertheless, dual infections do occur. In 1989, 19 percent of HIV-infected Peruvian men and 5 percent of HIV-infected women were found to be HTLV-1 coinfected; and in men, dual infection was associated with a higher number of sexual partners compared with HIV-only infected patients (Phillips et al., 1991). Dual infection has also been reported in Trinidad (Bartholomew et al., 1987), Brazil (Cortes et al., 1989), and the United States (Pierik and Murphy, 1991). Several studies have suggested that patients with dual infection are at higher risk of developing AIDS

(Bartholomew et al., 1987). In a prospective study of HIV-positive intravenous drug users, patients infected with both viruses were three times more likely to die from AIDS during follow-up than those infected with HIV-I alone (Page et al., 1990). In a Peruvian study, the mortality rate was 63 percent in HIV-infected patients and 80 percent in dually-infected patients. Of 50 patients who died without receiving any antiretroviral treatment, survival time was 5.02 ± 3.27 months in patients with dual infection, shorter than that of patients with HIV alone (10.07 ± 4.42 months) (Gotuzzo et al., 1992).

Association of HTLV-1 with Tuberculosis

It is well known that the incidence and clinical picture of tuberculosis (TB) is adversely affected by HIV infection. Similarly, in a Brazilian study, patients with TB and HTLV-1 exhibited a worse clinical course and a poorer prognosis than those without HTLV-1. In a study among 131 inpatients with TB in Lima, Peru, those patients infected with HIV-1 or with HTLV-1 were more likely to die during hospitalization than seronegative TB patients (RR = 2.6 for HIV [95 percent confidence interval = 1.05–6.30] and RR = 5.8 for HTLV-1 [95 percent confidence interval = 2.3–14.3]). The association was particularly strong among patients infected with both HIV-1 and HTLV-1 (RR = 6.61, 95 percent confidence interval = 2.5–17.2) (Henriquez et al., 2002).

Association of HTLV-1 with Chronic Infective Dermatitis

The term infective dermatitis was proposed by Sweet in 1966 for a relapsing eczematous condition in Jamaican children, usually associated with cutaneous infections by *Staphylococcus aureus* or β-hemolytic *Streptococcus* (Sweet, 1966). In 1990, LaGrenade described an association between chronic infective dermatitis and infection with HTLV-1 (LaGrenade et al., 1990). This syndrome has also been described in Colombia (Blank et al., 1995). Chronic infective dermatitis is commonly seen in children and is rare in adults. This disease presents with symmetric lesions on the scalp, face, armpits, and groin. These lesions improve markedly with antibiotics, but usually relapse when antibiotics are stopped.

Conclusion

HTLV-1 produces three different clinical patterns: lymphoproliferative disease (ATLL), autoimmune syndromes (TSP), and infections associated with immunosuppression (strongyloidiasis, crusted scabies and others). The infection is endemic in several countries in Latin America. HTLV-1 is transmitted mainly through breastfeeding, transfusion of whole blood, and as a STD. These modes of transmission are vulnerable to simple and effective methods of control, such as screening of pregnant women and avoiding lactation in those infected, universal screening of blood donors, and promotion of condom use in sexual risk groups.

REFERENCES

Araujo AQ, Leite AC, Dultra SV, Andrada-Serpa MJ. 1995. Progression of neurological disability in HTLV-1-associated myelopathy/tropical spastic paraparesis (HAM/TSP). *Journal of the Neurological Sciences* 129:147–151.

Bartholomew C, Blattner W, Cleghorn F. 1987a. Progression to AIDS in homosexual men co-infected with HIV and HTLV-I in Trinidad. *Lancet* 2:1469.

Bartholomew C, Saxinger C, Clark JW, Gail M, Dudgeon A, Mahabir B, Hull-Drysdale B, Cleghorn F, Gallo RC, Blattner WA. 1987b. Transmission of HTLV-1 and HIV among homosexual men in Trinidad. *Journal of the American Medical Association* 257:2604–2608.

Blank A, Herrera M, Lourido MA, Rueda R, Blank M. 1995. Infective dermatitis in Colombia. *Lancet* 346:710.

Blattner WA. 1990. Epidemiology of HTLV-1 and associated diseases. In Human Retrovirology: HTLV-1, WA Blattner, ed. New York: Raven Press.

Blattner WA, Nomura A, Clark JW, Ho GY, Nakao Y, Gallo R, Robert-Guroff M. 1986. Modes of transmission and evidence for viral latency from studies of human T-cell lymphotropic virus type I in Japanese migrant populations in Hawaii. *Proceedings of the National Academies of Sciences USA* 83:4895–4898.

Bouzas MB, Zapiola I, Quiruelas S, Gorvein D, Panzita A, Rey J, Carnese FP, Corral R, Perez C, Zala C, et al. 1994. HTLV Type I and HTLV Type II infection among Indians and Natives from Argentina. *AIDS Research and Human Retroviruses* 10:1567–1571.

Brites C, Weyll M, Pedroso C, Badaro R. 2002. Severe and Norwegian scabies are strongly associated with retroviral (HIV/HTLV-1) infection in Bahia, Brazil [letter]. *AIDS* 16:1292–1293.

Caribbean Epidemiology Center. 1990. Public Health Implications of HTLV-1 in the Caribbean. *Weekly Epidemiological Record* 65:63–65.

Cartier L and Cartier E. 1996. HTLV-I/II in Chile. Pp. 150–158 in HTLV, Truths and Questions, V Zaninovic, ed. Cali, Colombia: Fundación MAR.

Cortes E, Detels R, Aboulafia D, Li XL, Moudgil T, Alam M, Bonecker C, Gonzaga A, Oyafuso L, Tondo M. 1989. HIV-1, HIV-2 and HTLV-I infection in high risk groups in Brazil. *New England Journal of Medicine* 320:953–958.

de Cabral MB, Vera ME, Samudio M, Arias AR, Cabello A, Moreno R, Zapiola I, Bouzas MB, Muchinik G. 1995. HTLV-I/II antibodies among three different Indian groups from Paraguay. *Journal of Acquired Immune Deficiency Syndromes and Human Retrovirology* 19:548–549.

Delaporte E, Peeters M, Durand JP, Dupont A, Schrijvers D, Bedjabaga L, Honore C, Ossari S, Trebucq A, Josse R, et al. 1989. Seroepidemiological survey of HTLV-1 infection among randomized population of western central African countries. *Journal of AIDS* 2:410–413.

Gabbai AA, Bordin JO, Vieira-Filho JP, Kuroda A, Oliveira AS, Cruz MV, Ribeiro AA, Delaney SR, Henrard DR, Rosario J, et al. 1993. Selectivity of human T lymphotropic virus type I (HTLV-I) and HTLV-II infection among different populations in Brazil. *American Journal of Tropical Medicine and Hygiene* 49:664–671.

Gessain A, Barin F, Vernant JC, Gout O, Maurs L, Calender A, de The G. 1985. Antibodies to human T-lymphotropic virus type-I in patients with tropical spastic paraparesis. *Lancet* 2:407–410.

Gotuzzo E, Escamilla J, Phillips IA, Sanchez J, Wignall FS, Antigoni J. 1992. The impact of human T lymphotropic virus type I/II infection on the prognosis of sexually acquired cases of acquired immunodeficiency syndrome. *Archives of Internal Medicine* 152:1429–1432.

Gotuzzo E, Yamamoto V, Kanna M, et al. 1996. Human T lymphotropic virus type I infection among Japanese immigrants in Peru. *International Journal of Infectious Diseases* 1:75–77.

Gotuzzo E, Terashima A, Alvarez H, Tello R, Infante R, Watts DM, Freedman DO. 1999. *Strongyloides stercoralis* hyperinfection associated with human T cell lymphotropic virus type-I infection in Peru. *American Journal of Tropical Medicine and Hygiene* 60:146–149.

Gradilone A, Zani M, Barillari G, Modesti M, Agliano AM, Maiorano G, Ortona L, Frati L, Manzari V. 1986. HTLV-1 and HIV infection in drug addicts in Italy. *Lancet* 2:753–754.

Guderian R, Guevara A, Cooper P, Rugeles MT, Arango C. 1994. HTLV-1 infection and tropical spastic paraparesis in Esmeraldas Province of Ecuador. *Transactions of the Royal Society of Tropical Medicine and Hygiene* 88:399–400.

Henriquez C, Gotuzzo E, Cairampoma, et al. Impact of infection with HIV and/or HTLV-1 on the outcome of hospitalization for tuberculosis in a public hospital in Peru. Abstract at the 4th World Congress on Tuberculosis, Washington, DC, June 3–5, 2002.

Hinuma Y, Nagata K, Hanaoka M, Nakai M, Matsumoto T, Kinoshita KI, Shirakawa S, Miyoshi I. 1981. Adult T cell leukemia antigen in an ATL cell line and detection of antibodies to the antigen in human sera. *Proceedings of the National Academy of Sciences USA* 78:6476–6480.

Jeffrey KJ, Usuku K, Hall SE, Matsumoto W, Taylor GP, Procter J, Bunce M, Ogg GS, Welsh KI, Weber JN, Lloyd AL, Nowak MA, Nagai M, Kodama D, Izumo S, Osame M, Bangham CR. 1999. HLA alleles determine human T-lymphotropic virus-I (HTLV-1) proviral load and the risk of HTLV-1-associated myelopathy. *Proceedings of the National Academy of Sciences USA* 96:3848–3853.

Kaplan JE, Osame M, Kubota H, Igata A, Nishitani H, Maeda Y, Khabbaz RF, Janssen RS. 1990. The risk of development of HTLV-1 associated myelopathy/tropical spastic paraparesis among persons infected with HTLV-1. *AIDS* 3:1096–1101.

Katamine S. 1999. Milk-borne transmission of human T-cell lymphotropic virus Type 1 (HTLV-1) and its intervention in Nagasaki. *Acta Medica Nagasakiensia* 44:1–6.

Khabbaz R, Darrow WW, Hartley TM, Witte J, Cohen JB, French J, Gill PS, Potterat J, Sikes RK, Reich R, et al.. 1990. Seroprevalence and risk factors for HTLV-1 infection among female prostitutes in the United States. *Journal of the American Medical Association* 263:60–64.

LaGrenade L, Hanchard B, Fletcher V, Cranston B, Blattner W. 1990. Infective dermatitis of Jamaican children: a marker for HTLV-1 infection. *Lancet* 336:1345–1347.

Larson C and Taswell H. 1988. Human T-cell leukemia virus (HTLV-1) and blood transfusion. *Mayo Clinic Proceedings* 63: 869–875.

Mani KS, Mani AJ, Montgomery, RD. 1969. A spastic paraplegic syndrome in South India. *Journal of the Neurological Sciences* 9:179–199.

Murphy EL, Hanchard B, Figueroa JP, Gibbs WN, Lofters WS, Campbell M, Goedert JJ, Blattner WA. 1989. Modelling the risk of adult T cell leukemia/lymphoma in persons infected with human T lymphotropic virus type I. *International Journal of Cancer* 43:250–253.

Murphy EL, Wilks K, Hanchard B, Cranston B, Figueroa JP, Gibbs WN, Murphy J, Blattner WA. 1996. A case-control study of risk factors for seropositivity to HTLV-1 in Jamaica. *International Journal of Epidemiology* 25:1083–1089.

Nakada K, Kohakura M, Komoda H, Hinuma Y. 1984. High incidence of HTLV antibody in carriers of *Strongyloides stercoralis* [letter]. *Lancet* 1:633.

Nakagawa M, Izumo S, Ijichi S, Kubota H, Arimura K, Kawabata M, Osame M. 1995. HTLV-1-associated myelopathy: analysis of 213 patients based on clinical features and laboratory findings. *Journal of Neurovirology* 1:50–61.

Nerurkar VR, Song KJ, Saitou N, Melland RR, Yanagihara R. 1993. Interfamilial genomic diversity and molecular phylogeny of human T-cell lymphotrophic virus type I from Papua New Guinea and the Solomon Islands. *Virology* 196:506–513.

Neva FA. 1986. Biology and immunology of human strongyloidiasis. *Journal of Infectious Diseases* 153:397–406.

Okochi K, Sata H, Hinuma Y. 1984. A retrospective study on transmission of adult T-cell leukemia virus via blood transfusion: seroconversion in recipients. *Vox Sanguinis* 46:245–253.

Page JB, Lai SH, Chitwood DD, Klimas NG, Smith PC, Fletcher MA. 1990. HTLV-I/II seropositivity and death from AIDS among HIV-1 seropositive intravenous drug users. *Lancet* 335:1439–1441.

Paterson WD, Allen BR, Beveridge GW. 1973. Norwegian scabies during immunosuppressive therapy. *British Medical Journal* 4:211–212.

Phillips I, Hyams KC, Wignall FS, Moran AY, Gotuzzo E, Sanchez J, Roberts CR. 1991. HTLV-1 co-infection in a HIV-1 infected Peruvian population. *Journal of Acquired Immune Deficiency Syndromes* 4:301–302.

Pierik LT and Murphy EL. 1991. The clinical significance of HTLV-I and HTLV-II infection in the AIDS epidemic. Pp. 41–57 in AIDS Clinical Review, P Volberding and MA Jacobson, eds. New York: Marcel Dekker.

Poiesz BJ, Ruscetti FW, Gadzar AF, Bunn PA, Minna JD, Gallo RC. 1980. Detection and isolation of type C retrovirus particles from fresh and cultured lymphocytes of a patient with cutaneous T cell lymphoma. *Proceedings of the National Academy of Sciences USA* 77:7415–7419.

Sanchez-Palacios C, Gotuzzo E, Vandamme AM, Maldonado Y. 2003. Seroprevalence and risk factors for human T-cell lymphotropic virus (HTLV-1) infection among ethnically and geographically diverse Peruvian women. *International Journal of Infectious Diseases* 7:132–137.

Sato Y, Shiroma Y, Kiyuna S, Toma H, Kobayashi J. 1994. Reduced efficacy of chemotherapy might accumulate concurrent HTLV-1 infection among strongyloidiasis patients in Okinawa, Japan. *Transactions of the Royal Society of Tropical Medicine and Hygiene* 88:59.

Seiki M, Hattori S, Hirayama Y, Yoshida M. 1983. Human adult T-cell leukemia virus: Completed nucleotide sequence of the provirus genoma integrated in leukemia cell DNA. *Proceedings of the National Academy of Sciences USA* 80:3618–3622.

Sheremata WA, Benedict D, Squilacote DC, Sazant A, DeFreitas E. 1993. High-dose zidovudine induction in HTLV-1-associated myelopathy: safety and possible efficacy. *Neurology* 43:2125–2129.

Sweet RD. 1966. A pattern of eczema in Jamaica. *British Journal of Dermatology* 78:93–100.

Tajima K and Hinuma Y. 1992. Epidemiology of HTLV-I/II in Japan and the world. *Gann Monograph on Cancer Research* 39:129–149.

Tajima K, Tominaga S, Suchi, Kawagoe T, Komoda H, Hinuma Y, Oda T, Fujita K. 1982. Epidemiological analysis of the distribution of antibody to adult T-cell leukemia-virus-associated antigen: possible horizontal transmission of adult T-cell leukemia virus. *Gann* 73:893–901.

Takatsuki K, Uchiyama J, Sagawa K, Yodoi J. 1977. Adult T-cell leukemia in Japan. Pp. 73–77 in Topics in Hematology, S Sano, F Takaku, S Irino, eds. Amsterdam: Excerpta Medica.

Tsugane S, Watanabe S, Sugimura H, Otsu T, Tobinai K, Shimoyama M, Nanri S, Ishii H. 1988. Infectious status of human T lymphotropic virus type I and hepatitis B virus among Japanese immigrants in the Republic of Bolivia. *American Journal of Epidemiology* 128:1153–1161.

Wignall FS, Hyams KC, Phillips IA, Escamilla J, Tejada A, Li O, Lopez F, Chauca G, Sanchez S, Roberts CR. 1992. Sexual transmission of human T-cell lymphotropic virus type I in Peruvian prostitutes. *Journal of Medical Virology* 38:44–48.

Zaninovic V, Sanzón F, López F, Velandia G, Blank A, Blank M, Fujiyama C, Yashiki S, Matsumoto D, Katahira Y, et al. 1994. Geographic independence of HTLV-I and HTLV-II foci in the Andes Highland, the Atlantic Coast, and the Orinoco of Colombia. *AIDS Research and Human Retroviruses* 10:97–101.

Zurita S, Costa C, Watts D, Indacochea S, Campos P, Sanchez J, Gotuzzo E. 1997. Prevalence of human retroviral infection in Quillabamba and Cuzco, Peru: a new endemic area for human T-cell lymphotropic virus type 1. *American Journal of Tropical Medicine and Hygiene* 56:561–565.

PROGRESSION OF HEPATITIS C VIRUS INFECTION WITH AND WITHOUT SCHISTOSOMIASIS

Sanaa Kamal, M.D.
Ain Shams University, Cairo, Egypt

Hepatitis C virus (HCV) infects an estimated 170 million persons world-wide, and is a major cause of morbidity in developed and developing countries. In the United States, nearly 2 percent of the population is infected with this positive strand RNA virus from the flavivirus family (Seeff, 1997; Alter, 1997). In other regions, the prevalence of HCV infection is even higher reaching up to 10 percent to 31 percent of the population in some countries (Abdel Aziz et al., 2000; Habib et al., 2001). Approximately 70 percent of infected persons will go on to develop chronic hepatitis, and 15 to 20 percent will eventually develop cirrhosis. HCV-related cirrhosis is also one of the major risk factors for the development of hepatocellular carcinoma (Seeff, 1997). Despite recent improvements in treating HCV infection using interferon-alpha and ribavirin, about half of infected individuals will fail treatment or cannot be treated due to contraindications (Poynard et al., 1996; Thevenot et al., 2001). Also, for many persons worldwide, antiviral therapy is out of reach due to its prohibitive costs. Therefore, the development of an effective vaccine to prevent the continued spread of HCV infection remains an urgent goal. Likewise, a better understanding of the immunopathogenesis of this infection may facilitate the development of immunotherapeutic strategies to treat infected persons.

CD4 Response to HCV Infection

The host immune response probably plays a critical role in both control of HCV replication and liver injury. HCV infection evokes CD4+, HLA class II-restricted (Cerny and Chisari, 1999; Diepolder et al., 1996) and CD8+ (CTL) HLA class I-restricted T-cell response (Lechner et al., 2000; He et al., 1999). In the absence of an appropriate small animal model, studying the immunological events that occur in the earliest stages of infection in patients with acute hepatitis C infection thus offers the unique opportunity to identify efficient immune mechanisms of virus control and to characterize the factors determining the eventual outcome of disease. Several studies in individuals who experienced complete virologic recovery have found a significant association between a strong and maintained HCV-specific CD4+ T-cell response and viral clearance in acute hepatitis C (Gerlach et al., 1999; Kamal et al., 2001). As HCV-specific cellular immune responses are present in chronic infection, the other consideration is that the cytokine response may be qualitatively different in individuals with chronic infection as compared with acute resolved HCV. Analysis of the cytokine profile of bulk cultures as well as CD4+ T-cell clones from patients with hepatitis C revealed that viral clearance is more likely in cases displaying a T-helper 1 profile (Koziel, 1999). However, most studies are based on few individuals who recovered infection either spontaneously or after interferon therapy (Gerlach et al., 1999; Lohr et al., 1998). Thus longitudinal prospective studies analyzing the early antiviral immune responses in acute hepatitis C infection are crucial for understanding the pathogenesis of the disease and potentially in vaccine design. Once chronic infection is established HCV-specific CD4+ T-cells compartmentalize in the liver and differ functionally and clontypically from those in the peripheral blood (Schirren et al., 2000; Bertoletti et al., 1997). The significance of the intrahepatic CD4+ responses and their relation to liver injury have not been comprehensively investigated since most studies focus on the peripheral compartment due to the difficulty in obtaining liver biopsies.

CD8 Response to HCV Infection

The CD8+ T-cell response is thought to play a crucial role in the course of HCV infection. In humans and in chimpanzees, a strong and broadly directed HCV-specific CTL response has been associated with viral clearance during acute HCV infection. In contrast, individuals with chronic infection are often found to have a relatively weak and narrowly directed CD8+ T-cell response against HCV (Lechner et al., 2000; He et al., 1999). Whether these responses in chronic disease are still beneficial in containing viral replication or whether they are mediators of hepatic injury and disease is unclear. In several studies, the magnitude of the HCV-specific CD8+ T-cell response has been correlated to HCV viral load and to liver histology, but the results of these studies have been controversial. Overall, the levels of responses detected by most investigators have been fairly low, using a variety of methods, compared to those found in many other viral infections.

CTL Response to HCV Infection

Despite an occasionally broadly directed CTL response, virus persists within the liver, demonstrating the typical lack of effective clearance of infected hepatocytes by this response (Cerny and Chisari, 1999; Lechner et al., 2000; He et al., 1999). In fact, CTL have been hypothesized to contribute to liver pathology, perhaps by chronic secretion of cytokines that may enhance the development of cirrhosis. The reasons that the CTL response is unable to clear infection remain unclear. Possible mechanisms include escape of the virus from CTL epitopes, dysfunctional CTL, or direct inhibition of CTL through the virus.

Schistosomiasis and HCV Infection

Schistosomiasis is a chronic helminthic disease infecting more than 200 million people worldwide (Chitsulo et al., 2000). Infection with *Schistosoma mansoni* is endemic in Egypt with a prevalence range of 17.5 percent to 42.9 percent (El-

Khoby et al., 2000; Hammam et al., 2000). Morbidity in humans infected with *S. mansoni* results primarily from deposition of parasite ova in the portal areas inducing a T-cell-dependent granulomatous response which progresses to irreversible fibrosis and severe portal hypertension in more than 60 percent of cases. *S. mansoni* infection in mice is characterized by a strong Th2-associated immune response coupled with a defect in Th1-cell effector function (Sabin and Pearce, 1995). Although a predominant Th2 profile was shown to be beneficial in polyparasitism, where mice infected with *S. mansoni* are capable of eliminating *Trichuris muris* infection more efficiently than non-infected mice (Curry et al., 1995), it is assumed to be harmful in most viral infections.

Concomitant schistosomiasis and HCV infection is common in Egypt and other developing countries (Kamal et al., 2000a; Angelico et al., 1997; Pereira et al., 1995). Patients with concomitant HCV and schistosomiasis exhibit a unique clinical, virological, and histological pattern manifested by virus persistence with high HCV RNA titers, higher necroinflammatory and fibrosis scores in their liver biopsies and poor response to interferon therapy (Kamal et al., 2000a; Angelico et al., 1997; Pereira et al., 1995; Kamal et al., 2000b). This results in a markedly accelerated disease course once chronic HCV infection has been established. Our understanding of the pathomechanisms leading to this accelerated disease progression in HCV/*S. mansoni* coinfection is still extremely limited. This coinfection should be a valuable model to study the effect of one pathogen on the pathogenesis of the other agent, especially the influence of an altered T helper cell response on the other arms of the immune response as well as the clinical outcome. The model of HCV/*S. mansoni* coinfection also offers a unique opportunity to define the role of HCV-specific T-cells in viral control as well as the pathogenesis of HCV-related liver disease.

Comprehensive study of the different aspects of HCV/*S. mansoni* coinfection has been conducted and the data were presented in several publications. These studies, described below, provide insight into the mechanisms through which infection with one pathogen can influence the immunopathogenesis and the clinical course of another.

- **Chronic HCV and *S. mansoni* coinfection is associated with more severe disease** (Kamal et al., 2000a). One hundred and twenty-six patients with either chronic hepatitis C (group A), chronic schistosomiasis (group B), and chronic hepatitis C and schistosomiasis (group C) were enrolled and prospectively followed for 67.2 ± 22 months. HCV RNA titers were significantly higher in the coinfected group. Patients with coinfection showed higher fibrosis scores in their liver biopsies. Hepatocellular carcinoma was detected only in patients with coinfection. During follow-up, the mortality due to liver-related causes was 2 percent, 3 percent, and 48 percent in groups A, B, and C, respectively. In conclusion, patients with concomitant HCV and schistosomiasis are characterized through more advanced liver disease, higher HCV RNA titers, higher incidence of cirrhosis and hepatocellular carcinoma as well as higher incidence of liver-related morbidity and mortality.

• **HCV and *S. mansoni* coinfection is associated with poor response to interferon therapy** (Kamal et al., 2000b). Sixty-two patients (28 with chronic HCV and 34 patients with HCV and *S. mansoni*) were treated with interferon α-2b. The end of treatment response was 20 percent in coinfected patients versus 36 percent in monoinfected patients. The sustained response rate was 3 percent in coinfected patients versus 20 percent in monoinfected patients. In conclusion, patients with chronic hepatitis C coinfected with schistosomiasis respond poorly to interferon therapy and have higher relapse rates compared to patients with chronic HCV monoinfection.

• **Patients with HCV and *S. mansoni* coinfection fail to mount signifi-cant HCV-specific CD4+ T-cell responses and show alteration in the cytokine milieu along with more severe liver disease** (Kamal et al., 2001a). To define if immunological mechanisms are responsible for this alteration in the natural his-tory of HCV, the HCV-specific peripheral CD4+ T-cell responses and cytokines were analyzed in patients with chronic hepatitis C monoinfection, patients with *S. mansoni* monoinfection and patients with hepatitis C virus and *S. mansoni* coinfection. HCV-specific CD4+ proliferative responses to at least one HCV an-tigen were detected in 73.3 percent patients with HCV monoinfection compared to 8.6 percent coinfected with *S. mansoni*. Stimulation with HCV antigens pro-duced a type 1 cytokine profile in patients with HCV monoinfection compared to type 2 predominance in patients with coinfection. In contrast, there was no differ-ence in response to schistosomal antigens in patients with *S. mansoni* infection compared to those with coinfection. These findings suggest that the inability to generate HCV-specific CD4+/Th1 T-cell response plays a role in the persistence and severity of HCV infection in patients with coinfection.

• **Patients with acute hepatitis C and schistosomiasis coinfection cannot clear viremia and show rapid progression once chronic infection is estab-lished** (Kamal et al., 2001b). Immune responses during the first few months of acute HCV infection seem crucial for viral control, but the relationship of these responses to natural history is poorly characterized. We prospectively investi-gated the HCV-specific CD4+ and cytokine responses in patients with acute HCV hepatitis with or without *S. mansoni* coinfection, a parasitic infection with T helper (Th) 2 immune bias. HCV-specific CD4+ proliferative responses and cytokine production in peripheral blood mononuclear cells (PBMCs) were correlated with liver biopsy results at six months and end of follow-up. Whereas 5 of 15 patients with HCV alone recovered from acute HCV, all (17/17) patients with *S. mansoni* coinfection progressed to histologically proven chronic hepatitis. Coinfected pa-tients had either absent or transient weak HCV-specific CD4+ responses with Th0/Th2 cytokine production. The magnitude of the HCV-specific CD4+ re-sponse at week 12 was inversely correlated with the HCV RNA titers and the fibrosis progression rate in chronically infected patients.

We are currently conducting comprehensive and sensitive analysis of HCV-specific CTL and CD4+ responses in PBMCs and liver-infiltrating lymphocytes of patients coinfected with HCV and *S. mansoni* versus HCV-monoinfected patients.

Conclusion

In summary, HCV infection is a worldwide problem for which there has been insufficient success with treatment options presently available. The lack of a clear understanding of the immunological events during acute and chronic infection has hampered vaccine development and immunotherapeutic approaches to treatment. From an immunological point of view the interplay between T helper cell responses and CTL has been difficult to assess in humans, and infection with *S. mansoni* offers the unique situation of studying the impact of an altered response on the outcome and progression of HCV-related liver disease.

REFERENCES

Abdel Aziz F, Habib M, Mohamed M, Abdel Hamid M, Gamil F, Madkour S, Mikhail N, Thomas D, Fix A, Strickland T, Anwar W, Ismail S. 2000. Hepatitis C virus infection in a community in the Nile Delta: population description and HCV prevalence. *Hepatology* 32:111–115.
Alter MJ. 1997. Epidemiology of hepatitis C. *Hepatology* 26:62S–65S.
Angelico M, Renganathan E, Gandin C, Fathy M, Profili MC, Refai W, De Santis A, Nagi A, Amin G, Capocaccia L, Callea F, Rapicetta M, Badr G, Rocchi G. 1997. Chronic liver disease in Alexandria governorate, Egypt: contribution of schistosomiasis and hepatitis virus infections. *Journal of Hepatology* 26:236–243.
Bertoletti A, D´Elios MM, Boni C, De Carli M, Zignego AL, Durazzo M, Missale G, Penna A, Fiaccadori F, Del Prete G, Ferrari C. 1997. Different cytokine profiles of intrahepatic T cells in chronic hepatitis B and hepatitis C virus infections. *Gastroenterology* 112:193–199.
Cerny A and Chisari FV. 1999. Pathogenesis of chronic hepatitis C: immunological features of hepatic injury and viral persistence. *Hepatology* 30:595–601.
Chitsulo L, Engels D, Montresor A, Savioli L. 2000. The global status of schistosomiasis and its control. *Acta Tropica* 77:41–51.
Curry AJ, Else KJ, Jones F, Bancroft A, Grencis RK, Dunn DW. 1995. Evidence that cytokine-mediated immune interactions induced by *Schistosoma mansoni* alter disease outcome in mice concurrently infected with *Trichuris muris*. *The Journal of Experimental Medicine* 181:769–774.
Diepolder HM, Zachoval R, Hoffmann RM, Jung MC, Gerlach T, Pape GR. 1996. The role of hepatitis C virus specific CD4+ T lymphocytes in acute and chronic hepatitis C. *Journal of Molecular Medicine* 74:583–588.
El-Khoby T, Galal N, Fenwick A, Barakat R, El-Hawey A, Nooman Z, Habib M, Abdel Wahab F, Gabr NS, Hammam HM, Hussein MH, Mikhail NN, Cline BL, Strickland GT. 2000. The epidemiology of schistosomiasis in Egypt: summary of findings in nine governorates. *The American Journal of Tropical Medicine and Hygiene* 62:88–99.
Gerlach T, Diepolder H, Jung M, Gruner N, Schraut W, Zachoval R, Hoffman R, Schirren A, Santantonio T, Pape G. 1999. Recurrence of hepatitis C virus after loss of virus specific CD4+ T-cell response in acute hepatitis C. *Gastroenterology* 117:993–941.

Habib M, Mohamed MK, Abdel-Aziz F, Magder LS , Abdel-Hamid M, Gamil F, Madkour S, Mikhail NN, Anwar W, Strickland GT, Fix AD, Sallam I. 2001. Hepatitis C virus infection in a community in the Nile Delta: risk factors for seropositivity. *Hepatology* 33:248–253.

Hammam HM, Allam FA, Moftah FM, Abdel-Aty MA, Hany AH, Abd-El-Motagaly KF, Nafeh MA, Khalifa R, Mikhail NN, Talaat M, Hussein MH, Strickland GT. 2000. The epidemiology of schistosomiasis in Egypt: Assiut governorate. *The American Journal of Tropical Medicine and Hygiene* 62:73–79.

He XS, Rehermann B, Lopez-Labrador FX, Boisvert J, Cheung R, Mumm J, Wedemeyer H, Berenguer M, Wright TL, Davis MM, Greenberg HB. 1999. Quantitative analysis of hepatitis C virus-specific CD8(+) T cells in peripheral blood and liver using peptide-MHC tetramers. *Proceedings of the National Academy of Sciences USA* 96:5692–5697.

Kamal SM, Madwar MA, Bianchi L, EL Tawil A, Fawzy R, Peters T, Rasenack JW. 2000a. Clinical, virological and histopathological features: long-term follow-up in patients with chronic hepatitis C co-infected with *Schistosoma mansoni*. *Liver* 20:281–289.

Kamal SM, Madwar MA, Peters T, Fawzy R, Rasenack J. 2000b. Interferon therapy in patients with hepatitis C and schistosomiasis. *Journal of Hepatology* 32:172–174.

Kamal SM, Bianchi L, Al Tawil A, Koziel M, El Sayed Khalifa K, Peter T, Rasenack JW. 2001a. Specific cellular immune response and cytokine patterns in patients coinfected with hepatitis C virus and *Schistosoma mansoni*. *The Journal of Infectious Diseases* 184:972–982.

Kamal SM, Rasenack JW, Bianchi L, Al Tawil A, El Sayed Khalifa K, Peter T, Mansour H, Ezzat W, Koziel M. 2001b. Acute hepatitis C with and without schistosomiasis: correlation with hepatitis C-specific CD4+ T-cell and cytokine response. *Gastroenterology* 121:646–656.

Koziel MJ. 1999. Cytokines in viral hepatitis. *Seminars in Liver Disease* 19:157–169.

Lechner F, Wong D, Dunbar R, Chapman R, Chung R, Dohrenwend P, Robins G, Phillips R, Klenerman P, Walker B. 2000. Analysis of successful immune responses in persons infected with hepatitis C virus. *Journal of Experimental Medicine* 1499–1512.

Lohr HF, Gerken G, Roth M, Weyer S, Schlaak JF, Meyer zum Buschenfelde KH. 1998. The cellular immune responses induced in the follow-up of interferon-alpha treated patients with chronic hepatitis C may determine the therapy outcome. *Journal of Hepatology* 29:524–532.

Pereira LM, Melo MC, Saleh MG, Massarolo P, Koskinas J, Domingues AL, Spinelli, Mies S, Williams R, McFarlane IG. 1995. Hepatitis C virus infection in *Schistosomiasis mansoni* in Brazil. *Journal of Medical Virology* 45:423–428.

Poynard T, Leroy V, Conhard M. 1996. Meta-analysis of interferon randomized trials in the treatment of viral hepatitis C: effects of dose and duration. *Hepatology* 24:278–289.

Sabin EA and Pearce EJ. 1995. Early IL-4 production by non-CD4+ cells at the site of antigen deposition predicts the development of a T helper 2 cell response to *Schistosoma mansoni* eggs. *Journal of Immunology* 155:4844–4855.

Schirren CA, Jung MC, Gerlach JT, Worzfeld T, Baretton G, Mamin M, Hubert Gruener N, Houghton M, Pape GR. 2000. Liver-derived hepatitis C virus (HCV)-specific CD4+ T cells recognize multiple HCV epitopes and produce interferon gamma. *Hepatology* 32:597–603.

Seeff LB. 1997. Natural history of hepatitis C. *Hepatology* 26:21S–28S.

Thevenot T, Rigimbeau C, Ratziu V, Leroy V, Opolon P, Poynard T. 2001. Meta-analysis of interferon randomized trials in the treatment of viral hepatitis C in naive patients: 1999 update. *Journal of Viral Hepatitis* 8:48–62.

INTERACTIONS OF MULTIPLE INFECTIOUS AGENTS IN MALARIA-ENDEMIC AREAS: CONCURRENT HIV/AIDS AND MALARIA

Altaf A. Lal, Ph.D.
Division of Parasitic Diseases, National Center for Infectious Diseases
Centers for Disease Control and Prevention, Atlanta, GA

Establishment of microorganisms in human host populations requires structural, biologic, and molecular compatibilities between the host and pathogen. In situations where multiple infectious organisms coexist in an individual, the resulting polyparasitism could lead to increased infectivity, altered pathogen load, and modulation in pathogenesis. Burkitt's lymphoma, which is commonly found in areas with malaria transmission, is a good example of coinfections. It has been proposed that malaria-induced immune activation may be associated with the development of these lymphomas (Whittle et al., 1984).

The introduction of HIV-1 in the human population has altered the epidemiology of several infectious diseases. A number of these organisms, termed together as opportunistic infectious agents, cause significant morbidity and mortality. HIV-1 is now a firmly established infectious agent and the potential to interact with parasitic, viral, fungal, and bacterial infectious agents is very high.

The progression from HIV-1 infection to AIDS is associated with a decline in the CD4 T-cell count and an increase in HIV-1 viral load. Although several factors may be responsible for the variability in HIV-1 disease progression, immune activation appears to be an important determinant. Immune activation leads to up-regulation of viral co-receptors, decreased β chemokine secretion, enhanced viral entry and integration, viral assembly and/or release of the viral particles, changes in the cytokine environment and various degrees of immune dysfunction, hyporesponsiveness, and apoptosis. Because all systemic and/or local concurrent infections cause various degrees of immune activation, it is very likely that they may enhance HIV infection, increase HIV replication and viral load, and even promote progression of the disease.

Several studies have focused on the interaction between HIV/AIDS and three major infectious diseases, namely malaria, sexually transmitted diseases (STDs), and tuberculosis (TB) (Bentwich et al., 2000; Chandramohan and Greenwood, 1998). The main impact of STDs has been to facilitate HIV-1 transmission, and the interaction of TB and HIV-1 has been an increase in the burden of an already major cause of morbidity and mortality. As far as malaria is concerned, although early studies did not reveal a definite interaction between malaria and HIV, there is increasing evidence now that suggests these two pathogens interact, thus modifying the pathogenesis of each disease (Bentwich et al., 2000; Chandramohan and Greenwood, 1998; Corbett et al., 2002). This presentation will focus on the interactions between HIV/AIDS and malaria.

Malaria, TB, and HIV/AIDS are important public health problems in sub-Saharan Africa and some parts of Asia. Both HIV and malaria exert their heaviest toll in sub-Saharan Africa, where the progression of HIV-related disease is considered to be most rapid. The interaction between HIV/AIDS and malaria can be viewed in the mechanistic context, where immunomodulation by one organism can impact the natural course of infection of the co-existing pathogen, and in programmatic context, where the treatment for one disease may have beneficial impact on the other disease and/or the treatment for one disease may not be effective in the presence of the co-infecting pathogen.

Initial studies of the interactions between HIV and malaria focused on the ability of malaria parasites to act as opportunistic organisms in immunosuppressed HIV-positive persons. As recent reviews demonstrate, most of the earlier studies, conducted primarily in adults, did not show an effect of HIV infection on the prevalence or severity of malaria (Chandramohan and Greenwood, 1998; Corbett et al., 2002).

Earlier studies conducted in Zaire, Uganda, Rwanda, and Zambia, showed no or marginal effect of HIV infection on malaria parasitemia (Simooya et al., 1988; Chattopadhya et al., 1991; Greenberg, 1992). However, recent studies conducted in Malawi reported increased prevalence rates of malaria parasitemia and parasite density in HIV-infected pregnant women (Chandramohan and Greenwood, 1998). The higher prevalence of malaria parasitemia was seen in HIV-infected women of all gravidities, indicating that the parity-specific immunity to malaria, which is normally associated with multigravidae, was impaired in HIV-infected women (Chandramohan and Greenwood, 1998). More importantly, these studies revealed that infants born to HIV- and malaria-positive mothers were at a significantly higher risk for low birth weight. Increased prevalence of peripheral parasitemia and placental malaria has also been seen in HIV-positive pregnant women in western Kenya, which has higher rates of malaria transmission than Malawi (Chandramohan and Greenwood, 1998). The increased prevalence of parasitemia in HIV-positive women seemed to be pregnancy associated, because parasitemia in HIV-positive women reduced to the level seen in HIV-negative women 2–6 months postpartum.

HIV infection has been shown to induce poor responses to antimalarial treatment with sulfadoxine-pyrimethamine (S/P) in pregnant women. A recent study conducted in western Kenya indicated that although a standard two-dose S/P regimen worked well in controlling peripheral parasitemia and placental malaria during pregnancy in HIV-negative women, it failed to prevent peripheral and placental parasitemia in HIV-infected women. Poor response to S/P antimalarial treatment was also reported in pregnant Malawian women with HIV-1 infection. Because parasitemia was reduced drastically after each treatment and monthly S/P dosing worked well in both HIV-positive and HIV-negative women, it is possible that the poor treatment response was due to rapid re-infection rather than delayed parasite clearance. No difference in quinine treatment failure was seen between HIV-positive and HIV-negative children with malaria in Kinshasa, Zaire (Chandramohan and Greenwood, 1998; Corbett et al., 2002).

Conflicting results have been reported about the effect of HIV infection on malaria antibody responses in *Plasmodium falciparum*-endemic areas. Earlier studies conducted in Zambia and India showed no differences between HIV-positive and HIV-negative persons in terms of the prevalence of antimalarial antibodies (Simooya et al., 1988; Chattopadhya et al., 1991). Very few HIV-positive persons, however, were involved in these studies, and no attempts were made to compare the titers of antibody response, although one did compare the optical density (OD) (Chattopadhya et al., 1991).

In contrast, a study conducted in Uganda demonstrated consistent reduction in mean OD of antibodies to synthetic peptides from the ring-infected erythrocyte surface antigen (RESA) and circumsporozoite protein (CSP) of *P. falciparum* and CSP of *P. malariae*. In addition, HIV-positive persons with AIDS had significantly lower antibody levels (mean OD) of RESA antibodies than asymptomatic HIV-positive persons (Wabwire-Mangen et al., 1989). Cellular immune responses to malaria are seemingly also affected by HIV-1 infection. Compared with HIV-negative persons, AIDS patients in Burkina Faso had lower proliferation of PBMCs to stimulation with merozoite surface protein-1 (MSP-1) and parasite culture supernatant. They also had reduced in vitro production of IFN-γ and IL-2. The immune suppression induced by HIV was probably general, because PBMCs of AIDS patients also respond poorly to phytohaemagglutinin, tuberculin purified protein derivative, and lipopolysaccharide (Migot et al., 1996).

We have recently evaluated the influence of HIV-1 on malaria antigen specific antibody responses during pregnancy. These studies have revealed that maternal and neonatal antibody levels against blood stage and sporozoite stage antigenic determinants are significantly lower among HIV-infected women compared with HIV-uninfected women. We also observed reduced maternal-fetal transplacental antibody transfer in dually infected women. In another recent study conducted in Kenya, we found elevated production of IFN-γ by maternal placental (intervillous blood) mononuclear cells (IVBMC) from multigravidae to be associated with protection against placental malaria (Moore et al., 2000). A protective role for IFN-γ in controlling infection has been demonstrated both in human studies and with animal models. Mechanistically, this cytokine has been proposed to be important in mediating asexual blood-stage parasite clearance, perhaps via its regulatory influence on phagocytic cells. The importance of this cytokine in protection against placental malaria is further supported by our recent finding that IVBMC from HIV-positive women have impaired antigen-specific IFN-γ and IL-4 responses (Moore et al., 2000). Since these cytokines are produced primarily by T-cells, we conclude that this loss of cytokine responsiveness may play a role in the increased susceptibility of HIV-positive women to placental malaria.

It has been suggested that the progression from HIV-1 infection to AIDS is more rapid in sub-Saharan African patients than in persons living in developed countries (Gilks, 1993; Mulder et al., 1994; Grant et al., 1997). In addition to the lack of access to health care and treatment, chronic immune stimulation from increased exposure to other infectious agents are probable co-factors of immune activation. Earlier investigations of the relationship between HIV-1 and malaria focused mainly on the effect of HIV-1 infection on malaria. Only one study examined the effect of malaria on HIV-1 infection, and failed to detect any effect of malaria infection on HIV-1 progression. No measurements of changes in CD4+ T-cell counts and viral load, which are two current predictors of HIV disease progression, were done in this study.

Recent in vitro and in vivo studies, nevertheless, indicate that malaria can potentially affect the course of HIV infection in several aspects. The initial evidence of a possible effect of malaria on HIV-1 infection came from a retrospective analysis of data from a cohort study of mothers and infants in rural Malawi. It was demonstrated that infants born to mothers with both placental malaria and HIV-1 infection had post-neonatal mortality 4.5 times higher than infants born to mothers with only placental malaria, and 2.7–7.7 times higher than infants born to mothers with only HIV-1 infection (Chandramohan and Greenwood, 1998; Corbett et al., 2002). This increased mortality in infants born to mothers with dual HIV and malaria was attributed to the increased transmission of HIV from mothers to infants, although no HIV testing was conducted in these infants.

Because immune activation is an important prerequisite for efficient HIV infection and viral replication, we evaluated the effect of malarial antigen stimulation on HIV-1 infection. Stimulation with soluble malarial antigens or malarial pigment from *P. falciparum* enhanced HIV-1 replication in PBMC from naive donors by 10- to 100-fold. The malarial antigen-upregulated HIV-1 replication was mediated through induction of TNF-α via the activation of long terminal repeat (LTR)-directed viral transcription (Xiao et al., 1998). Preliminary studies conducted with PBMC from HIV-positive individuals residing in western Kenya indicated that recall immune responses induced by soluble malarial antigens can increase HIV-1 replication (Xiao et al., unpublished observation). PBMC from 3 of 10 HIV-1 infected individuals showed active in vitro viral production after the antigen stimulation.

These in vitro observations have been confirmed by the result of a recent prospective, cohort study of 47 HIV-positive adults with active falciparum malaria and 42 HIV-positive adults without malaria in Malawi. It was shown that HIV-positive individuals with active malaria had a mean plasma HIV-1 viral load 7-fold higher than HIV-positive individuals without malaria (Hoffman et al., 1999). Plasma HIV-1 RNA concentrations did not correlate significantly with *P. falciparum* parasite density or the duration of fever. However, antimalarial chemotherapy with S/P resulted in a small (37 percent) but significant reduction in

HIV-1 RNA load by week 4 post-treatment in individuals with HIV and malaria coinfection.

Another potential interaction between HIV and malaria is at the invasion stage of both pathogens. HIV-1 has been recently shown to bind erythrocytes from Caucasian persons through the Duffy antigen receptor for chemokines (DARC), a receptor that is also used by the invasion of *P. vivax* merozoites into reticulocytes (Lachgar et al., 1998). It has been proposed that erythrocytes may function as a reservoir for HIV-1, and this binding to CD4 (–) cells via DARC by HIV may be used as a mechanism for the entry of HIV-1 into endothelial cells and neurons (Lachgar et al., 1998). Because *P. falciparum*-infected erythrocytes adhere to brain endothelial cells and cause brain hemorrhage, it is conceivable that the sequestration of parasitized erythrocytes in the brain with HIV viral particles attached may facilitate the entry of HIV into neurons in individuals that are DARC-positive. This may promote the occurrence of neurologic disorders, which are frequently seen in AIDS patients.

Programmatic concerns for interactions between malaria and HIV/AIDS are mainly at the level of diagnosis and treatment. Earlier diagnostic studies showed false positivity of blood samples from malaria-affected individuals during HIV testing (Biggar et al., 1996). This was probably due to nonspecificity of the early HIV diagnostic kits, because antigen cross-reactivity between retroviruses and malaria parasites has been reported (Lal et al., 1994). As far as treatment of uncomplicated and complicated malaria is concerned, blood transfusion for the treatment of severe malarial anemia and presumptive treatment of febrile illness have emerged as two important problems. Recent studies have shown that many of the presumed malarial febrile illnesses were actually the result of primary HIV-1 infection (Nwanyanwu et al., 1997). This problem may be more severe in areas with high prevalence of HIV and malaria, leading to unnecessary use of antimalarials for the treatment of fever. This overuse of antimalarials may contribute to the rapid emergence of drug resistance. As far as the transfusion-related transmission of HIV is concerned, earlier studies clearly revealed that use of unscreened blood for the treatment of severe malarial anemia was a factor in the transmission of HIV.

While this paper provides an account of published work on the interaction between malaria and HIV/AIDS, there is compelling evidence of interaction between other microorganisms and HIV/AIDS. It is likely that the interactions between several microorganisms present together in an individual may modulate the pathogenesis and transmission of major infectious agents.

From a mechanistic point of view, however, a common thread that seems to tie this interaction together is immune activation induced by infectious agents prevalent in malaria-endemic areas. Therefore, removing risk factors of immune activation (i.e., co-infectious agents) by effective use of drugs, physical interventions to interrupt transmission, such as bednets for malaria, and other prevention methods should have the dual effect of reduced risk of rapid progression of HIV-related disease (by elimination or suppression of viral activating factors) and reduced morbidity and mortality by a co-infecting pathogenic organism.

The schematics of our current knowledge and the likely outcomes of the interaction between HIV and malaria are shown in Figure 2-1. It is very likely that multiple enteric, respiratory, bloodborne, vectorborne, and waterborne and foodborne agents may induce immunologic changes (even in asymptomatic infections) that promote infection, transmission, and clinical manifestation of illnesses of the co-infectious pathogens. It is therefore important to capture all morbidity data and conduct extensive diagnostic work in future studies so that the analysis can be controlled for the effect of different co-infectious agents.

In the context of HIV/AIDS and malaria, the available data should be considered in:

1. Promoting the development of and implementation of intervention guidelines and policies for prompt treatment of malaria with effective antimalarials; treatment would reduce the frequency of malaria-related illness and reduce the risk of rapid progression and transmission of HIV.

2. Incorporating prevention methods, such as the use of insecticide-impregnated bednets and environmental modifications in controlling malaria transmission.

3. Implementing blood screening guidelines in anemia-related blood transfusions.

Because of the increasing prevalence of major infectious diseases in many countries, even a small impact of coinfection-mediated increase in pathogenesis and transmission could have unparalleled human health consequences. Therefore, from a global health perspective, there is a need to raise awareness at the national level to the consequences of interactions of multiple infections in malaria-endemic regions of the world. These efforts need to be complemented by political commitment and funding at the national and international level for research and disease control and prevention programs for infectious diseases in malaria-endemic settings.

REFERENCES

Bentwich Z, Maartens G, Torten D, Lal AA, Lal RB. 2000. Concurrent infections and HIV pathogenesis. *AIDS* 14:2071–2081.

Biggar RJ, Miotti PG, Taha TE, Mtimavalye L, Broadhead R, Justesen A, Yellin F, Liomba G, Miley W, Waters D, Chiphangwi JD, Goedert JJ. 1996. Perinatal intervention trial in Africa: effect of a birth canal cleansing intervention to prevent HIV transmission. *Lancet* 347:1647–1650.

Chandramohan D and Greenwood BM. 1998. Is there an interaction between human immunodeficiency virus and Plasmodium falciparum? *International Journal of Epidemiology* 27:296–301.

Chattopadhya D, Kumari S, Chatterjee R, Verghese T. 1991. Antimalarial antibody in relation to seroreactivity for HIV infection in sera from blood donors. *Journal of Communicable Diseases* 23:195–198.

	Effect of HIV on Malaria	
Pathogen	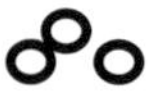 HIV	
Target cell	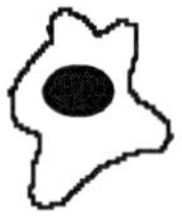 Macrophage and dendritic cell	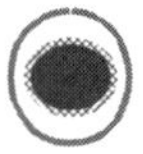 CD4 and CD8 T cell
Immunologic changes	1. Reduced production of NO and other reactive oxygen intermediates and phagocytosis 2. Reduced antigen-presenting function 3. Reduced antigen-dependent cellular cytotoxicity (ADCC) activity 4. Production of proinflammatory cytokines	1. Reduced number of CD4 T lymphocytes 2. Reduced T-helper activity, cytotoxic T cell activity, antigen-driven IFN-γ production, and memory responses 3. Exhaustion of certain T cell repertoire clones 4. Polyclonal B cell activation
Possible effect	1. Reduced antibody and cytokine responses because of malarial infection 2. Reduced killing of malarial parasites 3. Fever associated with primary HIV infection masqueraded as malaria	
Likely outcome **Mother**	1. Increased prevalence of peripheral malarial parasitema and placental malaria 2. Reduced transfer of anti-malarial antibodies 3. Poor response to antimalarial prophylaxis 4. Misuse of antimalarials in the treatment of HIV-associated fever	
Infant	1. Increased susceptibility to malarial infection 2. Rapid reinfection by malarial parasites (decreased time to reinfection) 3. Delayed development of antimalarial immunity 4. Increased severity of malaria 5. Poor response to antimalarial treatment	
Adolescent	1. Loss of antimalarial immunity 2. Delayed clearance of malarial parasitemia 3. Increased occurrence of severe malarial anemia and cerebral malaria	

FIGURE 2-1 Current knowledge and likely outcomes of the interaction between HIV and malaria.

	Effect of Malaria on HIV	
Pathogen	Malarial parasites	
Target cell	Macrophage and dendritic cell	CD4 and CD8 T cell
Immunologic changes	1. Activation of monocytes and dendritic cells 2. Production of proinflammatory cytokines 3. Upregulated expression of chemokine receptors (HIV-coreceptors)	1. Activation of T lymphocytes 2. Immunosuppression 3. Production of inflammatory cytokines 4. Upregulated expression of chemokine receptors
Possible effect	1. Increased susceptibility of mononuclear cells to HIV infection 2. Increased viral replication in HIV-infected cells 3. Pathologic and immunologic changes in the placenta 4. Use of antimalarials, which are immunosuppressive and may increase viral replication	
Likely outcome		
Mother	1. Increased HIV viral load 2. Increased vertical transmission of HIV 3. Lower birthweight of infants born from dually infected mothers	
Infant	1. Increased HIV transmission because of blood transfusion 2. Persistent, high HIV viral load 3. Possibility of increased HIV disease progression 4. Possibility of rapid death of HIV-infected infants	
Adolescent	1. Possibility of increased HIV viral load 2. Possibility of accelerated HIV disease progression	

Corbett EL, Steketee RW, ter Kuile FO, Latif AS, Kamali A, Hayes RJ. 2002. HIV-1/AIDS and the control of other infectious diseases in Africa. *Lancet* 359:2177–2187.

Gilks CF. 1993. The clinical challenge of the HIV epidemic in the developing world. *Lancet* 342:1037–1039.

Grant AD, Djomand G, De Cock KM. 1997. Natural history and spectrum of disease in adults with HIV/AIDS in Africa. *AIDS* 11:S43–S54.

Greenberg AE. 1992. Pp. 143–148 in *AIDS in the World,* TW Netter, J Mann, DJM Tarantola, eds. Boston: Harvard University Press.

Hoffman IF, Jere CS, Taylor TE, Munthali P, Dyer JR, Wirima JJ, Rogerson SJ, Kumwenda N, Eron JJ, Fiscus SA, Chakraborty H, Taha TE, Cohen MS, Molyneux ME. 1999. The effect of Plasmodium falciparum malaria on HIV-1 RNA blood plasma concentration. *AIDS* 13:487–494.

Lachgar A, Jaureguiberry G, Le Buenac H, Bizzini B, Zagury JF, Rappaport J, Zagury D. 1998. Binding of HIV-1 to RBCs involves the Duffy antigen receptors for chemokines (DARC). *Biomedicine and Pharmacotherapy* 52:436–439.

Lal RB, Rudolph D, Alpers MP, Sulzer AJ, Shi YP, Lal AA. 1994. Immunologic cross-reactivity between structural proteins of human T-cell lymphotropic virus type I and the blood stage of Plasmodium falciparum. *Clinical and Diagnostic Laboratory Immunology* 1:5–10.

Migot F, Ouedraogo JB, Diallo J, Zampan H, Dubois B, Scott-Finnigan T, Sanou PT, Deloron P. 1996. Selected P. falciparum specific immune responses are maintained in AIDS adults in Burkina Faso. *Parasite Immunology* 18:333–339.

Moore JM, Ayisi J, Nahlen BL, Misore A, Lal AA, Udhayakumar V. 2000. Immunity to placental malaria. II. Placental antigen-specific cytokine responses are impaired in human immunodeficiency virus-infected women. *Journal of Infectious Diseases* 182:960–964.

Mulder DW, Nunn AJ, Wagner HU, Kamali A, Kengeya-Kayondo JF. 1994. HIV-1 incidence and HIV-1-associated mortality in a rural Ugandan population cohort. *AIDS* 8:87–92.

Nwanyanwu OC, Kumwenda N, Kazembe PN, Jemu S, Ziba C, Nkhoma WC, Redd SC. 1997. Malaria and human immunodeficiency virus infection among male employees of a sugar estate in Malawi. *Transactions of the Royal Society of Tropical Medicine and Hygiene* 91:567–569.

Simooya OO, Mwendapole RM, Siziya S, Fleming AF. 1988. Relation between falciparum malaria and HIV seropositivity in Ndola, Zambia. *British Medical Journal* 297:30–31.

Wabwire-Mangen F, Shiff CJ, Vlahov D, Kline R, Serwadda D, Sewankambo NK, Mugerwa RD, Quinn TC. 1989. Immunological effects of HIV-1 infection on the humoral response to malaria in an African population. *The American Journal of Tropical Medicine and Hygiene* 41:504–511.

Whittle HC, Brown J, Marsh K, Greenwood BM, Seidelin P, Tighe H, Wedderburn L. 1984. T-cell control of Epstein-Barr virus-infected B cells is lost during P. falciparum malaria. *Nature* 312:449–450.

Xiao L, Owen SM, Rudolph DL, Lal RB, Lal AA. 1998. Plasmodium falciparum antigen-induced human immunodeficiency virus type 1 replication is mediated through induction of tumor necrosis factor-alpha. *Journal of Infectious Diseases* 177:437–445.

3

Obstacles and Opportunities for Framing Future Research

OVERVIEW

Humans exist in complex milieus, and their association with disease is affected both by the environment in which they live and by their genetic susceptibility to particular diseases. People live in concert with microbial agents that may or may not cause disease in particular individuals, depending on their environment and their genetics.

There are substantial obstacles to identifying organisms associated with a particular chronic disease. First, organisms can act in a "hit and run" manner, in which they cause disease initially but then are either resolved due to natural immunity or are successfully eliminated with antibiotics. The damage has been done, however, resulting in chronic disease. For some chronic diseases of this type, such as Reiter's syndrome, Guillain-Barré syndrome, or rheumatic heart disease, it is very difficult to find a fingerprint of the organism in the disease tissue. Second, organisms can be latent at the time of diagnosis. They may not be actively replicating, so there is no active RNA transcription. Third, chronic latent or recurrent infection may be involved in the pathogenesis so that, again, the organism may not be active at the time of diagnosis. Fourth, organisms may need a particular predisposing environment or a host with a particular genetic susceptibility, so the simple presence or absence of the organism may be misleading.

To address these problems, evidence is assembled in a number of ways: from epidemiological studies, from microbiological assessment of pathogenesis and etiology, from studies that mimic the disease process in vitro or in animals, and from clinical treatment trials.

Patrick Moore described how the discovery of new pathogens will require the talents of multiple disciplines, including epidemiology, clinical medicine, molecular biology, and pathology. Moore used the example of the identification of the virus that causes Kaposi's sarcoma, which often strikes gay men, to discuss general issues in causality and to illustrate the limits of current approaches for determining causality for a newly discovered agent and disease. The causative agent, named Kaposi's sarcoma-associated herpesvirus (KSHV), was identified using a genetic technique called representational difference analysis. Once the virus was identified, in 1994, events moved rather quickly—a fact that speaks to the importance of new pathogen discovery. The virus's genome has been sequenced, serologic tests have been developed, and studies have been initiated to understand its epidemiology and to test possible treatments. Moreover, the virus has since been found to cause at least two other types of disease. Based on this experience, Moore pointed to the need for researchers to move beyond Koch's postulates or other traditional guidelines in their efforts to determine disease causality for suspect microbes. Researchers are attempting to do this by applying various new techniques emerging from molecular biology and biotechnology. It seems clear as well that epidemiologists developing new criteria for causality will have to incorporate new pathogenic mechanisms that are not accounted for in current disease models.

Mikhail Pletnikov discussed the importance of expanding research to better understand the interplay of genetic and environmental factors in the causation of a number of important developmental behavioral disorders. Among methodological problems of studying the gene-environment interplay is the difficulty in firmly defining environmental factors and making them quantifiable. In this context, virus infections provide a promising research avenue, because of their etiologic connection to several neurodevelopmental disorders, including autism and schizophrenia, and because of the reliability of quantification of viral effects on brain and behavior. In particular, Pletnikov described work using an animal model to study gene-environmental interactions that occur during neonatal infection with Borna disease virus (BDV). Neonatal BDV infection in rats has been shown to produce distinct neuroanatomical, neurochemical, and behavioral abnormalities that resemble pathological and clinical features of some human developmental disorders. The significance of studying neonatal exposure derives from the fact that the effects of many genetic and environmental risk factors are evident either prior to or around the time of birth, and the interaction between them often is apparent well before the onset or diagnosis of the chronic disease condition. Thus, studying the effects of neonatal BDV infection across the entire postnatal period in genetically different strains of rats will aid in understanding the course and time-dependent character of the interaction of genetic background features and the virus infection. In this way, the model system may allow study of some tremendously complex mechanisms relevant to developmental disorders.

David Persing provided an overview of recent research in the area of infection, cancer, and the immune response. Current evidence suggests that inherited predisposition to cancer probably accounts for only a subset of total cancer patients, and in most models of the development of neoplasia, an underlying assumption is the contribution of an array of intrinsic and extrinsic factors within a multistep process. A basic prerequisite of many models is an increase in the baseline proliferation rates of essentially normal cell populations that leads to dysregulation of normal growth control mechanisms. Since many infectious processes often lead, directly or indirectly, to increased cell turnover and proliferation, certain agents are now widely regarded as carcinogens. Some of the pathogens that have been linked to cancer include human papillomaviruses (cervical cancer and other skin cancers), human T-cell leukemia viruses (adult T-cell leukemias and lymphomas in endemic areas), hepatitis B virus (liver cancer), Epstein-Barr virus (Burkitt's lymphoma and nasopharyngeal carcinoma), and *Helicobacter pylori* infection (gastric carcinoma and MALT lymphoma).In addition, new disease associations are being made with respect to previously known pathogens, such as the association of chronic hepatitis C virus infection with non-Hodgkin's lymphoma in certain populations.

In a separate presentation, Persing described recent and continuing advances in the development and application of techniques for identifying pathogens that cause chronic diseases. Although a paper on these subjects does not appear in this chapter, the following paragraph notes the highlights.

The ability to detect and manipulate nucleic acid molecules in microorganisms has created a powerful means for identifying previously unknown microbial pathogens and for studying the host-pathogen relationship. Although a paper on these subjects does not appear in the ensuing text, the highlights of his presentation are discussed here. Among the new technologies that Persing described is broad-range polymerase chain reaction, which has proved instrumental in linking a growing number of pathogens with chronic diseases, and representational difference analysis, which is an efficient means for finding differences between complex genomes and for identifying specific DNA sequences from the genomes of unknown pathogens. Researchers also are making use of sophisticated new DNA microarrays and biosensors that, among other things, can monitor host response as an indicator of the presence of infection or inflammation. In addition, new methods for generating "libraries" of genetic information from very small amounts of material are making it easier to conduct very specific and sensitive serologic tests. Equipped with these and other advanced tools, researchers are becoming better able to move beyond the limitations of Koch's postulates and to link infectious agents with chronic diseases more precisely and with greater confidence than ever before.

In the ensuing discussions, participants began to sketch in some of the characteristics of a comprehensive and coordinated effort that would enhance efforts both to identify links between infectious microorganisms and chronic diseases and to develop and implement interventions to minimize their health consequences. The goal was not to set specific priorities, but to identify opportunities. Highlighting a selection of the traits identified may provide a glimpse of the overall picture envisioned.

Participants agreed, for example, on the need to develop standardized definitions of infections and disease, to enable comparisons across studies and conclusions about causality, and on the need to ensure that laboratory assays maintain universally high standards of specificity, sensitivity, and reproducibility. New laboratory technology also is needed that can meet such performance standards while handling high throughput rates, in order to handle analyses of large cohorts in a reasonable amount of time, a trait that likely will be required in many future projects. Comparable efforts are needed to ensure that epidemiological studies are conducted with vigor and in an appropriate manner. One step will involve linking of databases that are designed (or modified) to be compatible. Peer review journals can reinforce performance standards if publication depends on the use of sound laboratory assays and epidemiologic design capable of supporting the conclusions.

Continued studies are needed to define temporal relationships between infections and disease—that is, what stage of infection determines outcome (e.g., first infection, reinfection, persistent infection, coinfection, or subsequent cross-reacting infection). Studies also are needed to clarify at which stage infection must be prevented or treated in order to minimize or eliminate chronic sequelae. It will be important to determine the expected benefit of actions, to ensure that the benefits will outweigh any possible risks. In other words, intervention should decrease chronic disease burden without unduly endangering the people who receive care.

There is a need to better understand the natural history, especially the earliest stages, of chronic diseases of unknown or incompletely known origins. What makes this task especially important is the hit-and-run nature of some diseases in which microbes set adverse events in motion and then disappear, the increased difficulty of imputing causation to microbes detected late in the course of disease, and the increased ease of treating or preventing disease at early time points. Toward this aim, clinicians should be increasingly encouraged to identify patients who have recently developed or seem to be developing various suspect chronic diseases, to collect in an orderly manner a range of clinical specimens, and then to follow the course of the disease in order to identify tell-tale early clinical features.

Calls were made for more effort devoted to developing animal models of chronic diseases, and to teaching health professionals about their value and their limitations. Animal models can be powerful tools when the etiology or pathogenesis of a disorder is unknown. Psychiatric modeling with animals may present an especially ripe area for probing a variety of important questions, yet many practitioners in the field are not accustomed to working with such models.

Increased emphasis should be placed on longitudinal studies, as well as on follow-up studies and "look back" studies of cohorts and surveillance results that have been generated in the past. Longitudinal studies may prove particularly valuable given that rapid advances in the field may mean that we might not know today which pieces of evidence will be needed in the future. Human specimen collections, such as the National Children's Study that will begin in 2004, may be especially important for longitudinal research.

Participants identified a number of specific populations that should receive additional attention. One such group includes people who move from rural areas into cities, both in the developing and the developed world. Studies are needed to see whether they bring new infections with them, or whether they prove to be susceptible to new infections that they previously had not encountered. With the world's changing demographics, gathering such information may provide a window into pathogenesis of a number of chronic diseases.

Efforts are needed to address problems related to informed consent. Many workshop participants expressed concern that current regulations and guidelines are too complex, too uncertain, or too restrictive to allow for meaningful sharing of data—and sometimes all three. There was general agreement that informed consent is and must remain an important part of research involving human subjects. But participants also agreed that all parties—from government, academia, and private funding agencies—need to work together to develop a more standardized method for gaining patient consent, for gathering identifying information, and for being able to use this identifying information in the future. This may be an opportunity for multiple institutions and multiple governments, domestic and foreign, to cooperate in devising a system of patient consent that operates more smoothly, protects patient rights, and allows for expanded research on infections and chronic diseases.

Given the magnitude of the outstanding scientific questions, and of the health consequences at stake, an increasing share of future research likely will involve groups of investigators representing a variety of disciplines, or groups of institutions working collaboratively. Although there remains a clear role for individual investigators, it is becoming apparent that large multidisciplinary projects often can best marshal the critical mass needed to address the thorniest biological problems. In many cases, these large projects will include a multinational component, in order to ensure that sufficient attention is paid to multiracial, multiethnic, and multicultural differences.

Participants called on the overall scientific community to evaluate whether it is organized and structured properly to address these issues, and whether its various components communicate effectively. The community also should mount a concerted effort to identify gaps in current knowledge about the etiology of chronic diseases, pinpoint what needs to be done to close those gaps, chart the obstacles that stand in the way, and then identify and provide the necessary financial resources (monetary and human) to drive progress.

Government can play an important role by reorienting its funding priorities. Indeed, the time is ripe. The government is now investing nearly $1 billion in rebuilding the nation's public health system, and part of the money will go toward linking state health departments more closely with local health departments than has historically been the case. At the same time, government research centers are launching major new interdisciplinary projects, and universities, which often have been in competition with one another, are beginning to join in collaborations. Thus, foundations are beginning to be built for bridges linking public health, clinical medicine, and research. But these promising efforts need to be nurtured to ensure continued cooperation.

PATHOGENS AND DISEASE: ISSUES IN DETERMINING CAUSALITY

Patrick S. Moore
University of Pittsburgh
Pittsburgh, PA

Successful new pathogen discovery requires the talents of multiple disciplines, including epidemiology, clinical medicine, molecular biology, and pathology. In this paper, the identification of Kaposi's sarcoma-associated herpesvirus (KSHV) illustrates general issues in causality and shows the limits on our ability to determine a causality for a newly discovered agent and disease (Moore and Chang, 1998).

The mysterious outbreak of Kaposi's sarcoma among gay men was the harbinger of the AIDS epidemic. It is now clear, however, that the AIDS-associated Kaposi's sarcoma epidemic was actually due to the collision of two independent viruses in a susceptible population: HIV and a new virus, KSHV or HHV8, which was found using molecular techniques (O'Brien et al., 1999).

Over 20 different agents had been put forward as the cause of KS before 1994. To look for the "KS agent" (Beral et al., 1990), Yuan Chang used representational difference analysis (RDA) to compare DNA from a Kaposi's sarcoma lesion to uninvolved, sterile-site tissue from the same patient on the assumption that the two samples would be genetically identical except for the presence of the putative agent's genome (Chang et al., 1994).

As shown in Figure 3-1, RDA is a subtractive hybridization technique in which PCR adapters are ligated onto digested DNA from the KS tissue (tester) (Lisitsyn et al., 1993). The tester DNA was then rehybridized back to a ten-fold excess of uninvolved sample DNA (driver) that had been identically digested. For human genomic fragments present in the KS sample, 90 percent of these fragments will form pairs with the corresponding antisense strand lacking the adapter from the normal tissue DNA. PCR with a primer specific to this adapter linearly amplifies these common sequences and, of course, there was no amplification of the DNA rehybridized from the driver alone. Sequences that were unique to the KS lesion, however, reanneal to each other and have adaptors on both ends, so that amplification occurs exponentially. The initial PCR products are then

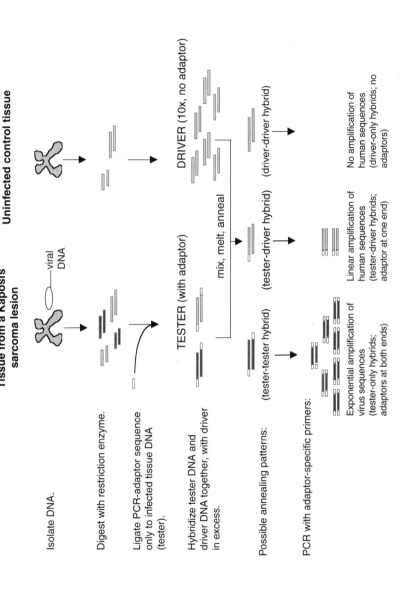

FIGURE 3-1 Representational differential analysis comparing DNA from a Kaposi's sarcoma lesion to sterile-site tissue from the same patient.

rehybridized again to the adapter-less healthy tissue DNA and the process is repeated, each time selectively enriching for the unique sequences found only in the KS lesion (Gao and Moore, 1996).

Four RDA fragments were generated by this process, two of which were found to be specific for the KS agent. Although these two fragments account for less than 1 percent of the entire 145-kilobase viral genome, the few base-pairs worth of unique information they provided made it possible to develop enough tools to identify the agent.

The two fragments were used as Southern hybridization probes and tested against KS lesions, showing that about three-quarters of the KS lesions were positive for viral DNA. Using internal specific primers from the KS 330 band, a PCR assay was developed that showed 25 out of 27, or 93 percent, of the initial KS lesions tested positive. Moreover, the negative samples were equally telling: one of the two negatives had degraded DNA and was not amplifiable by using cellular primers, and the other one was mislabeled normal human kidney.

KSHV is a gamma herpesvirus belonging to the same class as Epstein-Barr virus (EBV). It is associated with three different major proliferative diseases: Kaposi's sarcoma, primary effusion lymphoma (PEL) (Cesarman et al., 1995a), a monoclonal B cell lymphoma, and multicentric Castleman's disease (Soulier et al., 1995), which is a polyclonal hyperplasia caused by a virus-encoded cytokine expressed by KSHV (Parravicini et al., 1997). Nearly all KS and PEL patients have KSHV infection, but only about half of HIV-negative, multicentric Castleman's disease patients are positive for KSHV infection indicating that this disease has a heterogeneous pathogenesis.

The two aforementioned RDA fragments of the KSHV genome facilitated the identification of infected cell lines to serve as source material for viral DNA and as a reagent for biologic studies (Cesarman et al., 1995b). Genomic library walking was performed using cosmid and lambda libraries from one of these cell lines allowing sequencing of the remainder of the genome (Russo et al., 1996). Using this information, various techniques were used to identify likely antigens and generate serologic tests (Gao et al., 1996a,b; Kedes et al., 1996; Simpson et al., 1996). While identification of high-titered infected cell lines sped up this process, isolating the agent was not essential for developing tools to detect it. Molecular biology has reached the point where it is straightforward to identify a new agent, sequence its genome and develop serologic tests for it without ever having actually purified, living sample of the agent. The virus does not have to be grown in order to apply traditional techniques for determining whether or not an agent is present.

The virus itself is a tremendously interesting scientific problem. It has a long unique coding region containing all of the viral open reading frames. Unlike most viruses, KSHV has pirated cellular genes over its evolution and the viral genes are recognizable homologues to cellular genes of known function. Many of these genes provide new insights into tumor virology through their control of the cell cycle, prevention of apoptosis, or immune evasion properties.

One might conclude that this virus is completely different from other viruses and not much can be learned from it to extend to other viruses. In fact, the opposite is true. EBV, for example, induces cellular cyclin D2 to drive the cell through the G1/S cell cycle checkpoint; KSHV encodes its own version of a cyclin D with an analogous function. Other examples of functional correspondence between the KSHV homologues and viral genes encoded by even distantly related viruses can be readily seen (Moore and Chang, 1998a, 2001). For this reason KSHV might be considered something like a molecular Rosetta stone because by using it, we can begin to interpret the language of molecular virology in terms of cell biology for many different viruses.

The importance of new pathogen discovery is illustrated by a timeline of KS research. This would be equally true also for hepatocellular carcinoma and hepatitis C or a wide range of diseases where a new pathogen has been found. The point is that things change quite rapidly once the agent is finally found. Moritz Kaposi initially described the disorder in 1873, but not until 70 years later was there a suggestion of an infectious etiology. In 1981, the onset of the AIDS epidemic brought a tremendous increase in scientific interest in this cancer. There was still, however, little known about the pathogenesis of this disorder in 1993 when there were over 200,000 cases of AIDS in the United States. At that time over 20 different agents had been proposed at one time or another as the causal agent for Kaposi's sarcoma.

The description of KSHV was first published in 1994 and within two years its viral genome was completely sequenced (Neipel et al., 1997; Russo et al., 1996). By that time it was known that the virus was found in all forms of Kaposi's sarcoma (Boshoff et al., 1995; Chang et al., 1996; Moore and Chang, 1995), serologic tests had been developed (Gao et al., 1996a,b; Kedes et al., 1996; Miller et al., 1996; Simpson et al., 1996) and studies initiated to understand the epidemiology of this virus in KS (Moore et al., 1996; Whitby et al., 1995). Shortly thereafter, studies were performed to see whether ganciclovir, a specific antiviral agent, could be used to treat KS (Martin et al., 1999). At the present, there have been over 2,000 papers published on KSHV and its role in malignancy.

Finding a new pathogen also can benefit other fields. When KSHV was first described, only two other related rhadinoviruses had been described in new world primates. Although we live in North America, humans are still considered old world apes. One was herpesvirus saimiri from squirrel monkeys and the other herpesvirus ateles from spider monkeys. Researchers at the University of Washington began to look for other primate KSHV-like viruses (Rose et al., 1997). Using consensus PCR, two were found in rhesus macaques, and subsequently in all the various branches of the primates, both lower and higher primates. This suggests that the viral ancestor of KSHV evolved with us over time. Even more interesting, another group found a closely-related but distinctly different virus in rhesus macaques (Desrosiers et al., 1997). It was named rhesus rhadinovirus (RRV) and belongs to a second lineage of rhadinoviruses. RRV was initially only found in the lower primates, but last year an RRV was found in chimps (Greensill et al., 2000; Lacoste et al., 2000; Lacoste et al., 2001). The implication is that there is an ancestral KSHV/RRV-like virus split off in the primate evolution and has followed through with the different primate lineages, probably including humans. Thus, it is almost certain that there is an undiscovered HHV 9.

An issue in new pathogen discovery is making the step from finding a new DNA sequence to determining whether or not it causes a specific disease. Applying Koch's postulates (Koch, 1942) can elucidate the process:

- The agent occurs in every case of disease.
- The agent never occurs as a fortuitous or non-pathogenic strain.
- The agent can be isolated from the lesion, grown in pure culture, induce disease in a susceptible host and can be re-isolated from an infected susceptible host.

These were postulates that Koch developed for determining the cause of tuberculosis at a time when not much was known of viruses or the carrier state. This was a brilliant attempt to develop a scientific rationale for determining whether an agent is causal for disease or not.

Bradford Hill also developed epidemiologic criteria for causality which are shown here for KSHV and KS (Hill, 1965). Though developed specifically for cigarette smoking, most epidemiologists now use these criteria to determine causality:

- Is the infection present in cases; do all types of the disease involve infection? Is it reproducible in multiple settings?
- Does infection precede disease?
- Is the infection specific to the disease or is it ubiquitous infection among humans?
- Is the virus localized to the tumor (one interpretation of a biologic gradient)?
- Do the epidemiologic studies make sense (are they coherent?)?
- Is it biologically reasonable and do experiments confirm the relationship?

With regard to KSHV, the answers to these questions are largely true. KSHV is present in more than 95 percent of KS lesions. It can be said that the remaining negative 5 percent is probably spurious due to technical difficulties in detection or misdiagnosis, and in fact the virus is absolutely necessary for disease. Though this cannot be proven at present, it can be argued that the situation is very similar to that of papillomavirus and cervical cancer 5 years ago. Is it generalizable? Yes. All types of KS are infected as far as is known. It also appears to have the correct temporal association in that cohort studies show that patients are infected before developing disease, and not afterwards.

But specificity is an important question. KSHV is not singly associated with Kaposi's sarcoma. It is also associated with two other diseases. However, the epidemiology of these two diseases makes some sense in terms of Kaposi's sarcoma, so multiple outcomes are not too worrisome. Depending on the assay that is used, some researchers suggest that the infection rate in the general population for this virus is much higher than alluded to here, but careful studies suggest that less that 5 percent of Americans are infected with KSHV.

Is there a biologic gradient? Yes, there is. Are the epidemiologic findings coherent? Yes, a wide range of epidemiologic studies seem to come to exactly the same set of conclusions. Is it biologically plausible? Yes, there are multiple oncogenes in this virus, related viruses cause cancers, and there are blinded clinical trials which seem to suggest that treatment with ganciclovir prevents the development of Kaposi's sarcoma.

KSHV and KS was a relatively easy case even though it took two years and seven or eight different studies before these conclusions could be reached. Nonetheless, the case for causality was relatively easy.

Now let's consider issues where causality is more problematic. First, KSHV has been claimed not only to cause Kaposi's sarcoma, but also a wide variety of diseases that don't fit its epidemiologic pattern, such as multiple myeloma and sarcoidosis. Although studies supporting these associations were published in reputable journals, they were based on PCR or had other problems and remain questionable in terms of contemporary epidemiological knowledge. In the age of PCR, it is difficult for the casual observer to sort out what is true and what is not.

Assuming that the problem of poor laboratory technique can be solved, there are three more fundamental problems in determining causality. First, causality is relative and should not be thought of as being cast in stone. Causality depends on pathogenic assumptions. That is where Koch's postulates fall down and also where Hill's criteria fall down as well.

For example, if a virus is associated with autoimmune disorders, it can be assumed that one would have an immune response against that virus. In that case the individual may actually clear the virus, so a reverse association would be seen from what would normally be expected following Hill's criteria. The criteria simply do not apply in this case, even though it is a reasonable possibility.

Second, causality is normative. Researchers can get together and study the data but only a few agree to particular conclusions. When the studies describing KSHV as the cause of KS were completed, it was thought that the issue of causality would be resolved. However, it still required a great deal of interpretation. There were many contradictory studies that were ignored because they were not considered valid. But others might disagree, and this is true for just about any contentious issue. An agent is only considered causal for a disease when a majority of scientists agree and it is passed on as received wisdom to others. By then, few scientists probably know the actual studies that were actually used to determine causality.

Third, no agent causes disease alone. There are some fairly convincing examples, HIV as well as rabies virus. Simply not enough is understood about the epidemiology of rabies virus to know whether or not there are people who have been exposed to it who have not developed disease. But with the possible exception of those two viruses, virtually every other infection can have a symptomatic infection, and disease is determined by other factors than the virus alone.

There are several examples where current methods of determining causality break down. One is the role of EBV in nasopharyngeal carcinoma (NPC). There is extremely strong evidence that EBV is the cause of nasopharyngeal carcinoma, but EBV is a near ubiquitous infection. So Hill's criteria cannot be used to determine that EBV causes nasopharyngeal carcinoma since it is likely to be a composite risk factor and additional causal factors have to be used in conjunction with EBV infection. These factors are unknown for NPC, but it is easy to see that rather than using EBV infection alone as an exposure variable, it may be more valuable to measure exposure as EBV infection at a certain susceptible age or EBV infection in a cell having a specific mutation.

EBV and NPC shows another problem with Hill's criteria for causality. Raab-Traub developed an assay for EBV terminal repeat monoclonality and using this assay found that in NPC tumors, the precursor cell forming the monoclonal tumor was infected with a monoclonal form of the virus (Raab-Traub and Flynn, 1986). For molecular biologists and virologists, this is overwhelming proof that the virus causes the tumor since the odds of this happening by chance are so small. It is extremely unlikely that a healthy cell was first infected with the virus, and by chance the same cell independently became transformed into an expanding tumor cell population with EBV growing inside of it as a passenger virus. However, this does not neatly fit Hill's criteria and epidemiologists have no way of weighing the importance of this "overwhelming" piece of molecular evidence, especially in comparison to contradicting evidence such as the ubiquity of EBV infection among humans.

Multicentric Castleman's disease (MCD) illustrates additional problems related to determining causality for different diseases which look identical. About half of MCD tumors are positive for KSHV and so it seems that there are actually two diseases, not just one, under the label of MCD. KSHV is only considered necessary for the KSHV positive form. Now that it is known what to look for, there may be subtle clinical and pathologic clues that can distinguish the two forms of MCD. Analogous situations can be drawn for hepatocellular carcinoma and hepatitis virus C positive hepatocellular carcinoma, or for meningitis and any of the many causes of meningitis. While hepatitis virus C is not necessary for all liver cancers, it is obviously necessary for hepatitis virus C positive tumors. By defining a subset of diseases associated with a viral infection post-hoc, the causality argument becomes circular even though we now have good reasons for splitting up a disease manifestation into different diseases with different manifestations.

It is likely that in the future, improved knowledge of pathogenic mechanisms will reveal novel causal relationships. For example, not too long ago the idea that a bacteria could cause stomach ulcers would have been considered laughable. *Helicobacter pylori* and peptic ulcer disease had a pathogenic mechanism that was poorly understood and thus there was no framework to gauge whether or not a bacteria was the possible cause. In fact, pathologists had seen bacteria associated with ulcers for decades but didn't remark on them because there was no way to measure their significance.

New ways of determining causality that go beyond Hill's criteria and Koch's postulates need to be developed if new and complex mechanisms for disease are to be understood. Researchers have attempted to do this by taking into consideration new techniques of molecular biology (Fredericks and Relman, 1996). It seems clear that epidemiologists developing new criteria for causality will have to incorporate new pathogenic mechanisms that are not currently accounted for.

Unfortunately, no one can predict what new pathogenic mechanisms will be discovered and therefore there are no universal criteria for causality that will not need future revisions. In the end, it cannot be absolutely proved that an agent causes disease, only that it does not. Instead, while criteria such as Hill's or Koch's postulates are enormously helpful in guiding our thinking, we should not be constrained by them as has happened in cases like EBV and nasopharyngeal carcinoma. In this case, both science and public health have suffered from rigid adherence to abstract criteria. For cases where established criteria break down, all that can be done is to develop a detailed pathogenic model which can be tested using epidemiologic studies and further modified. In essence, to use the scientific method which is employed by scientists every day.

REFERENCES

Beral V, Peterman TA, Berkelman RL, Jaffe HW. 1990. Kaposi's sarcoma among persons with AIDS: a sexually transmitted infection? *Lancet* 335:123–128.

Boshoff C, Whitby D, Hatziioannou T, Fisher C, van der Walt J, Hatzakis A, Weiss R, Schulz T. 1995. Kaposi's sarcoma-associated herpesvirus in HIV-negative Kaposi's sarcoma. *Lancet* 345:1043–1044

Cesarman E, Chang Y, Moore PS, Said JW, Knowles DM. 1995a. Kaposi's sarcoma-associated herpesvirus-like DNA sequences in AIDS-related body-cavity-based lymphomas. *New England Journal of Medicine* 332:1186–1191.

Cesarman E, Moore PS, Rao PH, Inghirami G, Knowles DM, Chang Y. 1995b. In vitro establishment and characterization of two acquired immunodeficiency syndrome-related lymphoma cell lines (BC-1 and BC-2) containing Kaposi's sarcoma-associated herpesvirus-like (KSHV) DNA sequences. *Blood* 86:2708–2714.

Chang Y, Cesarman E, Pessin MS, Lee F, Culpepper J, Knowles DM, Moore PS. 1994. Identification of herpesvirus-like DNA sequences in AIDS-associated Kaposi's sarcoma. *Science* 265:1865–1869.

Chang Y, Ziegler JL, Wabinga H, Katongole-Mbidde E, Boshoff C, Schulz T, Whitby D, Maddalena D, Jaffe HW, Weiss RA, Moore PS. 1996. Kaposi's sarcoma-associated herpesvirus and Kaposi's sarcoma in Africa. *Archives of Internal Medicine* 156:202–204.

Desrosiers RC, Sasseville VG, Czajak SC, Zhang X, Mansfield KG, Kaur A, Johnson RP, Lackner AA, Jung JU. 1997. A herpesvirus of rhesus monkeys related to the human Kaposi sarcoma-associated herpesvirus. *Journal of Virology* 71:9764–9769.

Fredericks DN and Relman DA. 1996. Sequence-based identification of microbial pathogens: A reconsideration of Koch's postulates. *Clinical Microbiology Reviews* 9:18–33.

Gao SJ and Moore PS. 1996. Molecular approaches to the identification of unculturable infectious agents. *Emerging Infectious Diseases* 2:159–167.

Gao SJ, Kingsley L, Hoover DR, Spira TJ, Rinaldo CR, Saah A, Phair J, Detels R, Parry P, Chang Y, Moore PS. 1996a. Seroconversion to antibodies against Kaposi's sarcoma-associated herpesvirus-related latent nuclear antigens before the development of Kaposi's sarcoma. *New England Journal of Medicine* 335:233–241.

Gao SJ, Kingsley L, Li M, Zheng W, Parravicini C, Ziegler J, Newton R, Rinaldo CR, Saah A, Phair J, Detels R, Chang Y, Moore PS. 1996b. KSHV antibodies among Americans, Italians and Ugandans with and without Kaposi's sarcoma. *Nature Medicine* 2:925–928.

Greensill J, Sheldon JA, Murthy KK, Bessonette JS, Beer BE, Schulz TF. 2000. A chimpanzee rhadinovirus sequence related to Kaposi's sarcoma-associated herpesvirus/human herpesvirus 8: increased detection after HIV-1 infection in the absence of disease. *AIDS* 14:F129–135.

Hill AB. 1965. Environment and disease: association or causation? *Proceedings of the Royal Society of Medicine* 58:295–300.

Kedes DH, Operskalski E, Busch M, Kohn R, Flood J, Ganem D. 1996. The seroepidemiology of human herpesvirus 8 (Kaposi's sarcoma-associated herpesvirus): distribution of infection in KS risk groups and evidence for sexual transmission. *Nature Medicine* 2:918–924.

Koch R. 1942. The aetiology of tuberculosis (translation of Die Aetiologie der Tuberculose [1882]). Pp. 392–406 in Source Book of Medical History, DH Clark, ed. New York: Dover Publications, Inc.

Lacoste V, Mauclere P, Dubreuil G, Lewis J, Georges-Courbot MC, Gessain A. 2000. KSHV-like herpesviruses in chimps and gorillas. *Nature* 407:151–152.

Lacoste V, Mauclere P, Dubreuil G, Lewis J, Georges-Courbot MC, Gessain A. 2001. A novel gamma 2-herpesvirus of the Rhadinovirus 2 lineage in chimpanzees. *Genome Research* 11:1511–1519.

Lisitsyn NA, Rosenberg MV, Launer GA, Wagner LL, Potapov VK, Kolesnik TB, Sverdlov ED. 1993. A method for isolation of sequences missing in one of two related genomes. *Molekuliarnaia Genetika, Mikrobiologiia, i Virusologiia* 3:26–9

Martin DF, Kuppermann BD, Wolitz RA, Palestine AG, Li H, Robinson CA. 1999. Oral ganciclovir for patients with cytomegalovirus retinitis treated with a ganciclovir implant. *New England Journal of Medicine* 340:1063–1070.

Miller G, Rigsby MO, Heston L, Grogan E, Sun R, Metroka C, Levy JA, Gao SJ, Chang Y, Moore P. 1996. Antibodies to butyrate-inducible antigens of Kaposi's sarcoma-associated herpesvirus in patients with HIV-1 infection. *New England Journal of Medicine* 334:1292–1297.

Moore PS and Chang Y. 1995. Detection of herpesvirus-like DNA sequences in Kaposi's sarcoma lesions from persons with and without HIV infection. *New England Journal of Medicine* 332:1181–1185.

Moore PS and Chang Y. 1998a. Antiviral activity of tumor-suppressor pathways: clues from molecular piracy by KSHV. *Trends in Genetics* 14:144–150.

Moore PS and Chang Y. 1998b. The discovery of KSHV (HHV 8). *Epstein-Barr Virus Report* 5:1–3.

Moore PS and Chang Y. 2001. Kaposi's sarcoma-associated herpesvirus. Pp. 2803–2833 in Fields Virology, DM Knipe and P Howley, eds. Philadelphia: Lippincott, Williams & Wilkins.

Moore PS, Kingsley LA, Holmberg SD, Spira T, Gupta P, Hoover DR, Parry JP, Conley LJ, Jaffe HW, Chang Y. 1996. Kaposi's sarcoma-associated herpesvirus infection prior to onset of Kaposi's sarcoma. *AIDS* 10:175–180.

Neipel F, Albrecht JC, Fleckenstein B. 1997. Cell-homologous genes in the Kaposi's sarcoma-associated rhadinovirus human herpesvirus 8: determinants of its pathogenicity?. [Review]. *Journal of Virology* 71:4187–4192.

O'Brien TR, Kedes D, Ganem D, Macrae DR, Rosenberg PS, Molden J, Goedert JJ. 1999. Evidence for concurrent epidemics of human herpesvirus 8 and human immunodeficiency virus type 1 in US homosexual men: rates, risk factors, and relationship to Kaposi's sarcoma. *Journal of Infectious Diseases* 180:1010–1017.

Parravinci C, Corbellino M, Paulli M, Magrini U, Lazzarino M, Moore PS, Chang Y. 1997. Expression of a virus-derived cytokine, KSHV vIL-6, in HIV-seronegative Castleman's disease. *American Journal of Pathology* 151:1517–1522.

Raab-Traub N and Flynn K. 1986. The structure of the termini of the Epstein-Barr virus as a marker of clonal cellular proliferation. *Cell* 47:883–889.

Rose TM, Strand KB, Schultz ER, Schaefer G, Rankin GW Jr, Thouless ME, Tsai CC, Bosch ML. 1997. Identification of two homologs of the Kaposi's sarcoma-associated herpesvirus (human herpesvirus 8) in retroperitoneal fibromatosis of different macaque species. *Journal of Virology* 71:4138–4144.

Russo JJ, Bohenzky RA, Chien MC, Chen J, Yan M, Maddalena D, Parry JP, Peruzzi D, Edelman IS, Chang Y, Moore PS. 1996. Nucleotide sequence of the Kaposi sarcoma-associated herpesvirus (HHV8). *Proceedings of the National Academy of Sciences* 93:14862–14867.

Simpson GR, Schulz TF, Whitby D, Cook PM, Boshoff C, Rainbow L, Howard MR, Gao SJ, Bohenzky RA, Simmonds P, Lee C, de Ruiter A, Hatzakis A, Tedder RS, Weller IV, Weiss RA, Moore PS. 1996. Prevalence of Kaposi's sarcoma associated herpesvirus infection measured by antibodies to recombinant capsid protein and latent immunofluorescence antigen. *Lancet* 348:1133–1138.

Soulier J, Grollet L, Oksenhendler E, Cacoub P, Cazals-Hatem D, Babinet P, d'Agay MF, Clauvel JP, Raphael M, Degos L. 1995. Kaposi's sarcoma-associated herpesvirus-like DNA sequences in multicentric Castleman's disease. *Blood* 86:1276–1280.

Whitby D, Howard MR, Tenant-Flowers M, Brink NS, Copas A, Boshoff C, Hatzioannou T, Suggett FE, Aldam DM, Denton AS, et al. 1995. Detection of Kaposi's sarcoma-associated herpesvirus (KSHV) in peripheral blood of HIV-infected individuals predicts progression to Kaposi's sarcoma. *Lancet* 364:799–802.

EXPLORING THE GENETIC BACKGROUND–ENVIRONMENT INTERPLAY IN AN ANIMAL MODEL OF NEURODEVELOPMENTAL DISORDERS: A MULTIDISCIPLINARY APPROACH

Mikhail V. Pletnikov, M.D., Ph.D.*

Departments of Psychiatry and Behavioral Sciences, Johns Hopkins University
School of Medicine, Baltimore, MD
and
Laboratory of Pediatric and Respiratory Viral Diseases, Center for Biologics
Evaluation and Research, U.S. Food and Drug Administration, Bethesda, MD

Data from family, twin, and adoption studies convincingly show evidence of a substantial genetic contribution to most neurodevelopmental disorders in humans. Moreover, recent improvements in molecular and genetic technologies have resulted in the implication of genes at several chromosomal loci and a search for candidate genes continues. However, multiple examples of deviation of complex developmental disorders from clear-cut Mendelian transmission cannot be fully explained by incomplete penetrance, variable expressivity, or polygenic etiology. A growing body of evidence suggests an important role of environmental factors in the causation of some developmental behavioral disorders. Unfortunately, environmental studies have been carried out with the same concept in mind, i.e., a search for relevant risk factors that would be self-sufficient to explain the pathogenesis of human conditions. Very little, if any, theoretical or methodological interaction between genetic linkage analysis and environmental (e.g., toxicology or teratology) studies has been undertaken. However, it is the gene-environment interaction that determines variable disease outcomes and responses to treatment and must be addressed in future research approaches.

Although it is clear that there are critical interactions between genes and environment to produce disease phenotypes, this concept has not been a focus of extensive consideration that the important role of environmental factors becomes more apparent in the setting of interaction with genetic determinants. Separating the search for genetic determinants vs. environmental disease etiologies was, in part, based on the assumption that genes and environmental sources are mainly additive in their effects, with the outcome reflecting the sum of their influences. However, the evidence is now clear that genes and environment are interactive as well, and several important issues of the gene-environment interaction are illustrated here with data obtained on the animal model of neurodevelopmental damage in rats neonatally infected with an experimental teratogen, Borna disease virus (BDV).

Among methodological problems of studying the gene-environment interplay is the difficulty in firmly defining environmental factors and making them

---

*This work was supported by the National Institutes of Health, grant 2RO1 MH 48948-08A1.

quantifiable. In this context, virus infections provide a promising research avenue because of their clear etiologic connection to several human neurodevelopmental disorders and because of reliability of quantification of viral effects on brain and behavior (Johnson, 1998). For example, in the BDV model, neonatal infection of the rat's brain with this 8.9-kb non-segmented, negative-strand, enveloped RNA virus (Briese et al., 1994; Cubitt et al., 1994) produces distinct neuroanatomical, neurochemical and behavioral abnormalities that resemble pathological and clinical features of human developmental disorders (Carbone et al., 1991; Carbone and Pletnikov, 2000; Bautista et al., 1994, 1995; Dittrich et al., 1989; Pletnikov et al., 1999, 2000, 2001; Hornig et al., 1999; Eisenman et al., 1999; Gonzalez-Dunia et al., 2000; Weissenbock et al., 2000).

Considering gene-environmental interaction may also help us to better understand the nature of some environmental risk factors. For example, in adult infected Lewis rats, BDV-induced brain damage is primarily mediated by T-cell inflammatory response, causing generalized encephalitis and meningitis (Narayan et al., 1983; Hirano et al., 1983). This global damage significantly hampers studies of other pathogenic mechanisms of viral neurotoxicity. In contrast, in different genetic settings (e.g., black hooded rats or tree shrews), adult BDV infection does not appear to evoke significant inflammatory response, providing new insights into the mechanisms of chronic BDV-associated neurobehavioral deficits (Herzog et al., 1991; Sprankel et al., 1978).

Similar methodological advantages are demonstrated by neonatal rat BDV infection serving as an animal model of neurodevelopmental damage, while also emphasizing a neurodevelopmental perspective in studying the gene-environment interaction. The significance of the neurodevelopmental perspective is substantiated by the fact that effects of many genetic and environmental risk factors are evident either prior to or around the time of birth, and the interaction between them is apparent well before the identified onset/diagnosis of the classical, chronic disease condition. For this reason, we study effects of neonatal BDV infection across the entire postnatal period in genetically different strains of rats in order to understand the course and time-dependent character of the interaction of genetic background features and the virus infection.

In the newer view on the gene-environment interaction, wherein environmental factors are considered to have variable effects on individuals with different genotypes, gene-environment interactions result from genetically-mediated differences in sensitivity to environmental factors. This issue clearly underlines a need for searching for genes that mediate susceptibility to environmental factors rather than genes that directly determine specific chronic conditions. From a pathogenesis point of view, if environmental effects are mainly observed in vulnerable individuals, there is also a need in understanding what pathogenic role individual characteristics may play in modulating differential responses to the environment, variable disease outcome, and sensitivity to treatments. Obviously, such studies must be complex and multidisciplinary, simultaneously addressing alterations in brain structure, chemistry, endocrine function and behaviors in genetically different settings.

Here, using our BDV neonatal rat model of neurodevelopmental damage, we present the data of the developmental analysis of the pathogenic role of baseline (i.e., strain-related) differences in physiology, neurochemistry, and behaviors between two inbred rat strains, Lewis and Fisher344 rats in determining BDV-induced (i) brain damage, (ii) alterations in monoamine systems, (iii) behavioral deficits, and (iv) responses to pharmacological treatment.

Our data show that basic virus infection in both strains is comparable, e.g., similar virus replication and distribution in brain parenchyma in BDV-infected Fisher344 and Lewis rats throughout the postnatal period and similar inhibition of body weight gain in both rat strains. However, the outcome of this virus infection in these two different strains is not identical. Neonatal BDV infection produces a more profound thinning of the neocortex in Fisher344 rats compared to Lewis rats, while a similar reduction in granule cells in the dentate gyrus of the hippocampus and the comparable hypoplasia of the cerebellum was observed in two rat strains (Pletnikov et al., 2002a).

Neurochemical studies indicated regional and strain-specific monoamine alterations in tissue content, turnover and density of post- and presynaptic receptors in developing and adult BDV-infected Lewis and Fisher344 rats at postnatal day (PND) 30 and 120.

The observed strain-specific brain pathology and neurochemical alterations may explain differential behavioral deficits and responses to ameliorative pharmacological treatments in BDV-infected Lewis and Fisher344 rats. For example, when assessed by the prepulse inhibition of the acoustic startle paradigm, neonatal BDV infection impaired sensorimotor gating in Fisher344 but not in Lewis rats at PND 30 and 120 (Pletnikov et al., 2002a). Also, neonatal BDV infection produced greater hyperactivity in Fisher344 rats compared to Lewis rats. The difference in hyperactivity was especially evident at PND 30.

Effects of the interaction of genetic background and environmental insult were further observed in responses of diseased animals to ameliorative pharmacological treatments. Novelty-induced hyperactivity remained unaffected by injections of a serotonin (5-HT) A1 receptors agonist 8-OH-DPAT in BDV-infected Lewis rats, while 8-OH-DPAT significantly decreased novelty-induced hyperactivity in BDV-infected Fisher344 rats. In contrast, novelty-induced hyperactivity was significantly depressed by a selective serotonin reuptake inhibitor (SSRI), fluoxetine, in BDV-infected Lewis rats and remained unaffected in BDV-infected Fisher344 rats (Pletnikov et al., 2002b).

In conclusion, it is likely that the interaction between genetic background and environmental insult contributes to the variability seen in chronic human conditions. The specific mechanisms and processes involved in the genotype-environment interaction remain largely unknown and are only just beginning to be explored. In the present work, some theoretical and methodological aspects of the gene-environmental interaction are discussed and illustrated with the data from the analysis of effects of different genetic background on neurodevelopmental damage and responses to treatment in two rat strains following the neonatal BDV infection.

REFERENCES

Bautista JR, Schwartz GJ, de la Torre JC, Moran TH, Carbone KM. 1994. Early and persistent abnormalities in rats with neonatally acquired Borna disease virus infection. *Brain Research Bulletin* 34:31–40.

Bautista JR, Rubin SA, Moran TH, Schwartz GJ, Carbone KM. 1995. Developmental injury to the cerebellum following perinatal Borna disease virus infection. *Brain Research. Developmental Brain Research* 90:45–53.

Briese T, Schneemann A, Lewis AJ, Park YS, Kim S, Ludwig H, Lipkin WI. 1994. Genomic organization of Borna disease virus. *Proceedings of the National Academy of Sciences* 91:4362–4366.

Carbone K and Pletnikov M. 2000. Borna again, starting from the beginning. *Molecular Psychiatry* 5:577.

Carbone KM, Park SW, Rubin SA, Waltrip RW II, Vogelsang GB. 1991. Borna disease: association with a maturation defect in the cellular immune response. *Journal of Virology* 65:6154–6164.

Cubitt B, Oldstone M, de la Torre JC. 1994. Sequence and genome organization of Borna disease virus. *Journal of Virology* 68:1382–1396.

Dittrich W, Bode L, Kao M, Schneider K. 1989. Learning deficiencies in Borna disease virus-infected but clinically healthy rats. *Biological Psychiatry* 26:818–828.

Eisenman LM, Brothers R, Tran MH, Kean RB, Dickson GM, Dietzschold B, Hooper DC. 1999. Neonatal Borna disease virus infection in the rat causes a loss of Purkinje cells in the cerebellum. *Journal of Neurovirology* 5:181–189.

Gonzalez-Dunia DM, Watanabe S, Syan M, Mallory E, de la Torre JC. 2000. Synaptic pathology in Borna disease virus persistent infection. *Journal of Virology* 74:3341–3448.

Herzog S, Frese K, Rott R. 1991. Studies on the genetic control of resistance of black hooded rats to Borna disease. *Journal of General Virology* 72:535–540.

Hirano N, Kao M, Ludwig H. 1983. Persistent, tolerant or subacute infection in Borna disease virus-infected rats. *Journal of General Virology* 64:1521–1530.

Hornig M, Weissenbock H, Horscroft N, Lipkin WI. 1999. An infection-based model of neurodevelopmental damage. *Proceedings of the National Academy of Sciences* 96:12102–12107.

Johnson RT. 1998. Viral infections of the nervous system. Philadelphia: Lippincott-Raven.

Narayan OS, Herzog K, Frese H, Rott R. 1983. Behavioral disease in rats caused by immunopathological responses to persistent Borna virus in the brain. *Science* 220:1401–1403.

Pletnikov MV, Rubin SA, Vasudevan K, Moran TH, Carbone KM. 1999. Developmental brain injury associated with abnormal play behavior in neonatally Borna Disease Virus (BDV)-infected Lewis rats: A model of autism. *Behavioral Brain Research* 100:30–45.

Pletnikov MV, Rubin SA, Schwartz GJ, Carbone KM, Moran TH. 2000. Effects of neonatal rat Borna disease virus (BDV) infection on the postnatal development of monoaminergic brain systems. *Brain Research. Developmental Brain Research* 119:179–185.

Pletnikov MV, Rubin SA, Carbone KM, Moran TH, Schwartz GJ. 2001. Neonatal Borna disease virus infection (BDV)-induced damage to the cerebellum is associated with sensorimotor deficits in developing Lewis rats infection on the postnatal development of monoaminergic brain systems. *Brain Research. Developmental Brain Research* 126:1–12.

Pletnikov MV, Rubin SA, Vogel MW, Moran TH, Carbone KM. 2002a. Effects of genetic background on neonatal Borna disease virus infection-induced neurodevelopmental damage. I. Brain pathology and behavioral deficits. *Brain Research* 944:97–107.

Pletnikov MV, Rubin SA, Vogel MW, Moran TH, Carbone KM. 2002b. Effects of genetic background on neonatal Borna disease virus infection-induced neurodevelopmental damage. II. Neurochemical alterations and responses to pharmacological treatments. *Brain Research* 944:108–123.

Sprankel H, Richard K, Ludwig H, Rott R. 1978. Behavior alterations in tree shrews (Tupaia glis, Diard 1820) induced by Borna disease virus. *Medical Microbiology and Immunology* 26:1–18.

Weissenbock H, Hornig M, Hickey WF, Lipkin WI. 2000. Microglia activation and neuronal apoptosis in bornavirus infected neonatal Lewis rats. *Brain Pathology* 10:260–272.

INFECTION, CANCER, AND THE IMMUNE RESPONSE

David H. Persing, M.D., Ph.D.
Corixa Corporation and the Infectious Disease Research Institute, Seattle, WA
and
Franklyn G. Prendergast, M.D., Ph.D.
Department of Pharmacology and the Mayo Clinic Cancer Center,
Rochester, MN

During the past decade, the scientific community has witnessed a virtual explosion of information regarding the genetic basis of disease, especially of inherited disorders and human cancers. Much of the effort of the Human Genome Initiative has been focused on genetic abnormalities that arise during the development of neoplasia and upon congenital predispositions to cancer that are associated with the inheritance of mutations within tumor suppressor genes and other loci. These studies are of critical importance to our understanding of genetic and cellular processes contributing to neoplasia. However, to date the evidence suggests that inherited predisposition to cancer probably accounts for only a subset of total cancer patients and appears to be insufficient to explain the sporadic cases currently comprising the majority.

In most models of the development of neoplasia, an underlying assumption is the contribution of an array of intrinsic and extrinsic factors within a multi-step process. A basic prerequisite of many models is an increase in the baseline proliferation rates of essentially normal cell populations, accompanied by genotypic and phenotypic alterations leading to dysregulation of normal growth control mechanisms. Accordingly, preneoplastic conditions are often associated with an increase in the proliferation of tissues, and some cancer predisposing conditions result from inherited predispositions toward increased mitotic rate (e.g., familial polyposis). However, virtually any condition leading to increased cellular proliferation, whether by a direct or indirect mechanism, might potentiate the development of malignancy. Since many infectious processes often lead, directly or indirectly, to increased cell turnover and proliferation, certain agents are now widely regarded as carcinogens (Rosenthal and Purtilo, 1997).

In 1991, zur Hausen estimated that a significant fraction of all human cancers worldwide are associated with infections due to viruses, including human papillomaviruses (cervical cancer and other skin cancers), human T-cell leukemia viruses (adult T-cell leukemias and lymphomas in endemic areas), hepatitis B virus (liver cancer), and Epstein-Barr virus (Burkitt's lymphoma and nasopharyngeal carcinoma) (zur Hausen, 1991). The estimate of the influence of infection may now need to be revised in light of the fact that new viral associations have been discovered and that other, nonviral associations have been uncovered (Rosenthal and Purtilo, 1997). These include a common bacterial pathogen (*Helicobacter pylori* infection with gastric carcinoma and MALT lymphoma), and new viruses (hepatitis C virus with liver cancer, HHV-6 with non-Hodgkin's lymphoma, HHV-8 [a.k.a. KSHV]) with Kaposi's sarcoma, Castleman's disease, and body cavity lymphomas (Mueller, 1995). In addition, new disease associations are being made with respect to previously known pathogens, such as the association of chronic hepatitis C virus infection with non-Hodgkin's lymphoma in certain populations (Luppi et al., 1996). The following sections will summarize briefly some of the established and emerging associations between chronic infections and human cancer, as reflected in Table 3-1.

Chronic Bacterial Infections Associated with Human Malignancy

Helicobacter pylori

After many years of unwarranted skepticism, the medical establishment in the United States and worldwide generally now recognizes *Helicobacter pylori* as the most common cause of diffuse superficial gastritis and gastric and duodenal ulcers (McGowan et al., 1996). Infections caused by *H. pylori* persist within the gastric mucosa for many years, and the incidence of infection is associated with lower economic status and increasing age. Consistent with the step-wise elucidation of the role of the etiologic agent, the treatment for gastric and duodenal ulcer has evolved from a surgical approach (gastrectomy), to medical management of gastric hyperacidity (H2 blockers), and most recently toward antibiotic therapy directed against *H. pylori* (McGowan et al., 1996).

Inflammation associated with *H. pylori* infection may progress to chronic atrophic gastritis, which is a known predisposing condition for the development of gastric carcinoma. Accordingly, *H. pylori* infection has been linked epidemiologically to gastric adenocarcinoma; many studies involving thousands of participants have now shown an increased risk of gastric cancer in persons with elevated antibodies to *Helicobacter pylori* and in known *H. pylori* carriers (Uemura et al., 2001). It is probable that host genetic factors (blood type, HLA type, other immunogenetically determined factors) as well as microbial virulence factors (particularly the presence of the *cagA* virulence factor) contribute to tissue burden of organisms, persistence of infection, and the nature of the inflammatory response,

TABLE 3-1 Infectious Agents Associated with Malignancies

Infectious Agent	Neoplasm
BACTERIA	
Helicobacter pylori	Gastric adenocarcinoma, intestinal type MALT lymphoma, non-Hodgkin's lymphoma
Fusobacterium fusiforme and *Borrelia vincentii*	Squamous cell carcinoma arising from tropical phagedenic ulcer
Vibrio cholerae	Possible associations with immunoproliferative small intestinal disease (IPSID), non-Hodgkin's lymphoma
VIRUSES	
Epstein-Barr virus	Burkitt's lymphoma, nasopharyngeal carcinoma, and reversible lymphoproliferative diseases in immunodeficient patients
Human T-lymphotropic viruses I and II	Adult T-cell leukemia, T-cell lymphoma
Human papillomavirus	Cutaneous and mucosal papillomas and carcinomas
Hepatitis B and C viruses	Hepatitis, chronic active hepatitis and hepatocellular carcinoma
Human herpesvirus-8 (KSHV)	Kaposi's sarcoma, body cavity lymphoma
Human immunodeficiency virus	Kaposi's sarcoma, and non-Hodgkin's lymphoma, cutaneous and mucosal papillomas and carcinomas
SV-40	Possible associations with mesothelioma and ependymoma
PROTOZOA	
Strongyloides stercoralis	T-cell leukemia (with HTLV)
Plasmodium falciparum[a]	Burkitt's lymphoma
Schistosoma hematobium	Squamous cell carcinoma of the urinary bladder
S. mansoni, S. japonicum	Colonic carcinomas
Clonorchis sinensis	Cholangiocarcinoma
Opisthorchis viverrini	Cholangiocarcinoma

[a]*Plasmodium falciparum* is a cofactor for development of Burkitt's lymphoma in endemic regions.

all of which may contribute directly or indirectly to the development of carcinoma (Delchier et al., 2001). The association of *H. pylori* infection with gastric cancer was an important landmark, because it provided the first definitive link between a chronic bacterial infection, chronic inflammation originating within the target tissue, and the ultimate development of a human cancer.

Perhaps even more provocative has been the association of *H. pylori* with lymphoproliferative disease. *H. pylori* infection is associated with a proliferative response of mucosa-associated lymphoid tissues (MALT). This polyclonal or oligoclonal lymphocytic proliferation, which consists mostly of B cells, appears to be predisposed toward the subsequent development of malignant lymphomas of the non-Hodgkin's type (Delchier et al., 2001). Several studies have now demonstrated regression of early MALT lymphomas by antibiotic treatment directed against *H. pylori* (Fischbach et al., 1997; Weber et al., 1994). This suggests further that the maintenance of the MALT lesion is directly associated with *H. pylori* infection, and may in fact be due to an antigen (or perhaps superantigen) and/or cytokine-driven proliferative response. Non-Hodgkin's lymphomas harboring *bcl2* rearrangements may emerge years after regression of the underlying MALT lymphoma by antibiotic therapy directed against *H. pylori* (Horstmann et al., 1994); it has been proposed that malignant cells may already be present in small numbers within the late-stage MALT lymphoma population prior to antibiotic treatment and may emerge thereafter as an antigen-independent lymphoproliferative disease (Graham et al., 1994; Thijs et al., 1995).

An important implication of these findings is the potential for cancer chemoprevention directed against the underlying infectious agent. Treatment of *H. pylori* in early stages of infection could result in lower risk of developing complications of chronic infection (Thijs et al., 1995). However, because *H. pylori* infections are common, and the development of cancer is an uncommon complication of infection, further work should be done to identify at-risk populations in order to better target chemoprevention efforts (Graham et al., 1994).

Other Bacterial Infections

If *H. pylori* can serve as an infectious trigger of a lymphoproliferative disease, might other chronic bacterial infections also be involved? Small intestinal lymphomas have been described as a complication of chronic infection with *Tropheryma whippeli,* the Whipple's disease-associated bacillus, which has been documented to persist for many years (Gillen et al., 1993). Unrecognized cases of Whipple's disease may be more common than previously suspected, based on findings of several recent studies employing detection methods based on the polymerase chain reaction (PCR) (Ramzan et al., 1997). A disease known as immunoproliferative small intestinal disease (IPSID) has been associated epidemiologically with enteric infection possibly due to *Vibrio cholerae*, primarily in developing countries (Isaacson, 1994). Hyperplastic lymphoid tissue develops in the small bowel in association with the disease, converting to malignant lymphoma at later stages. Consistent with the experience of regression of MALT lymphoma in *H. pylori*-infected patients, tetracycline treatment sometimes causes regression of IPSID lesions in patients with early lesions, and is often used in conjunction with chemotherapy in later stage lesions (Trotman et al., 1999). Finally, tropical phagedenic ulcer is a chronic persistent dermatological infection of developing countries caused by coinfection with *Fusobacterium* and a spirochete, *Borrelia vincentii* (Robinson et al., 1988). This infection leads to the development squamous cell carcinoma within the depigmented margins of the ulcerative lesion. Antibiotic treatment is effective for eliminating the bacterial infection and presumably also for reducing cancer risk.

Taken together, it seems that chronic bacterial infections other than *H. pylori* may also predispose to the development of malignancy, especially non-Hodgkins lymphoma, by virtue of direct or indirect stimuli of target cell proliferation. Given the increasing incidence of non-Hodgkin's lymphoma in the US, and the fact that the inciting organisms might be detectable in cancer patients at the time of presentation suggests that pathogen discovery efforts aimed at well-defined patient populations might well be productive. More importantly, effective chemoprevention strategies may depend upon the identification of microbial, environmental, and host determinants in the development of neoplasia.

Parasitic Infections Associated with Malignancy

Some infections with protozoa are associated with malignancy in humans. Burkitt's lymphoma is thought to arise from the convergence of two pathogens in the same host—Epstein-Barr virus and the malarial parasite, *Plasmodium falciparum*. Clustered cases of Burkitt's lymphoma match the geographic distribution of holoendemic malaria (Facer and Playfair, 1989). The well-known immunosuppressive effects of chronic malarial infection are thought to predispose the host to the transforming effects of EBV, perhaps by a mechanism similar to that described for EBV-related malignancies in immunosuppressed hosts (Lam et al., 1991). Another possible virus/parasite interaction in the development of malignancy is the possible association of *Strongyloides stercoralis* in the development of HTLV-associated leukemia which is mentioned below (Plumelle et al., 1997).

Schistosomiasis, a helminth infection with a wide geographic distribution, is associated with carcinoma of the urinary bladder (Rosin et al., 1994). Chronic infection with *S. hematobium* causes chronic inflammation, fibrosis, and increased proliferation of squamous cells; malignant squamous cell carcinomas usually arise from this premalignant proliferative lesion. In contrast, most malignant tumors of the bladder that arise outside of the context of infection with *S. hematobium* in endemic areas are transitional cell carcinomas. A similar mechanism of increasing cell turnover may apply to the development of cholangiocarcinoma during chronic biliary tract infection with *Clonorchis sinensis* and *Opisthorchis viverrini* (Shin et al., 1996). Infection with both of these organisms is associated with chronic inflammation and proliferation of the biliary epithelium. Chronic inflammation of the bile duct epithelium due to infection with the newly recognized protozoa *Septata intestinalis* and *Cryptosporidium parvum* have been recognized in this country, but it is not yet known whether these infections are associated with malignancy.

Viruses Associated with Human Malignancies

Although malignancies associated with viral infection have been studied in animal models for decades, clear evidence of involvement of viral infection in human malignancies has been lacking until about the past decade. A growing number of viral infections have been associated with various human malignancies including carcinomas and adenomas of the cervix and upper airways, liver cancer, and lymphomas and leukemias. As mentioned above, it is estimated that approximately 15 percent of all malignancies worldwide are associated with known viral infections. This estimate is based on associations with already known viral infections. However, recent history has documented that there are likely to be many viral infections of humans that are still to be uncovered.

Malignancy associated with viral infection has in some cases been attributed to direct effects of viral gene products, as described above for the human papillomavirus, or it may be associated with increased cellular proliferation of a target tissue, as described for the bacterial infections above. In both settings, host immune responses are likely to play an important role in the tolerance of persistent viral infection.

The Gamma-herpesviruses, EBV and KSHV

Since its discovery in the early 1960s in an African Burkitt's lymphoma cell line, Epstein-Barr virus has become widely regarded as an oncogenic virus, especially in the immunocompromised host. It is also highly prevalent in the US and worldwide, with 80–90 percent seroconversion by young adulthood in most countries. Most childhood infections are clinically silent, but primary EBV infection in older children or young adulthood is the major cause of acute mononucleosis. During primary infection a polyclonal expansion of B cells occurs resulting in the formation of heterophile antibodies as well as EBV-specific cellular and humoral immune responses. Latency is established in a subset of B cells which can be interrupted under certain conditions to produce reactivation of infection (Goldschmidts et al., 1992).

In the mid-1950s, missionary doctor Denis Burkitt described a unique malignant lymphoma of childhood usually involving the jaw and viscera. He later identified the distribution of cases of the lymphoma to areas of Africa that are endemic for malaria (the "lymphoma belt"). To this day, Burkitt's lymphoma remains one of the most dreaded diseases in sub-Saharan Africa. EBV can be found in nearly 100 percent of endemic lymphomas, in contrast to its lower prevalence in non-endemic Burkitt-type malignancies. In both endemic and non-endemic tumor types, translocation of the *c-myc* cellular oncogene to an expressed locus downstream from the immunoglobulin G promoter (IgG-P) occurs by gene rearrangement. However, the IgG-P/*c-myc* breakpoints in endemic cases occur within a more tightly clustered region, suggesting stereotypic recombinational patterns in the malaria-associated cases. Whether this pattern of recombination occurs directly in response to malarial infection is currently unknown (Facer and Playfair, 1989), but an attractive hypothesis is that immunoglobulin gene rearrangement driven by expansion of *Plasmodium*-specific B-cells participates in the development of malignant clones. Differences in EBV subtypes have been observed in endemic and non-endemic cases; endemic cases contain EBV subtype 2, in contrast to non-endemic cases which usually harbor EBV subtype 1 (Magrath et al., 1992). Mechanisms for the possible pathogen interaction between EBV and Plasmodium are poorly understood; the well known immunosuppressive effects of malarial infection have been proposed by several investigators to activate EBV-associated lymphoproliferation (Lam et al., 1991). The combination of immunosuppression with antigen-specific proliferation may, in this model, lead to the development of a unique type of cancer.

EBV is also associated with nasopharyngeal carcinoma (NPC), a malignancy that represents the most common tumor of males in southern China. Additional environmental exposures to salted fish containing nitrosodimethylamines, and perhaps inhaled herbal extracts have been implicated as possible cofactors in the development of this malignancy. Latent forms of the EBV genome can be detected by in situ hybridization. Immunologic predisposition may also contribute, as reflected in relative overrepresentation of certain HLA types in patients with NPC along with evidence of intrafamilial case clustering. In addition, an atypical immune response as determined by the presence of IgA to certain EBV proteins suggests that an aberrant immune response to the virus may underlie cancer risk (Hsu et al., 2001). This EBV-specific IgA response may be an indirect, albeit diagnostically important, indication of EBV infection on mucosal surfaces which itself serves as a proferative stimulus of epithelial cell populations accompanied by lymphocytic infiltration (lymphoepithelioma).

A recent report implicated EBV in the development of human breast cancer (Magrath and Bhatia, 1999); various studies have detected up to a 51 percent prevalence of EBV in breast cancer tissues, depending on the methods used. Since the known EBV-associated carcinomas are lymphoepitheliomas, and since most breast carcinomas are not lymphoepitheliomas, these findings have been controversial and indeed many studies fail to confirm the initial findings (Chu et al., 2001). A critical link to be established here would be the demonstration of unusual immunological responses to EBV proteins as demonstrated for NPC.

In the developed world, the most common EBV-associated tumor is non-Hodgkin's lymphoma associated with immunosuppression. Most non-Hodgkin's lymphomas originating in the context of HIV infection are associated with EBV, and CNS lymphomas in AIDS patients are nearly exclusively EBV positive (Knowles, 1996). In transplant recipients, EBV-associated tumors often originate as polyclonal or oligoclonal proliferations, occasionally evolving into monoclonal populations (Ambinder, 1990). Reversal of immunosuppression often leads to regression of polyclonal lymphoproliferative disease, consistent with the control of direct proliferative effects of EBV by cytotoxic T-cell responses. Once the tumor has become predominantly monoclonal, however, reversal of immune suppression often has no effect. The progression of non-Hodgkin's lymphomas in immunosuppressed patients is reminiscent of the development of MALT lymphoma, in which an initial polyclonal lymphoproliferative response is followed by the evolution of more aggressive tumors that are apparently less subject to immune surveillance.

A new member of the gamma-herpesvirus family was recently discovered by the application of nucleic acid-based pathogen discovery techniques to Kaposi's sarcoma (KS). KS had long been suspected to have an infectious etiology because of its peculiar epidemiology (Chang and Moore, 1996). The newly recognized virus, which has been called human herpesvirus 8 or KS-associated herpesvirus (KSHV), has been found in HIV-associated cases as well as in non-HIV associated endemic KS in Mediterranean and African men (Moore and Chang, 1995). A similar virus of primates, *Herpesvirus samirai*, causes an aggressive T-cell lymphoma and polyclonal B-cell proliferation in an experimental model of primate infection (Trimble and Desrosiers, 1991). Current epidemiologic evidence suggests that KSHV is necessary but not sufficient for development of most cases of KS. Defects in immune surveillance may contribute to the evolution of KSHV-associated lesions in a manner similar to its more highly prevalent cousin, EBV; these defects may be acquired or intrinsic in nature.

Recently, KSHV was recognized in dendritic cells of the bone marrow from patients with multiple myeloma and a smaller number of patients with monoclonal gammopathy of unknown significance (MGUS), a paraproteinemia which often predisposes to myeloma (Beksac et al., 2001; Rettig et al., 1997). Multiple myeloma is a malignancy of B-cells which represents the second most frequently diagnosed hematologic malignancy in the US. These findings were and still are controversial, especially from an epidemiologic perspective, and subsequent studies have failed to detect an association with KSHV infection in myeloma patients (Ablashi et al., 2000).

Human Retroviruses

The human retroviruses, human T cell leukemia viruses type I and II, infect millions of persons worldwide and are associated with various neoplastic manifestations and immunologic abnormalities. HTLV infects approximately one million people in the Japanese islands and localized populations within the Caribbean basin and South America. HTLV-related lymphomas are common in these areas, and approximately 400 patients develop HTLV associated leukemia yearly in Japan. The fact that only a small subset of HTLV infected patients develop malignant manifestations clearly implicates other factors, either environmental or genetic, that may predispose patients to neoplasia within the multi-step pathway. In the tropics, the high frequency of HTLV-associated malignancies in areas endemic for other protozoal diseases has suggested that coinfection with the latter may play a role in their pathogenesis. Recently, infection with *Strongyloides stercoralis* was found to be an independent risk factor for development of HTLV-associated leukemia in Jamaica (Plumelle et al., 1997). The increasingly recognized immunosuppressive effects of HTLV infection on the cytotoxic T cell response may also be implicated in the development of other cancers, such as carcinoma of the cervix (Strickler et al., 1995).

Perhaps because it is only rarely associated with lymphomagenesis in the United States, relatively less attention has been paid to this virus compared to its distant cousin, HIV. However, many valuable lessons have been learned about the transforming ability of human retroviruses in the development of HTLV-related neoplasia. Furthermore, with the advent of powerful new pathogen discovery techniques, it is possible that additional human retroviruses will be found and that experience gained from evaluation of HTLV-associated cases could be extrapolated to other diseases. Indeed, given the wide variety of exogenous and endogenous retroviruses found within other higher primate species, this seems likely. Several novel endogenous retroviruses have been isolated and identified in patients with autoimmune diseases and malignances. In the case of human seminoma, elevated antibody titers to retroviral *gag* proteins from a novel human endogenous retrovirus (strain K10) that was originally isolated from a seminoma tumor cell line are found in patients and very infrequently in healthy controls (Sauter et al., 1995). Antigens crossreactive with Jaagsiekte virus, a known causative agent in the development of lung adenocarcinoma of sheep, have been detected in human lung carcinoma specimens (Palmarini et al., 1999). Sequences related to known oncogenic retroviruses have also been detected in human breast cancers (Liu et al., 2001). Phylogenetic analyses of other (presumably) exogenous and known endogenous retroviruses have shown that some are related to vertebrate oncoviruses found in mice (mouse mammary tumor virus) as well as to primate endogenous retroviruses. Further work will be necessary to determine whether the sequences of these exogenous and endogenous viruses play a significant role in human cancers or other malignancies.

Malignancies associated with HIV infection include increased susceptibility to cervical dysplasia, squamous cell carcinoma, B cell lymphomas, Kaposi's sarcoma, and possibly seminomas and testicular cancer. It is interesting that in most examples of increased frequency of malignancy in HIV patients, viral cofactors have been directly implicated in the progression of neoplasia. Epstein-Barr virus plays an important role in the evolution of B cell lymphomas in these patients, Kaposi's sarcoma virus participates in the tumorigenesis of Kaposi's sarcoma, and human papillomavirus infection contributes to the development of carcinomas of the skin and cervix. A reduction in levels of antigen-specific cytotoxic T cell responses are associated with activation of infection or disease progression in all of these cases, and a reduction in the efficiency of immune surveillance has been proposed as a factor in tumorigenesis. Consistent with this hypothesis, patients on immunosuppressive therapy following transplantation appear to be at increased risk for the same spectrum of malignancies with the exception of a lower incidence of KS; accordingly, KSHV appears to be much less prevalent in transplant patients compared to HIV patients, presumably because of the risk factors associated with the predominantly sexual transmission of KSHV (Chang and Moore, 1996) .

Hepatitis B Virus

Primary infection with hepatitis B virus usually follows an acute and convalescent course in immunocompetent hosts with ultimate resolution of disease. However, in approximately 5 to 10 percent of adults, and in most infants born to infected carrier mothers, primary infection leads to chronic active hepatitis which may progress to cirrhosis of the liver and hepatocellular carcinoma (Kew, 1996). Continuous proliferation of hepatocytes, which may be present for the life of the host, is a prominent feature of chronic active hepatitis; in such patients, the relative risk of developing hepatocellular carcinoma is increased 20–40 fold. Because of the large number of carriers of hepatitis B virus (HBV), approximately 200 million persons worldwide, hepatocellular carcinoma is one of the most common cancers in the world and is the most common cancer in HBV-endemic areas of the Far East and sub-Saharan Africa. The development of hepatocellular carcinoma probably depends upon direct effects of certain viral determinants along with chronic persistent proliferation of hepatocytes. HBV-related hepatocellular carcinomas often contain defective HBV genomes expressing one or more viral open reading frames; the viral X gene, which is often expressed in malignant tissues, is a transcriptional transactivator of host promoter sequences including those associated with oncogene expression and integrated viral genomes can activate host proto-oncogenes. There is little doubt that continuous proliferation of hepatocytes is also an important contributor to the development of neoplastic disease, since other disorders associated with chronic hepatitis and hepatocyte turnover (such as chronic alcoholism or hereditary hemochromatosis) may also lead to an increased predisposition to liver cancer, and the effects of alcohol ingestion and viral infection may well be synergistic in this regard (Brechot et al., 1996).

Hepatitis C Virus

A rapidly emerging association of chronic viral infection with malignancy is the development of hepatocellular carcinoma associated with chronic hepatitis C virus infection. In the United States, HCV infection is projected to become the major cause of liver cancer, due in part the large number of chronic carriers in this country, currently estimated at 3.5 million persons. In the case of HCV infection, a major determinant of development of hepatocellular cancer appears to be duration of infection and the degree of persistent liver injury (Zein and Persing, 1996). Several studies have associated certain HCV subtypes with differences in liver disease severity, interferon responsiveness, and duration of infection. Viral subtypes that appear to have been in the U.S. population for longer periods of time are dramatically overrepresented among patients with liver cancer. Specifically, subtype 1b, which is present in 15–20 percent of cases nationwide, is present in 90 percent or more of liver cancer patients in several studies conducted at different centers (Zein et al., 1996). Since presence of genotype 1b appears to be a marker of longer duration of infection in U.S. patients, it is possible that other genotypes will be more commonly implicated in cases of hepatocellular carcinoma in other countries, and that the overrepresentation of genotype 1b in the United States will decline over time. Additional factors such as alcohol consumption may contribute independently to risk of neoplasia, even in patients with more recent infections (Brechot et al., 1996). As for HPV infection, host immunogenetic or other factors may play a role in susceptibility to viral infection as well as in determining the severity of infection (see below).

Recently, chronic HCV infection has been associated with the development of B-cell non-Hodgkin's lymphomas in an Italian population (Mele et al., 2003) and with the development of cryoglobulinemia and monoclonal gammopathy in the United States (Cacoub et al., 1994). The development monoclonal gammopathy is thought to presage the development of hematologic malignancies in a significant subset of cases; it is not yet known whether HCV-associated monoclonal gammopathy or mixed cryoglobulinemia is a predisposing variable for the development of such malignancies in the United States. One recent study suggests that HCV infection-associated lymphoproliferative disease might include multiple myeloma (Montella et al. 2001). It is possible that MGUS is a marker of an underlying benign, perhaps antigen driven lymphoproliferative process, which may after many years convert to a malignant process via somatic mutation. In this respect, the genesis of neoplasia may be similar to that described for *Helicobacter pylori*-related MALT lymphoma. The relative disparity in the frequency of non-Hodgkin's lymphoma associated with HCV infection in the United States compared to that in Europe may conceivably reflect differences in duration of infection within the population, immunogenetic differences, or exposure to other oncoviruses including KHSV.

Human Papillomavirus Infection

In the past decade, human papillomavirus (HPV) has emerged as the single most important risk factor for development of cervical carcinoma, and it may be associated with neoplasia in other tissues as well. To date, more than 80 HPV subtypes have been described in a wide variety of epithelial tissues, with some viral subtypes found exclusively in certain tissues; partial sequences of novel subtypes indicate that over 100 subtypes may exist in humans. It is estimated that approximately 95 percent of cervical cancers worldwide are associated with infection by certain human papillomavirus subtypes, usually types 16 or 18 but occasionally other types. HPV-associated cervical cancers typically harbor at least remnants of the HPV genome in the form of two viral oncogenes which are consistently expressed in malignant tissues. The viral E6 gene product binds to tumor suppressor protein p53, promoting its degradation, and the viral E7 product binds to the retinoblastoma gene product, resulting in a functional inactivation. In addition, the E6 and E7 oncoproteins stimulate cell proliferation by activating cyclins E and A. The combination of these effects is to immortalize keratinocytes in vitro. However, additional mutational events are apparently needed to provide the fully transformed phenotype, since immortalized keratinocytes do not form tumors in vivo (zur Hausen and Rosl, 1994). Nonetheless, the viral E6 and E7 genes and their products may become attractive diagnostic targets for monitoring metastatic disease and for the development of tumor-specific immunotherapeutic protocols.

The association of HPV infection with carcinomas of other tissues has been less clear cut, but is somewhat reminiscent of the early days of research on the association of HPV with cervical cancer in which a fundamental limitation in the detection of the large variety of HPV types led initially to great controversy. On the other hand, the inherent proneness of PCR technology to contamination problems, coupled with its ability to detect extremely small numbers of possibly incidental HPV contaminants, warrants a careful interpretation of the growing number of reports implicating this virus in malignancies of many types. Archetypal "oncogenic" subtypes of HPV appear capable of infecting different anatomical sites, and associations of HPV infection with squamous cell carcinomas of the head and neck are reasonably well established. The involvement of HPV in the pathogenesis of skin cancer, the most common malignancy in the world, was suggested recently and a new family of HPV types has now been described in recurrent squamous cell carcinomas of the skin in transplant patients (Shamanin et al., 1996). This finding seems consistent with the clinical experience in patients who are immunosuppressed by HIV infection, in which cervical dysplasia is highly prevalent (Sun et al., 1995).

The role of HPV infection in epithelial carcinomas of the bladder and lung are also being investigated. Studies of the bovine papilloma virus (BPV) have been shown to have an association with cancer of the bladder in cattle (Olson et al., 1965). Inoculation of BPV into newborn hamsters or mice has also been demonstrated to induce tumors (zur Hausen, 1996). Some human studies in recent years have suggested that relatively common HPV types can be detected in human transitional cell carcinoma (TCC) of the bladder in up to 34 percent of cases in certain patient populations (Smetana et al., 1995), but the presence of HPV in the neoplastic tissue has been difficult to demonstrate with consistency (Chetsanga et al., 1992). Interestingly, cases of rapidly progressive multifocal TCC of the bladder have been reported in patients following renal and cardiac transplantation, suggesting that HPV may play a more significant role in TCC of the bladder in immunosuppressed patients (Noel et al., 1994). Although smoking history is the leading risk factor in the development of squamous cell carcinoma of the lung, a recent study implicated the presence of HPV type 16 in an unexpectedly high number of cases of well-differentiated squamous cell carcinoma of the lung on the island of Okinawa (Kinoshita et al., 1995). However, although some studies have supported this finding (Hirayasu et al., 1996), others have failed to implicate HPV in lung cancer (Szabo et al., 1994). In this regard, it is interesting to note that risk of cervical cancer is linked epidemiologically to risk of carcinoma of the lung but not uterine or ovarian cancers, and that both of the former are linked to smoking (Anderson et al., 1997). Clearly, additional studies will be necessary which are designed to rule out the effects of incidental virus and DNA contamination, yet also designed to be capable of detection of the widest range of HPV types.

Recent studies of the natural history of HPV infection have suggested that the ability of the genetically heterogeneous papillomaviruses to exploit relative deficiencies in the immune response may represent an important determinant of the risk of developing chronic infection and subsequent neoplastic disease. Attention has focused recently on cytokine production in HPV-specific helper T lymphocyte populations in women with cervical cancer compared to women in whom the disease regresses spontaneously. Several studies have now indicated that failure to mount cytotoxic T cell (CTL) responses to human papillomavirus-infected cells may significantly predispose to the development of cervical cancer (Tsukui et al., 1996); this failure may be virus type-specific, such that the types represented most often in cervical cancer are those most successful at avoidance of CTL activity (Ellis et al., 1995). Conditions associated with reduced CTL activity, such as HIV and HTLV infection, oral contraceptive use, pregnancy, and immune suppression associated with transplantation have likewise been associated with increased HPV viral burden and acceleration of disease progression (Sun et al., 1995). Twin studies have suggested that risk factors for cervical cancer, as for another HPV-associated lesion, epidermoplasia verruciformis, may be inherited (Ahlbom et al., 1997). More recent studies have failed to detect an association with somatic mutations in the gene encoding p53, and have further explored associations with the immunoglobulin gene cluster (Cuzick et al., 2000). Understanding the contribution of the environmental, host somatic, and host immunogenetic factors to the development of HPV-related dysplasia is an area of intense research activity which may lead to direct practical benefits to patients in the form of improved immunomodulatory approaches to early and late stage lesions. Since the prevalence of HPV infection is so high, the use of routine testing for HPV is of questionable value (Stoler, 2001), except in patients with Pap smears containing atypical features (ASCUS). Clearly, if additional immunogenetic and other host susceptibility factors can be identified, the positive predictive power of HPV testing in cervical cancer screening programs may increase to acceptable levels (Klug et al., 2001).

The Role of Humoral and Cellular Immune Responses

As illustrated vividly by HIV infection, infection with one pathogen may lead to a predisposition toward other infectious processes as well as cancer; a key feature of the immune suppression associated with HIV infection and pharmacologically-produced immunosuppression following transplantation is a reduction of cytotoxic T-cell (CTL) and related T-helper type 1 responses (Spina and Tirelli, 1992). One important theme that recurs among the above mentioned programs, and in cancer research in general, is the relationship of T cell responses to the evolving tumor. A decline in cytotoxic immunity has been associated with virus-associated tumors in immunosuppressed patients, and relative deficits in the establishment of CTL responses during the initial stages of infection are associated with progression of infection in otherwise immunocompetent hosts. Relative differences in the ability to mount cytotoxic T-cell responses have been noted among mouse strains for several years, and recent evidence suggests that immunogenetic determinants in humans may play similar roles. From a teleological perspective, it is likely that viruses and other pathogens associated with chronic infections in humans have evolved means of avoiding CTL responses in at least some hosts in order to maximize reservoir capacity. An example is the recent documentation of point mutations within a dominant HLA B7-associated CTL epitope of the human papillomavirus E6 gene product; the presence of sequence variation has implications for vaccine design and immunotherapy, and overall, viral diversity must be taken into account in the design of therapeutic strategies.

Just as the suppression of cellular immune responses may relate to development of cancer, the development of humoral immune responses may be extremely useful for determining the history of exposure to the pathogen and for the serologic surveillance necessary to establish the etiologic role of a given pathogen. Serologic studies have been critical to the understanding of the role of *H. pylori* as an etiologic cofactor in various malignancies; when no such assays are available for a novel infectious agent, surrogate serologic assays can be used as proposed previously (Persing, 1997). Furthermore, since IgG antibody subclasses are generated on the basis of T-cell help, measurement of IgG subclasses may lead to an understanding of the role of T-cell responses (i.e., the proportional Th1 and Th2-type responses) in determining the resolution or persistence of a particular infection (Moro et al., 2001).

Role Reversal: The Cancer Cell as the Ultimate Eukaroytic Parasite

Independent of the etiologic roles of infectious agents in the development of human cancer, in more than one sense, the cancer cell itself represents the ultimate eukaryotic parasite. Cancer cells, like parasitic protozoa, use a variety of mechanisms to avoid immune surveillance including persistence in small numbers, active secretion of immunosuppressive substances, downregulation of MHC class 1-based recognition, and antigenic variation (Buchanan and Nieland-Fisher, 2001). Humoral immune responses to cancer-specific antigens often occur in cancer patients and are undetectable in patients without cancer (Disis et al., 1997), suggesting that immunologic tolerance can be broken and that many types of cancer-specific immune responses, in the form of tissue-specific autoimmune phenomena, can be tolerated in humans. Antibody responses in cancer patients have led to the discovery of many important cancer-specific antigens (Chen, 2000). At the same time, these studies point to the relative lack of efficacy of humoral immune responses in the control of a developing malignancy, much the same way that in chronic carriers of protozoan parasites, immune responses to pathogen-specific antigens happily coexist with the pathogens themselves. Indeed, many of the lessons learned from parasite immunology can be extrapolated to human cancer, especially in the development of new vaccine-based approaches to the treatment of both diseases.

Conclusions

In purely reductionistic terms, infectious diseases can be viewed as horizontally acquired genetic disorders, in which exogenously acquired nucleic acids of a pathogen integrate, either chromosomally, episomally, or extracellularly, with those of the host to disrupt normal cellular processes or produce inflammation. Developing a better understanding of the interactions of human microbial flora with their hosts, along with an understanding of other host and environmental determinants of pathogenicity, represents an increasingly important intersection of infectious disease research with the Human Genome Project. Illustrations of the latter concept are provided by the discovery of resistance to HIV infection by virtue of mutations within a gene encoding an HIV coreceptor (CCR-5) (Samson et al., 1996). Another important example is the inherited susceptibility to *Mycobacterium avium-intracellulare* infections in families carrying a mutant allele of the interferon-gamma (IFN-γ) receptor (Newport et al., 1996). The identification of such an allele within the human population has far-reaching implications, since it may be associated with a general reduction in the ability to mount cytotoxic T-cell responses during infections of many types. Genetic predisposition to papillomavirus infection appears to underlie the inherited skin disorder epideromodysplasia verruciformis (Majewski and Jablonska, 1995), in which cytotoxic T-cell responses apparently fail to develop against certain papillomavirus subtypes. Since early generation of such responses appears to be a critical step in the resolution of human papillomavirus infections, patients harboring functionally similar mutations may be uniquely predisposed to the development of cervical and other cancers linked to HPV infection. By focusing on unusually severe outcomes of relatively common infectious diseases, we may be able to identify critical immunogenetic factors in the formation of protective immune responses, and to tailor patient management and cancer chemoprevention efforts (in some cases directed against the pathogens themselves) in appropriate ways.

REFERENCES

Ablashi DV, Chatlynne L, Thomas D, Bourboulia D, Rettig MB, Vescio RA, Viza D, Gill P, Kyle RA, Berenson JR, Whitman JE. 2000. Lack of serologic association of human herpesvirus-8 (KSHV) in patients with monoclonal gammopathy of undetermined significance with and without progression to multiple myeloma. *Blood* 96:2304–2306.

Ahlbom A, Lichtenstein P, Malmstrom H, Feychting M, Hemminki K, Pedersen NL. 1997. Cancer in twins: genetic and nongenetic familial risk factors. *Journal of the National Cancer Institute* 89:287–293.

Ambinder RF. 1990. Human lymphotropic viruses associated with lymphoid malignancy: Epstein-Barr and HTLV-1. *Hematology Oncology Clinics of North America* 4:821–833.

Anderson KE, Woo C, Olson JE, Sellers TA, Zheng W, Kushi LH, Folsom AR. 1997. Association of family history of cervical, ovarian, and uterine cancer with histological categories of lung cancer—the Iowa women's health study. *Cancer Epidemiology, Biomarkers & Prevention* 6:401–405.

Beksac M, Ma M, Akyerli C, DerDanielian M, Zhang L, Liu J, Arat M, Konuk N, Koc H, Ozcelik T, Vescio R, Berenson JR. 2001. Frequent demonstration of human herpesvirus 8 (HHV-8) in bone marrow biopsy samples from Turkish patients with multiple myeloma (MM). *Leukemia* 15:1268–1273.

Brechot C, Nalpas B, Feitelson MA. 1996. Interactions between alcohol and hepatitis viruses in the liver. *Clinics in Laboratory Medicine* 16:273–287.

Buchanan J and Nieland-Fisher NS. 2001. Role of immune function in human papillomavirus infection. *Journal of the American Medical Association* 286:1173–1174.

Cacoub P, Fabiani FL, Musset L, Perrin M, Frangeul L, Leger JM, Huraux JM, Piette JC, Godeau P. 1994. Mixed cryoglobulinemia and hepatitis C virus. *American Journal of Medicine* 96:124–132.

Chang Y and Moore PS. 1996. Kaposi's Sarcoma (KS)-associated herpesvirus and its role in KS. *Infectious Agents & Disease* 5:215–222.

Chen YT. 2000. Cancer vaccine: identification of human tumor antigens by SEREX. *Cancer Journal* 6 (Suppl 3):S208–217.

Chetsanga C, Malmstrom PU, Gyllensten U, Morenolopez J, Dinter Z, Peterson U. 1992. Low incidence of human papillomavirus type 16 DNA in bladder tumour detected by polymerase chain reaction. *Cancer* 69:1208–1211.

Chu PG, Chang KL, Chen YY, Chen WG, Weiss LM. 2001. No significant association of Epstein-Barr virus infection with invasive breast carcinoma. *American Journal of Pathology* 159:571–578.

Cuzick J, Terry G, Ho L, Monaghan J, Lopes A, Clarkson P, Duncan I. 2000. Association between high-risk HPV types, HLA DRB1* and DQB1* alleles and cervical cancer in British women. *British Journal of Cancer* 82:1348–1352.

Delchier JC, Lamarque D, Levy M, Tkoub EM, Copie-Bergman C, Deforges L, Chaumette MT, Haioun C. 2001. Helicobacter pylori and gastric lymphoma: high seroprevalence of CagA in diffuse large B-cell lymphoma but not in low-grade lymphoma of mucosa-associated lymphoid tissue type. *American Journal of Gastroenterology* 96:2324–2328.

Disis ML, Pupa SM, Gralow JR, Dittadi R, Menard S, Cheever MA. 1997. High-titer HER-2/neu protein-specific antibody can be detected in patients with early-stage breast cancer. *Journal of Clinical Oncology* 15:3363–3367.

Ellis JR, Keating PJ, Baird J, Hounsell EF, Renouf DV, Rowe M, Hopkins D, Duggan-Keen MF, Bartholomew JS, Young LS et al. 1995. The association of an HPV16 oncogene variant with HLA-B7 has implications for vaccine design in cervical cancer. *Nature Medicine* 1:464–470.

Facer CA and Playfair JH. 1989. Malaria, Epstein-Barr virus, and the genesis of lymphomas. *Advances in Cancer Research* 53:33–72.

Fischbach W, Tacke W, Greiner A, Konrad H, Muller H. 1997. Regression of immunoproliferative small intestinal disease after eradication of Helicobacter pylori. *Lancet* 349:31–32.

Gillen CD, Coddington R, Monteith PG, Taylor RH. 1993. Extraintestinal lymphoma in association with Whipple's disease. *Gut* 34:1627–1629.

Goldschmidts WL, Bhatia K, Johnson JF, Akar N, Gutierrez MI, Shibata D, Carolan M, Levine A, Magrath IT. 1992. Epstein-Barr virus genotypes in AIDS-associated lymphomas are similar to those in endemic Burkitt's lymphomas. *Leukemia* 6:875–878.

Graham DY, Malaty HM, Go MF. 1994. Are there susceptible hosts to Helicobacter pylori infection? *Scandinavian Journal of Gastroenterology Supplement* 205:6–10.

Hirayasu T, Iwamasa T, Kamada Y, Koyanagi Y, Usuda H, Genka K. 1996. Human papillomavirus DNA in squamous cell carcinoma of the lung. *Journal of Clinical Pathology* 49:810–817.

Horstmann M, Erttmann R, Winkler K. 1994. Relapse of MALT lymphoma associated with Helicobacter pylori after antibiotic treatment [letter] [see comments]. *Lancet* 343:1098–1099.

Hsu MM, Hsu WC, Sheen TS, Kao CL. 2001. Specific IgA antibodies to recombinant early and nuclear antigens of Epstein-Barr virus in nasopharyngeal carcinoma. *Clinical Otolaryngology and Allied Sciences* 26:334–338.

Isaacson PG. 1994. Gastrointestinal lymphoma. *Human Pathology* 25:1020–1029.

Kew MC. 1996. Hepatitis B and C viruses and hepatocellular carcinoma. *Clinics in Laboratory Medicine* 16:395–406.

Kinoshita I, Dosaka-Akita H, Shindoh M, Fujino M, Akie K, Kato M, Fujinaga K, Kawakami Y. 1995. Human papillomavirus type 18 DNA and E6-E7 mRNA are detected in squamous cell carcinoma and adenocarcinoma of the lung. *British Journal of Cancer* 71:344–349.

Klug SJ, Wilmotte R, Santos C, Almonte M, Herrero R, Guerrero I, Caceres E, Peixoto-Guimaraes D, Lenoir G, Hainaut P, Walboomers JM, Munoz N. 2001. Tp53 polymorphism, hpv infection, and risk of cervical cancer. *Cancer Epidemiology Biomarkers and Prevention* 10:1009–1012.

Knowles DM. 1996. Etiology and pathogenesis of AIDS-related non-Hodgkin's lymphoma. *Hematology/Oncology Clinics of North America* 10:1081–1109.

Lam KM, Syed N, Whittle H, Crawford DH. 1991. Circulating Epstein-Barr virus-carrying B cells in acute malaria. *Lancet* 337:876–878.

Liu B, Wang Y, Melana SM, Pelisson I, Najfeld V, Holland JF, Pogo BG. 2001. Identification of a proviral structure in human breast cancer. *Cancer Research* 61:1754–1759.

Luppi M, Grazia Ferrari M, Bonaccorsi G, Longo G, Narni F, Barozzi P, Marasca R, Mussini C, Torelli G. 1996. Hepatitis C virus infection in subsets of neoplastic lymphoproliferations not associated with cryoglobulinemia. *Leukemia* 10:351–355.

Magrath I and Bhatia K. 1999. Breast cancer: a new Epstein-Barr virus-associated disease? *Journal of the National Cancer Institute* 91:1349–1350.

Magrath I, Jain V, Bhatia K. 1992. Epstein-Barr virus and Burkitt's lymphoma. *Seminars in Cancer Biology* 3:285–295.

Majewski S and Jablonska S. 1995. Epidermodysplasia verruciformis as a model of human papillomavirus-induced genetic cancer of the skin. *Archives of Dermatology* 131:1312–1318.

McGowan CC, Cover TL, Blaser MJ. 1996. Helicobacter pylori and gastric acid: biological and therapeutic implications. *Gastroenterology* 110:926–938.

Mele A, Pulsoni A, Bianco E, Musto P, Szklo A, Sanpaolo MG, Iannitto E, De RenzoA, Martino B, Liso V, Andrizzi C, Pusterla S, Dore F, Maresca M, Rapicetta M, Marcucci F, Mandelli F, Franceschi S. 2003. Hepatitis C virus and B-cell non-Hodgkin lymphomas: an Italian multicenter case-control study. *Blood*. 102(3):996–999.

Montella M, Crispo A, Frigeri F, Ronga D, Tridente V, De Marco M, Fabbrocini G, Spada O, Mettivier V, Tamburini M. 2001. HCV and tumors correlated with immune system: a case-control study in an area of hyperendemicity. *Leukemia Research* 25:775–781.

Moore PS and Chang Y. 1995. Detection of herpesvirus-like DNA sequences in Kaposi's sarcoma in patients with and without HIV infection [see comments]. *New England Journal of Medicine* 332:1181–1185.

Moro MH, Bjornsson J, Marietta EV, Hofmeister EK, Germer JJ, Bruinsma E, David CS, Persing DH. 2001. Gestational attenuation of Lyme arthritis is mediated by progesterone and IL-4. *Journal of Immunology* 166:7404–7409.

Mueller N. 1995. Overview: viral agents and cancer. *Environmental Health Perspectives* 103(Suppl 8):259–261.

Newport MJ, Huxley CM, Huston S, Hawrylowicz CM, Oostra BA, Williamson R, Levin M. 1996. A mutation in the interferon-gamma-receptor gene and susceptibility to mycobacterial infection. *New England Journal of Medicine* 335:1941–1949.

Noel JC, Thiry L, Verhest A, Deschepper N, Peny MO, Sattar AA, Schulman CC, Haot J. 1994. Transitional cell carcinoma of the bladder: evaluation of the role of human papillomaviruses. *Urology* 44:671–675.

O'Connor F, Buckley M, O'Morain C. 1996. Helicobacter pylori: the cancer link. *Journal of the Royal Society of Medicine* 89:674–678.

Olson C, Pamucku AM, Brobst DF. 1965. Papillomalike virus from bovine urinary tumours. *Cancer Research* 25:840–847.

Palmarini M, Sharp JM, de las Heras M, Fan H. 1999. Jaagsiekte sheep retrovirus is necessary and sufficient to induce a contagious lung cancer in sheep. *Journal of Virology* 73:6964–6972.

Persing DH. 1997. The cold zone: a curious convergence of tick-transmitted diseases. *Clinical Infectious Diseases* 25(Suppl 1):S35–42.

Plumelle Y, Gonin C, Edouard A, Bucher BJ, Thomas L, Brebion A, Panelatti G. 1997. Effect of Strongyloides stercoralis infection and eosinophilia on age at onset and prognosis of adult T-cell leukemia. *American Journal of Clinical Pathology* 107:81–87.

Ramzan NN, Loftus E, Burgart LJ, Rooney M, Batts KP, Wiesner RH, Fredricks DN, Relman DA, Persing DH. 1997. Diagnosis and monitoring of Whipple disease by polymerase chain reaction. *Annals of Internal Medicine* 126(7).

Rettig MB, Ma HJ, Vescio RA, Pold M, Schiller G, Belson D, Savage A, Nishikubo C, Wu C, Fraser J, Said JW, Berenson JR. 1997. Kaposi's sarcoma-associated herpesvirus infection of bone marrow dendritic cells from multiple myeloma patients. *Science* 276:1851–1854.

Robinson DC, Adriaans B, Hay RJ, Yesudian P. 1988. The clinical and epidemiologic features of tropical ulcer (tropical phagedenic ulcer). *International Journal of Dermatology* 27:49–53.

Rosenthal IJ and Purtilo DT. 1997. Neoplasms associated with infectious agents. P. 1707. In Pathology of Infectious Diseases, vol. II, DH Connor, FW Chandler, HJ Manz, DA Schwartz, EE Lack, eds. Stamford, CT: Appleton and Lange.

Rosin MP, Anwar WA, Ward AJ. 1994. Inflammation, chromosomal instability, and cancer: the schistosomiasis model. *Cancer Research* 54:1929s–1933s.

Samson M, Libert F, Doranz BJ, Rucker J, Liesnard C, Farber CM, Saragosti S, Lapoumeroulie C, Cognaux J, Forceille C, Muyldermans G, Verhofstede C, Burtonboy G, Georges M, Imai T, Rana S, Yi Y, Smyth RJ, Collman RG, Doms RW, Vassart G, Parmentier M. 1996. Resistance to HIV-1 infection in caucasian individuals bearing mutant alleles of the CCR-5 chemokine receptor gene [see comments]. *Nature* 382:722–725.

Sauter M, Schommer S, Kremmer E, Remberger K, Dolken G, Lemm I, Buck M, Best B, Neumann-Haefelin D, Mueller-Lantzsch N. 1995. Human endogenous retrovirus K10: expression of Gag protein and detection of antibodies in patients with seminomas. *Journal of Virology* 69:414–421.

Shamanin V, zur Hausen H, Lavergne D, Proby CM, Leigh IM, Neumann C, Hamm H, Goos M, Haustein UF, Jung EG et al. 1996. Human papillomavirus infections in nonmelanoma skin cancers from renal transplant recipients and nonimmunosuppressed patients [see comments]. *Journal of the National Cancer Institute* 88:802–811.

Shin HR, Lee CU, Park HJ, Seol SY, JM Chung, Choi HC, Ahn YO, Shigemastu T. 1996. Hepatitis B and C virus, Clonorchis sinensis for the risk of liver cancer: a case-control study in Pusan, Korea. *International Journal of Epidemiology* 25:933–940.

Smetana Z, Keller T, Leventon-Kriss S, Huszar M, Lindner A, Mitrani-Rosenbaum S, Mendelson E, Smetana S. 1995. Presence of human papilloma virus in transitional cell carcinoma in Jewish population in Israel. *Cellular & Molecular Biology* 41:1017–1023.

Spina M and Tirelli U. 1992. Human immunodeficiency virus as a risk factor in miscellaneous cancers. *Current Opinion in Oncology* 4:907–910.

Stoler MH. 2001. HPV for cervical cancer screening: is the era of the molecular Pap smear upon us? *Journal of Histochemistry and Cytochemistry* 49:1197–1198.

Strickler HD, Rattray C, Escoffery C, Manns A, Schiffman MH, Brown C, Cranston B, Hanchard B, Palefsky JM, Blattner WA. 1995. Human T-cell lymphotropic virus type I and severe neoplasia of the cervix in Jamaica. *International Journal of Cancer* 61:23–26.

Sun XW, Ellerbrock TV, Lungu O, Chiasson MA, Bush TJ, Wright T Jr. 1995. Human papillomavirus infection in human immunodeficiency virus-seropositive women. *Obstetrics & Gynecology* 85:680–686.

Szabo I, Sepp R, Nakamoto K, Maeda M, Sakamoto H, Uda H. 1994. Human papillomavirus not found in squamous and large cell lung carcinomas by polymerase chain reaction [see comments]. *Cancer* 73:2740–2744.

Thijs JC, Kuipers EJ, van Zwet AA, Pena AS, de Graaff J. 1995. Treatment of Helicobacter pylori infections. *QJM* 88:369–389.

Trimble JJ and Desrosiers RC. 1991. Transformation by herpesvirus saimiri. *Advances in Cancer Research* 56:335–355.

Trotman BW, Pavlick AC, Igwegbe IC, Goldstein MM. 1999. Immunoproliferative small intestinal disease: case report and literature review. *Journal of the Association for Academic Minority Physicians* 10:88–93.

Tsukui T, Hildesheim A, Schiffman MH, Lucci JR, Contois D, Lawler P, Rush BB, Lorincz AT, Corrigan A, Burk RD, Qu W, Marshall MA, Mann D, Carrington M, Clerici M, Shearer GM, Carbone DP, Scott DR, Houghten RA, Berzofsky JA. 1996. Interleukin 2 production in vitro by peripheral lymphocytes in response to human papillomavirus-derived peptides: correlation with cervical pathology. *Cancer Research* 56:3967–3974.

Uemura N, Okamoto S, Yamamoto S, Matsumura N, Yamaguchi S, Yamakido M, Taniyama K, Sasaki N, Schlemper RJ. 2001. Helicobacter pylori infection and the development of gastric cancer. *New England Journal of Medicine* 345:784–789.

Weber DM, Dimopoulos MA, Anandu DP, Pugh WC, Steinbach G. 1994. Regression of gastric lymphoma of mucosa-associated lymphoid tissue with antibiotic therapy for Helicobacter pylori. *Gastroenterology* 107:1835–1838.

Zein NN and Persing DH. 1996. Hepatitis C genotypes: current trends and future implications. [Review] [50 refs]. *Mayo Clinic Proceedings* 71:458–462.

Zein NN, Poterucha JJ, Gross J Jr, Wiesner RH, Therneau TM, Gossard AA, Wendt NK, Mitchell PS, Germer JJ, Persing DH. 1996. Increased risk of hepatocellular carcinoma in patients infected with hepatitis C genotype 1b. *American Journal of Gastroenterology* 91:2560–2562.

zur Hausen H. 1991. Viruses in human cancers. *Science* 254:1167–1173.

zur Hausen H. 1996. Roots and perspectives of contemporary papillomavirus research. *Journal of Cancer Research and Clinical Oncology* 122:3–13.

zur Hausen H and Rosl F. 1994. Pathogenesis of cancer of the cervix. Cold Spring Harbor Symposia on Quantitative *Biology* 59:623–628.

4

Opportunities to Prevent and Mitigate the Impact of Chronic Diseases Caused by Infectious Agents

OVERVIEW

The ultimate goal in identifying connections between infectious agents and chronic diseases is to find better ways to cure, or even prevent, those diseases. Various therapeutic approaches may prove fruitful and deserve continued attention. Several of these areas were explored during the workshop, along with ways to most effectively move therapeutic methods from the laboratory into widespread practice. Discussion was somewhat limited, however, by time constraints and the availability of speakers.

Among therapeutic possibilities, vaccines hold a special attraction, given their unique record of totally eliminating or eradicating several target diseases. Recent advances in molecular biology and genetics have provided powerful new methods for vaccine development. Of particular importance is the possibility offered by the new sciences of genomics and proteomics to detect the relevant antigens and to identify specific aspects of immunity that should be enhanced by the vaccine. There also have been important advances made in understanding the processes of acquired immunity and the pathogenesis of various diseases (including the interplay between microbe and host). Collectively, these efforts may point the way to the eventual development of effective means to control at least some chronic diseases.

To underpin scientific efforts, sound planning and program management is a must. In order to most effectively develop and implement new prevention and intervention efforts—encompassing vaccines and a host of other means—there will need to be in place an overarching strategy to guide efforts across a range of fronts. This strategy will rely heavily on collaborations to enhance the productivity of independent investigators, to integrate rigorously executed laboratory techniques into well-designed epidemiologic studies and surveillance systems, and to complement short-term studies with long-term follow-up. It also will be necessary to develop funding mechanisms that recognize the value of such crosscutting efforts.

Helena Mäkelä described the recent advances that are raising promise for the development of vaccines to fight chronic diseases, either by preventing acute infection or by curing established persistent infection. The possibility of developing a vaccine to fight cardiovascular disease, one of the major killers in the United States and worldwide, served as an example. The vaccine would target *Chlamydia pneumoniae*, which has been linked to atherosclerosis by several lines of evidence, though its causative role has not been conclusively established. Among efforts to date, researchers have developed an experimental model of *C. pneumoniae* in the mouse, and work with this system is yielding fundamental lessons. Also, a number of candidate vaccines have been prepared and tested for prevention of acute infection, and several of them have proved to afford at least partial protection.

Siobhán O'Conner presented a blueprint for the strategic approach that will be needed to integrate laboratory research, epidemiology, and surveillance. This blueprint is based on several basic tenets that stress the importance of standardized or comparable case definitions—for the infection as well as the outcome—and universally high standards of specificity, sensitivity, and reproducibility of laboratory assays. As the field advances, a number of crosscutting issues also will require continuous attention. One such issue will be the need to provide adequate medical education (both academic training and continuing education) so that health professionals will be able to capitalize on the benefits afforded by confirmed and newly discovered links between infectious agents and chronic diseases, while at the same time protecting the well-being of their patients. O'Connor concluded that although the links between microbial infections and chronic diseases can be complex and multifactorial, they can be characterized—and beneficial interventions against infection can be designed.

DEVELOPING VACCINES FOR PREVENTION OF CHRONIC DISEASE

P. Helena Mäkelä, M.D., Ph.D. *
National Public Health Institute, Helsinki, Finland

The potential of vaccination as an intervention is undeniable. Vaccines have

*I wish to thank warmly colleagues whose contribution to this paper have been essential: Jenni M. Vuola, Mirja Puolakkainen, Tuula Penttilä, Anne Sarén, Anu Haveri, and Laura Mannonen from the Institute or Department of Virology, Haartman Institute, University of Helsinki.

the unique record of totally eliminating or eradicating their target disease—smallpox in the recent past, polio likely to happen in the near future.

The important point is that vaccination has a target separate and different from the human body, thus making it possible to destroy the microbe without harm to the host. Vaccination is an exciting novel concept for intervention in chronic diseases arising from the realization of a link of many chronic conditions with infectious agents.

A second aspect that sets vaccination apart from other interventions is that it is based on acquired immunity, the powerful defense system of the mammalian body. It provides a very sophisticated machinery for defense against the target microbe; what vaccination needs to do is to enhance its activity and direct it to the specified target.

Recent advances of molecular biology and genetics have provided vaccine development with very powerful methods of research. These include the possibilities offered by genomics and proteomics to detect the relevant antigens to include in the vaccine and to identify the branches of immunity that should be enhanced by the new vaccines. At least equally important are the advances recently made and to be made in understanding the processes of acquired immunity on one hand and of pathogenesis of the diseases—an interplay between the microbe and host—on the other. Also to be included here are new means of producing the desired vaccine antigens in a heterologous host, e.g., *E. coli* or yeast, thus bypassing difficulties of growing a fastidious microbe or purifying a specific protein. An even more sophisticated form of vaccination is administration, instead of a vaccine antigen, its gene inserted in the genome of a viral or bacterial vector or a naked piece of nucleic acid, relying on its expression in the vaccinated individual. The advances in immunology suggest possibilities of developing novel adjuvants to enhance or suppress selected responses. Increasing knowledge of mucosal immunity may allow the development of more specific vaccines according to the site of the microbial invasion to be prevented.

However, many problems and questions immediately arise:

1. How certain is the link of a chronic disease to the microbe suspected as the culprit? A major barrier to vaccine development is not knowing how great an investment is needed before a vaccine is on the market. Obviously the industry will want to closely assess all information about the link when making decisions of starting the development process or of continuing it throughout. The public sector might be less sensitive to this kind of uncertainty, but it does not as a rule have the capacity and know-how to carry out the full process of modern vaccine development. On the other hand, on the competitive market, early start of the development would be an important advantage.

2. What is known of the pathogenesis of the chronic disease and the infection behind it? Important questions with immediate relevance to vaccine development are whether or not the chronic disease is dependent on the continued pres-

ence and persistence, of the microbe (as seems to be the case with gastric ulcer associated with *Helicobacter pylori* infection) or mediated by a process once set in motion or fully carried out by the microbe that then disappears (the latter may be the case with juvenile diabetes due to destruction of islet cells associated with a viral infection).

3. How does acquired immunity affect the condition? In case of persistent infection we would need to know the characteristics of the immunity that allows the infection to persist—which component is missing and why, how could we change the situation to convert the persistence-associated immunity to a protective immunity? Would it be possible to affect this during the persistent state so that the persistence could be cured? For vaccine development, the characteristics of protective immunity for each infection would need to be known. Questions that can be asked to help this characterization include the role of antibodies (if yes, to which antigens? is high affinity essential? would some isotype be specifically needed?) and the role of T cells (and further, whether it is the CD4+ cells stimulated by antigenic peptide bound to the MCH class II molecules on the surface of antigen-presenting cells or the CD8+ cells stimulated by peptide bound to class I molecules, and whether it should be a Th 1- or Th 2-type response, each associated with its separate sets of cytokines).

4. Do we have an experimental animal model? The use of such a model is normally an essential part of vaccine development that helps to convert the theoretical findings at the laboratory bench to a form on which we can predict what can be expected of the vaccine's performance in humans. The better the model, the more we can learn about the candidate vaccine, and more importantly, about the pathogenesis of the infection, the disease, and the immunity. Nevertheless, it is also true that no animal experiments can replace final clinical trials in which the vaccine is evaluated in its real target population.

Of the problems listed, the question of persistent infection requires special attention as a feature not considered in the context of conventional vaccines. Again, there are more open questions than facts. In order to persist, the microbe will have to hide from both innate host defenses and the effector mechanisms of acquired immunity. This raises a series of questions. Where exactly does this take place? How can we identify—diagnose—a persistent infection? What are the host factors that induce persistence and/or allow it to continue? What about the microbe? Is it dormant, with only a few genes active? If so, which ones are they and what are their products (which might be the sought-after vaccine antigens)? The intracellular space is protected from antibodies, and indeed utilized by most persisting microbes. But then we need to ask in which cells, in which part of the body (e.g., Herpes viruses in the nuclei of the neurons in sensoric ganglia), and in which compartment of the cells? Intracellular bacteria most often enter via phagocytic vacuoles, but can then further modify their microenvironment by regulating the acidification of the vacuolar fluid, fusion with lysosomal granules, etc.

Strategies for Vaccination to Prevent Chronic Disease Associated with an Infectious Agent

The many varieties in which microbes may lead to chronic conditions suggest that different strategies of vaccination will be needed. These can be classified as one of two basic types: one, preventing the primary acute infection, and two, curing the persistent infection.

Prevention of acute infection has many advantages. It would not differ from the established concept of vaccination. Vaccine development would be straightforward up to and including the clinical efficacy trial, in which the prevention of the acute infection would be the outcome measured. Thus, one would not need to worry about the pathogenesis of the chronic disease. The success of this approach has indeed been demonstrated for the hepatitis B vaccine (reduction of chronic hepatitis and liver cancer in 10 years following vaccination in infancy [Lee and Ko, 1997]). This vaccine is now recommended by the World Health Organization for use in the infant immunization program all over the world. An effective vaccination program reaching a high coverage rate would also be likely to reduce the transmission of the infectious agent and thereby lead to herd immunity further enhancing the overall effect of the program. Vaccination of this type would seem very attractive for prevention of infections that lead to the chronic disease relatively early in life, e.g., for juvenile diabetes, if the connection to the infectious agent is established and a vaccine available.

For a vaccine of this type to succeed it would need to be highly efficacious, leading to full elimination of the infective agent and continued protection from eventual new encounters. Specifically it should not allow persistence to develop, and demonstration of this effect should be included in the final tests for vaccine licensure. From a programmatic point of view this type of vaccine should be administered before the infection is normally acquired, which usually means early in infancy. This would not cause problems as such since most vaccinations now take place within the infant immunization program, assuring an effective infrastructure for vaccine delivery and good access to a high proportion of all children born. However, the vaccine should be effective enough to provide protection up to an advanced age—preferably through life, a fairly strict requirement. Furthermore, the main problem may lie in motivating the inclusion of one more vaccine among the injections given to infants, if the intended benefits—prevention of a chronic disease—will only be seen decades later.

The second alternative, curing an already established persistent infection, would be an answer to the programmatic problem just described. The vaccine could be given later in life, at a time when individuals start to worry about the dangers of various chronic conditions affecting higher age groups. Motivation for vaccination would be especially high among those who have already experienced symptoms of the chronic disease. On the other hand, so far there is no established infrastructure or system for reaching the adults who should be vaccinated, although one is currently needed for efficient delivery of the annual influenza vaccine. However, the development of a vaccine capable of curing an established persistent infection is a formidable challenge, and no such vaccine exists as a model.

The Example of Cardiovascular Disease

The role of *Chlamydia pneumoniae* in atherosclerosis is supported by several lines of evidence but has not been conclusively established (Saikku, 1999; Grayston, 2000; O'Connor et al., 2001). This is a definite handicap for serious investment in vaccine development. On the other hand, the disease is so prevalent and well known as the major cause of death for those aged 40 years and above that the potential market for a vaccine would be very lucrative. Therefore, let us examine how a vaccine could be developed and used.

C. pneumoniae is an obligate intracellular gram-negative bacterium. It has a small genome of approximately 1.2 million nucleotides fully sequenced. Its primary mode of transmission is via the respiratory route from man to man, and the respiratory infection that develops is usually mild but can also progress to pneumonia. The first infection occurs in childhood and in early adolescence, repeated infections are common. Fifty to seventy percent of adults are seropositive. There is little accurate information about acquired immunity in man; antibody responses are easily demonstrated to several antigens, and the same is true of T-cell responses. However, the immunity following infection does not prevent repeated infections and allows the development of persistent infection. It is not clear whether or not the immunity itself plays a critical role in the pathogenesis of the cardiovascular disease.

There is quite a bit of evidence for persistence of *C. pneumoniae* after infection: it has been identified in peripheral blood mononuclear cells and in vascular plaques of individuals with other osclerotic disease. The role and mechanisms of action of the persistent bacteria in the pathogenesis of cardiovascular disease is open—potential mechanisms suggested include local reactivation of the bacteria with resulting local inflammation, activation of the blood coagulation system, and induction of various cytokines either directly by the bacteria or their components (especially lipopolysaccharide) or in conjunction with immune cells and/or antibodies.

An experimental model of *C. pneumoniae* infection has been developed in the mouse (Kaukoranta-Tolvanen et al., 1993; Penttilä et al., 1998). The acute infection resulting from intranasal inoculation of moderate doses of *C. pneumoniae* (10^5–10^6 inclusion forming units [IFUs]) resembles the human infection in many ways. It is a pneumonia that is symptomatically mild. The bacteria are seen in the lungs inside epithelial cells and macrophages; their numbers stay high for 1–2 weeks and then decrease to undetectable (culture-negative) in 3–4 weeks. An immune response can be seen in antibody production and T-cell responses. Most importantly, the infection results in partial protection seen on reinfection when a similar intranasal inoculation results in a lower peak level of IFUs and their disappearance in 1–2 weeks.

The role of different branches of the immune system has been studied in the mouse model using gene-deleted mice as well as mice injected with antibodies to deplete specific immune cells or interferon (Penttilä et al., 1999; Rottenberg et al., 1999). These experiments have shown that the cure of the acute infection did not require antibodies or either CD4+ of CD8+ T-cells; however, in more severely deleted mice lacking both types of T cells cultivable bacteria continued to be present in the lungs in relatively high numbers. Interferon gamma (INF-γ) was identified as an important mediator. The protective immunity seen on reinfection would be more relevant from the vaccine development point of view. The experimental findings pointed at the central role of CD8+ cells in this protection: if they were depleted, the reinfection proceeded at the same kinetics as the primary infection. IFN-γ appeared to be a mediator of cure also in this phase. In summary, consistent with the intracellular multiplication of *C. pneumoniae*, T cells, and, especially CD8+ T cells, seem to have a key position in protective immunity.

A number of candidate vaccines have been prepared and tested for prevention of the acute infection (Penttilä et al., 2000; Svanholm et al., 2000; Murdin et al., 2000). Killed *C. pneumoniae* particles (EB, the infectious elementary bodies) afforded partial protection that was less strong than seen during recovery from a previous infection. Several *C. pneumoniae* genes given in the form of naked DNA vaccines have likewise provided partial protection but again less strong than seen in reinfection. The immune response to the products of the respective *C. pneumoniae* genes were easily measurable as both antibody and T-cell responses, including cytotoxic CD8+ lymphocytes (CTL). In the same approach, several other genes have failed to induce protection.

The key determinants of protection in the acute infection model are still not known. The prominent role of the intracellular life of *C. pneumoniae* is consistent with the importance of CD8+ cells in protective immunity. The vaccines that so far have given positive signals of protection have stimulated CD8+ cells. Then why only incomplete protection? Is it due to us not having identified the right antigen(s)? Quite possibly so: most of the *C. pneumoniae* gene products likely remain within the body of the gram-negative bacterium, which further resides within the intracellular vesicle known as inclusion body. Therefore only few proteins would be likely to reach the cytoplasm of the host cell, a primary requirement in order to be processed, associated with the nascent MHC class I molecules and presented by these on the cell surface essential for recognition by immune CTLs. These proteins would most likely be protein(s) purposely exported by the bacteria to interact with the host cell components and subvert these to the benefit of the microbe. In other gram-negative bacteria, such proteins are typically secreted by a specific "Type III Secretion" machinery, and evidence is accumulating for the importance of the Type III system also in *Chlamydiae* (Fields and Hackstadt, 2000; Bavoil et al., 2000).

In addition to hiding from the immune system by their intracellular lifestyle, *Chlamydiae* have also developed a sophisticated mechanism for thwarting the MHC-based immune recognition. This takes place by downregulation of the transcription of both MHC class I and class II molecules; the downregulation is mediated by specific degradation by *C. pneumoniae*-coded proteins of host cell factors promoting the transcription (Zhong et al., 1999, 2000). This is an entirely novel mechanism of immune evasion by pathogenic microbes, and certainly presents a formidable challenge for vaccine development.

The immune recognition and subsequent killing of the infected cells is not necessarily uniform for all cells; thus the infection may proceed or become persistent in only a part of the initially infected cells. Then we are faced with the likely possibility that antigen presentation in the persistently infected cells will differ from that seen during the acute phase. Very likely, therefore, a vaccine capable of preventing and curing the persistent infection will be different from the one preventing the acute infection. The mouse model may be suitable for studying the persistent infection, too. *C. pneumoniae*-specific DNA can be detected by PCR for at least 2 months after cultures have turned negative, and the dormant infection can be reactivated by immunosuppressive treatment of the mice (Malinverni et al., 1995; Laitinen et al., 1996). Our experience with both methods of detection suggests that persistence develops in part of the animals only, a further point of resemblance to the human *C. pneumoniae* infection. Persistent infection can also be detected in vitro in cell cultures of *C. pneumoniae* (Byrne et al., 2001; Pantoja et al., 2001). Such a mode of growth can be induced by treatment of the culture with IFN-γ or sublethal doses of antibiotics or by depletion of tryptophan. The morphology of the inclusion bodies in which *C. pneumoniae* normally multiply and mature to the infectious EB forms changes and no EBs are seen.

Crucial questions on the path to the development of a vaccine aimed at curing the persistent *C. pneumoniae* infection then include:

- Which *C. pneumoniae* proteins are produced during persistence?
- Which of them reach the cytoplasm?
- Are these processed for MHC class I presentation?
- Are the processed epitopes presented on the cell surface or is the *C. pneumoniae*-mediated downregulation of MHC class I complete?
- Is the recognition by CD8+ cells efficient, leading to immunization?
- Is the recognition by specific CTLs efficient, leading to cell lysis or killing?
- Are there infected cells escaping the CTLs?

If we are lucky, answers to these questions as well as the large amount of work devoted to developing vaccines for other *Chlamydiae* (*C. trachomatis, C. psittaci*) may lead to the development of the desired vaccine for prevention of *C. pneumoniae*-associated cardiovascular disease (Igietseme et al., 2002). However, other questions remain. We would need to define how the vaccine will be used, the main alternative being incorporation in the infant immunization program or recommended to all at a certain age. If the former, who will pay for the cost of vaccination to prevent a disease perhaps 50 years later? If the latter, will the target be all individuals or only males, and at which age, 30 or 40 or 50 years?

REFERENCES

Bavoil PM, Hsia RC, Ojcius DM. 2000. Closing in on *Chlamydia* and its intracellular bag of tricks. *Microbiology* 146:2713–2731.

Byrne GI, Ouellette SP, Wang Z, Rao JP, Lu L, Beatty WL, Hudson AP. 2001. *Chlamydia pneumoniae* expresses genes required for DNA replication but not cytokinesis during persistent infection of HEp-2 cells. *Infection and Immunity* 69:5423–5429.

Fields KA and Hackstadt T. 2000. Evidence for the secretion of *Chlamydia trachomatis* CopN by a type III secretion mechanism. *Molecular Microbiology* 38:1048–1060.

Grayston JT. 2000. Background and current knowledge of *Chlamydia pneumoniae* and atherosclerosis. *The Journal of Infectious Diseases* 181:S402–410.

Igietseme JU, Black CM, Caldwell HD. 2002. Chlamydia vaccines. Strategies and status. *Biodrugs* 16:19–35.

Kaukoranta-Tolvanen S-SE, Laurila AL, Saikku P, Leinonen M, Liesirova L, Laitinen K. 1993. Experimental infection of *Chlamydia pneumoniae* in mice. *Microbial Pathogenesis* 15:293.

Laitinen K, Laurila AL, Leinonen M, Saikku P. 1996. Reactivation of *Chlamydia pneumoniae* infection in mice by cortisone treatment. *Infection and Immunity* 64:1488–1490.

Lee CL and Ko YC. 1997. Hepatitis B vaccination and hepatocellular carcinoma in Taiwan. *Pediatrics* 99:351–353.

Malinverni R, Kuo CC, Campbell LA, Grayston JT. 1995. Reactivation of *Chlamydia pneumoniae* lung infection in mice by cortisone. *The Journal of Infectious Diseases* 172:593–594.

Murdin AD, Dunn P, Sodoyer R, Wang J, Caterini J, Brunham RC, Aujame L, Oomen R. 2000. Use of a mouse lung challenge model to identify antigens protective against *Chlamydia pneumoniae* lung infection. *The Journal of Infectious Diseases* 181(Suppl 3):S544–551.

O'Connor S, Taylor C, Lee AC, Epstein S, Libby P. 2001. Potential infectious etiologies of atherosclerosis: A multifactorial perspective. *Emerging Infectious Diseases* 7:780–788.

Pantoja LG, Miller RD, Ramirez JA, Molestina RE, Summersgill JT. 2001. Characterization of *Chlamydia pneumoniae* persistence in HEp-2 cells treated with gamma interferon. *Infection and Immunity* 69:7927–7932.

Penttilä JM, Anttila M, Puolakkainen M, Laurila A, Varkila K, Sarvas M, Mäkelä PH, Rautonen N. 1998. Local immune responses to *Chlamydia pneumoniae* in the lungs of BALB/c mice during primary infection and reinfection. *Infection and Immunity* 66:5113–5118.

Penttilä JM, Anttila M, Varkkila K, Puolakkainen M, Sarvas M, Mäkelä PH, Rautonen N. 1999. Depletion of CD8+ cells abolishes memory in acquired immunity against *Chlamydia pneumoniae* in BALB/c mice. *Immunology* 97:490–496.

Penttilä T, Vuola JM, Puurula V, Anttila M, Sarvas M, Rautonen N, Mäkelä PH, Puolakkainen M. 2000. Immunity to *Chlamydia pneumoniae* induced by vaccination with DNA vectors expressing a cytoplasmic protein (Hsp60) or outer membrane proteins (MOMP and Omp2). *Vaccine* 19:1256–1265.

Rottenberg ME, Rotfuchs ACG, Gigliotti D, Svanholm C, Bandholtz L, Wigzell HJ. 1999. Role of innate and adaptive immunity in the outcome of primary infection with *Chlamydia pneumoniae*, as analyzed in genetically modified mice. *The Journal of Immunology* 162:2829–2836.

Saikku P. 1999. Epidemiology of *Chlamydia pneumoniae* in atherosclerosis. *American Heart Journal* 138:S500–503.

Svanholm C, Bandholtz L, Castanos-Velez E, Wigzell H, Rottenberg ME. 2000. Protective DNA immunization against *Chlamydia pneumoniae*. *Scandinavian Journal of Immunology* 51:345–353.

Zhong G, Fan T, Liu L. 1999. Chlamydia inhibits interferon γ-inducible major histocompatibility complex class II expression by degradation of upstream stimulatory factor 1. *The Journal of Experimental Medicine* 189:1931–1938.

Zhong G, Liu L, Fan T, Fan P, Ji H. 2000. Degradation of transcription factor RFX5 during the inhibition of both constitutive and interferon γ-inducible major histocompatibility complex class I expression in Chlamydia-infected cells. *The Journal of Experimental Medicine* 191:1525–1534.

TOWARD A STRATEGIC APPROACH: INTEGRATING EPIDEMIOLOGY, LABORATORY RESEARCH, AND SURVEILLANCE; SETTING PRIORITIES

Siobhán O'Connor, M.D., M.P.H.
Assistant to the Director of the National Center for Infectious Diseases
[For Infectious Causes of Chronic Diseases]
Centers for Disease Control and Prevention, Atlanta, GA

Evidence that microbes are at the root of chronic conditions such as peptic ulcer disease, Whipple's disease, hepatocellular carcinoma, and cervical cancer has transformed medicine. These examples underscore the plausibility that infectious agents might be linked to numerous other non-communicable chronic conditions. Indeed, research into speculative and as yet to be proposed associations can no longer be viewed as "fishing expeditions," despite the investigative challenges. Strategies that use collaborations to enhance the productivity of independent investigators, integrate rigorously executed laboratory techniques into well-designed epidemiologic studies and surveillance systems, and complement short-term studies with long-term follow-up can overcome the hurdles to create new prevention and intervention opportunities. Balancing research on potential infectious links for common chronic conditions, in which the contribution of microbes to overall burden could be minor, with that on less common diseases, perhaps likely to have a primary infectious cause, could benefit many.

The Basics

Certain basic tenets, however, are crucial to successfully defining, characterizing, and mitigating the burden of chronic diseases that is induced by infectious diseases. Widespread use of standardized or comparable case definitions—for the infection and the outcome—is needed for comparisons across studies and conclusions on causality. So, too, are universally high standards of specificity, sensitivity, and reproducibility in laboratory assays, applied to appropriate specimens and controls. Minimum performance criteria are feasible, even when investigator creativity enters uncharted territory or population and exposure differences impact reproducibility. Peer review journals can reinforce these standards if publication depends upon the use of sound epidemiologic design and laboratory assays capable of supporting the conclusions.

Building on the Basics

From these basics, integration and complementation of laboratory elements with epidemiologic studies and surveillance systems can clarify new and suspected associations. However, this will require greater investment in:

• Pathogen discovery activities that: identify novel agents, define which species of known agents impart chronic sequelae, and detect agents in alternative tissues;
• Development of new and improved laboratory technologies to advance pathogen discovery and the detection of known agents;
• Expansion of viral screening methodology; and
• Continued development of improved, more sensitive and specific laboratory diagnostic assays that can identify an infectious root of disease at the site of pathology or a distant site, and distinguish active from latent or past infection.

Demonstrated in HIV/AIDS, human herpesvirus 8-associated Kaposi's sarcoma and *Chlamydia trachomatis*-related reactive arthritis, among others, observational and applied (laboratory) epidemiology remain powerful tools by which to recognize infection-chronic disease associations. Therefore, just as vital will be a parallel investment in epidemiology that emphasizes:
• Linking of databases—for infection-chronic disease associations, infectious diseases, and chronic syndromes—designed or modified to be compatible;
• Observational epidemiology to identify clusters and trends;
• Application of validated pathogen discovery technology to further describe the epidemiology of infections and identify potential infection-chronic disease links;
• Achieving balance between cross-sectional studies and longitudinal cohorts of individuals affected and unaffected by a chronic disease, including those infected and uninfected;
• Longitudinal follow-up of infectious exposures through surveillance systems (e.g., state-based FoodNet surveillance) and cohorts of recently infected people; and
• Banking specimens for analysis with future technology and to study newly proposed etiologic associations.

As these options are considered, it will be important to plan, prioritize, and invest in research that addresses certain key issues, including studies that:

• Define temporal relationships between infection and disease, the stage of infection that determines chronic outcome (e.g., first infection, re-infection, persistent infection, co-infections, or a subsequent cross-reacting infection);
• Clarify the stage at which infection must be prevented or treated to minimize or eliminate chronic sequelae—intervention should decrease the chronic disease burden;
• Support multi-center/multi-investigator collaborations that pool findings with comparable case-definitions, study designs, and validated laboratory assays to increase the power and statistical significance of results;
• Initiate or expand existing multi-national and multi-racial/ethnic studies that can identify groups at high risk for infection-related chronic sequelae (because of genetic, environmental, cultural, or multifactorial predisposition); and
• As appropriate, expand cohorts and specimen sampling in established systems (e.g., NHANES) in order to study less common conditions and high risk populations OR establish new networks, building on systems such as managed care organizations.

Complementary to these issues will be questions of etiopathogenesis. By what process(es) does infection influence chronic sequelae? For some associations, it will be important to first identify the links and potential interventions, later elucidating the pathway from infection to disease. In other situations, understanding mechanisms of pathogenesis can spur research to consider microbial roots of disease. This is certain to be a dynamic area in which a balanced approach may be the most productive.

Overarching Issues

Strategies that build on fundamentals of sound science are likely to identify and clarify additional infectious disease-chronic disease links, confirming this arena to be both our challenge and our future. Some investments of today may yield early answers, while other returns may take years. That is the nature of the unknown and of chronic conditions. However, the potential benefits of these investments to populations and to individuals are great—greatest if investment begins now. As the field expands two additional, crosscutting issues call for continuous consideration:

• To capitalize on the benefits afforded by confirmed and newly discovered infection-chronic disease links, medical education (training and continuing education) must improve recognition of known and potential links, the attendant intervention opportunities, and the cautions against inappropriate therapies; and

• The potential changes that population migrations and individual travel impart on the distribution and character of even established associations create an ongoing need for surveillance.

Although the links between infectious diseases and chronic diseases can be complex and multifactorial, they can be characterized, and beneficial interventions against infection designed. Most fruitful is an approach that increases investments in the laboratory, epidemiology, and surveillance, emphasizing integration of these elements and collaborations that can increase the yield of research and medical science.

Appendix
A

Workshop Agenda

LINKING INFECTIOUS AGENTS AND CHRONIC DISEASES:

**Defining the Relationship, Enhancing the Research,
and Mitigating the Effects**

October 21–22, 2002
Room 100
The National Academies
500 Fifth Street, NW
Washington, DC 20001

AGENDA

MONDAY, OCTOBER 21, 2002

8:30 a.m. Continental Breakfast

9:00 **Welcome and Opening Remarks**
Adel Mahmoud, Chair, Forum on Microbial Threats
Stanley Lemon, Vice Chair, Forum on Microbial Threats

Session I
Case Studies of Infectious Agents Associated with Chronic Diseases

Evidence continues to mount implicating microorganisms as etiologic agents of chronic diseases that contribute to substantial mortality and morbidity. This session will examine definitive and emerging associations between infectious agents and chronic diseases with a range of pathogenic mechanisms and diversity in etiologic microbes. The review will explore advances in research, detection, and screening that have contributed to these discoveries and some of the challenges that remain.

9:15   **Human papillomavirus infection as the cause of**
            cervical cancer
            Eduardo Franco, McGill University

9:45   **Infectious agents and cardiovascular disease**
            Michael Dunne, Pfizer, Inc.

10:15   **Infectious agents and demyelinating diseases**
            Richard Johnson, Johns Hopkins University School of Medicine

10:45   **The role of infectious agents in schizophrenia, bipolar**
            disorder, and other serious neuropsychiatric diseases
            Robert Yolken and E. Fuller Torrey, Johns Hopkins University
            School of Medicine and Stanley Foundation

11:15   **BREAK**

11:30   **Common infections and uncommon disease: Elusive**
            associations of enteroviruses and type I diabetes mellitus
            Mark Pallansch, Centers for Disease Control and Prevention

12:00 p.m. **Chronic hepatitis B virus infections**
            William Mason, Fox Chase Cancer Center

12:30   **Retrovirus-induced lung cancer in sheep:**
            Perspectives on the human disease
            Hung Fan, University of California, Irvine

1:00   **LUNCH**

Session II
Challenges in Framing the Research

Identification and confirmation of the infectious causation of chronic diseases are complicated by several factors, which include detection of microbes at the time of diagnosis of the chronic condition, the lack of adequate methods to identify novel or rare microorganisms, and the influence of environmental and genetic factors on the etiology of the chronic diseases. This session will examine these challenges and identify existing and potential methods and technologies for overcoming these obstacles.

2:00   **Kaposi's sarcoma, KSHV and causality: Koch's postulates in the age of molecular biology**
        Patrick Moore, Mailman School of Public Health, Columbia University

2:30   **Microbial agents in chronic diseases: Guilt by association versus pathologic etiology**
        Thomas Quinn, Johns Hopkins University School of Medicine

3:00   **Novel diagnostic, therapeutic, and chemopreventive strategies**
        David Persing, Corixa Corporation

3:30   **BREAK**

Session III
Discussion Panel: Shaping the Research and Development Agenda

3:45   Panel members, Forum members, and the audience will comment on and respond to considerations such as the role of industry in developing diagnostics; possibilities for the coordination between basic and clinical scientists, pathologists, and epidemiologists in developing standardized specific case definitions and specimens and the development of comparable methods of analysis; the lessons that can be learned about the microbes from the chronic sequelae they produce; and methods for funding the research.

        David Morens, National Institute of Allergy and Infectious Diseases
        Ian Lipkin, University of California, Irvine, and Mailman School of Public Health, Columbia University
        Susan Swedo, National Institute of Mental Health

5:30   **Adjournment of the first day**

TUESDAY, OCTOBER 22, 2002

8:30 a.m.   Continental Breakfast

9:00   **Opening Remarks**

Session IV
Implications for Developing Countries

As researchers, clinicians, and policymakers have recognized the growing disease burden from chronic diseases in developing countries, understanding of the infectious etiology of these diseases becomes increasingly important in these areas where many infectious diseases still remain endemic. This session will review the consequences of highly prevalent infectious diseases linked to chronic diseases and explore the global and local response needed to combat these outcomes in resource-limited environments.

9:15   **Interaction of multiple infectious agents in endemic areas**
            Altaf Lal, Centers for Disease Control and Prevention

9:45   **Progression of hepatitis C virus infection with and without**
            schistosomiasis
            Sanaa Kamal, Ain Shams University, Cairo, Egypt

10:15   **Infectious agents and epilepsy**
            J.W.A.S. Sander, Institute of Neurology, University College,
            London

10:45   **Potential long-term consequences of early childhood enteric**
            and parasitic infections
            Richard Guerrant, University of Virginia School of Medicine

11:15   **HTLV-1: Clinical impact of chronic infection**
            Eduardo Gotuzzo, University of Peru, Lima, Peru

12:00 p.m. **LUNCH**

Session V
Barriers and Opportunities to Detect, Prevent, and Mitigate the Impact of Chronic Diseases Caused by Infectious Agents

The complexity of the relationship between infectious agents and chronic diseases requires a multi-disciplinary approach to reveal the implications of early detection and prevention of chronic diseases caused by infectious agents. This session will summarize the advances and gaps in collaborative research on detection and diagnostic technologies, their integration with epidemiological studies and surveillance that can forward the efforts in this important area, and the implications for clinical management practices and priorities.

1:00   **Testing the reliability of the causal relationship: Considering genetic and environmental susceptibility**
         Mikhail Pletnikov, Johns Hopkins University School of Medicine

1:30   **DNA sequence analysis of a stealth-adapted simian cytomegalovirus**
         W. John Martin, Center for Complex Infectious Diseases

2:00   **Development of vaccines to prevent chronic disease**
         P. Helena Mäkelä, National Public Health Institute, Helsinki, Finland

2:30   **Integrating epidemiology, laboratory research, and surveillance**
         Siobhán O'Connor, Centers for Disease Control and Prevention

3:00   **BREAK**

Session VI
Discussion Panel: The Next Steps for the Healthcare Community

Panel members, Forum members, and the audience will comment on and respond to considerations such as the role of industry and academic research in developing treatments; the implications for the health care and prevention community in detecting and treating these diseases; and the benefits of managing acute infections vs. chronic diseases—the argument for vaccines and antimicrobials.

3:15   **Kathryn Carbone,** FDA, Center for Biologics Evaluation and Research
         Thomas Shinnick, Centers for Disease Control and Prevention

5:00   **Closing Remarks / Adjournment**

Appendix
B

Information Resources

OVERVIEW

Danesh J, Newton R, Beral V. 1997. A human germ project? *Nature* 389:21–24.

Mueller N. 1995. Overview: viral agents and cancer. *Environmental Health Perspectives* 103:259–261.

Parsonnet J. 1995. Bacterial infection as a cause of cancer. *Environmental Health Perspectives* 103 Suppl 8:263–268.

Persing DH and Prendergast FG. 1999. Infection, immunity, and cancer. *Archives of Pathology & Laboratory Medicine* 123:1015–1022.

CAUSAL ASSOCIATIONS

Commission on Tropical Diseases of the International League Against Epilepsy. 1994. Relationship between epilepsy and tropical diseases. *Epilepsia* 35:89–93.

Durkin MS, Khan NZ, Davidson LL, Huq S, Munir S, Rasul E, Zaman SS. 2000. Prenatal and post-natal risk factors for mental retardation among children in Bangladesh. *American Journal of Epidemiology* 152:1024–1033.

El-Serag HB and Mason AC. 2000. Risk factors for the rising rates of primary liver cancer in the United States. *Archives of Internal Medicine* 160:3227–3230.

Epstein SE, Zhou YF, Zhu J. 1999. Infection and atherosclerosis: emerging mechanistic paradigms. *Circulation* 100:E20–E28.

Franco EL, Duarte-Franco E, Ferenczy A. 2001. Cervical cancer: epidemiology, prevention, and the role of human papillomavirus infection. *Canadian Medical Association Journal* 164:1017–1025.

Gilden DH, Burgoon MP, Kleinschmidt-DeMasters BK, Williamson RA, Ghausi O, Burton DR, Owens GP. 2001. Molecular immunologic strategies to identify antigens and β-cell repsonses unique to multiple sclerosis. *Archives of Neurology* 58:43–48.

Johnson RT. 1994. The virology of demyelinating diseases. *Annals of Neurology* 36 Suppl:S54–S60.

Lipkin WI, Hornig M, Briese T. 2001. Borna disease virus and neuropsychiatric disease—a reappraisal. *Trends in Microbiology* 9:295–298.

Maeda N, Palmarini M, Murgia C, Fan H. 2001. Direct transformation of rodent fibroblasts by jaaagsiekte sheep retrovirus DNA. *Proceedings of the National Academy of Sciences* 98:4449–4454.

Morris JA. 1995. Schizophrenia, bacterial toxins and the genetics of redundancy. *Medical Hypotheses* 46:362–366.

Roivainen M, Rasilainen S, Ylipaasto P, Nissinen R, Ustinov J, Bouwens L, Eizirik DL, Hovi T, Otonkoski T. 2000. Mechanism of coxsackievirus-induced damage to human pancreatic β-cells. *The Journal of Clinical Endocrinology and Metabolism* 85:432–440.

Scott MR, Will R, Ironside J, Nguyen HO, Tremblay P, DeArmond SJ, Prusiner SB. 1999. Compelling transgenetic evidence for transmission of bovine spongiform encephalopathy prions to humans. *Proceedings of the National Academy of Sciences* 96:15137–15142.

Stuver S. 1998. Towards global control of liver cancer? *Seminars in Cancer Biology* 8:299–306.

Swedo SE, Leonard HL, Garvey M, Mittleman B, Allen AJ, Perlmutter S, Lougee L, Dow S, Zamkoff J, Dubbert BK. 1998. Pediatric autoimmune neuropsychiatric disorders associated with streptococcal infections: clinical description of the first 50 cases. *American Journal of Psychiatry* 155:264–271.

Yolken RH, Karlsson H, Yee F, Johnston-Wilson NL, Torrey EF. 2000. Endogenous retroviruses and schizophrenia. *Brain Research Reviews* 31:193–199.

TOOLS FOR RESEARCH

Fredricks DN and Relman DA. 1996. Sequence-based identification of microbial pathogens: a reconsideration of Koch's postulates. *Clinical Microbiology Reviews* 9:18–33.

Lisitsyn NA. 1995. Representational difference analysis: finding the differences between genomes. *Trends in Genetics* 11:303–307.

Relman DA and Falkow S. 2001. The meaning and impact of the human genome sequence for microbiology. *Trends in Microbiology* 9:206–208.

IMPLICATIONS FOR DETECTION AND INTERVENTION

de The G. 1995. Viruses and human cancers: challenges for preventive strategies. *Environmental Health Perspectives* 103:269–273.

Humphrey RW, Davis DA, Newcomb FM, Yarchoan R. 1998. Human herpesvirus 8 (HHV-8) in the pathogenesis of Kaposi's sarcoma and other diseases. Leukemia and Lymphoma 28:255–264.

Makela PH. 1999. Is cardiovascular disease preventable by vaccination? *Annals of Medicine* 31:61–65.

Munoz N and Bosch FX. 1996. The causal link between HPV and cervical cancer and its implications for prevention of cervical cancer. *Bulletin of the Pan American Health Organization* 30:362–377.

Appendix C

Biosketches

MEMBERS OF THE FORUM ON MICROBIAL THREATS

ADEL A.F. MAHMOUD, M.D., Ph.D., *(Chair)*, is President of Merck Vaccines at Merck & Co., Inc. He formerly served Case Western Reserve University and University Hospitals of Cleveland as Chairman of Medicine and Physician-in-Chief from 1987 to 1998. Prior to that, Dr. Mahmoud held several positions, spanning 25 years, at the same institutions. Dr. Mahmoud and his colleagues conducted pioneering investigations on the biology and function of eosinophils. He prepared the first specific anti-eosinophil serum, which was used to define the role of these cells in host resistance to helminthic infections. Dr. Mahmoud also established clinical and laboratory investigations in several developing countries, including Kenya, Egypt, and The Philippines, to examine the determinants of infection and disease in schistosomiasis and other infectious agents. This work led to the development of innovative strategies to control those infections, which have been adopted by the World Health Organization (WHO) as selective population chemotherapy. In recent years, Dr. Mahmoud turned his attention to developing a comprehensive set of responses to the problems associated with emerging infections in the developing world. He was elected to membership of the American Society for Clinical Investigation in 1978, the Association of American Physicians in 1980, and the Institute of Medicine of the National Academy of Sciences in 1987. He received the Bailey K. Ashford Award of the American Society of Tropical Medicine and Hygiene in 1983, and the Squibb Award of the Infectious Diseases Society of America in 1984. Dr. Mahmoud is a member of the Institute of Medicine and its Board on Global Health. He also chairs the U.S. Delegation to the U.S.–Japan Cooperative Medical Science Program.

194

STANLEY M. LEMON, M.D., (*Vice-chair*), is Dean of the School of Medicine at the University of Texas Medical Branch at Galveston. He received his undergraduate degree in biochemical sciences from Princeton University *summa cum laude* and his M.D. with honors from the University of Rochester. He completed postgraduate training in internal medicine and infectious diseases at the University of North Carolina at Chapel Hill, and is board-certified in both areas. From 1977 to 1983, he served with the U.S. Army Medical Research and Development Command, directing the Hepatitis Laboratory at the Walter Reed Army Institute of Research. He joined the faculty of the University of North Carolina School of Medicine in 1983, serving first as Chief of the Division of Infectious Diseases, and then Vice Chair for Research of the Department of Medicine. In 1997, Dr. Lemon moved to the University of Texas Medical Branch as Professor and Chair of the Department of Microbiology & Immunology. He was subsequently appointed Dean *pro tem* of the School of Medicine in 1999, and permanent Dean of Medicine in 2000. Dr. Lemon's research interests relate to the molecular virology and pathogenesis of the positive-stranded RNA viruses responsible for hepatitis C and hepatitis A. He is particularly interested in the molecular mechanisms controlling replication of these RNA genomes and related mechanisms of disease pathogenesis. In addition, he has a longstanding interest in vaccine development. Dr. Lemon has published more than 180 papers and numerous textbook chapters related to hepatitis and other viral infections. He chaired the Anti-Infective Drugs Advisory Committee and the Vaccines and Related Biologics Advisory Committee of the U.S. Food and Drug Administration, as well as the Steering Committee on Hepatitis and Poliomyelitis of WHO's Programme on Vaccine Development. From 2000 to 2002, he chaired the Institute of Medicine (IOM) Committee on a Strategy for Minimizing the Impact of Naturally Occurring Infectious Diseases of Military Importance. At present, he is chairman of the U.S. Hepatitis Panel of the U.S.–Japan Cooperative Medical Science Program and cochair of the IOM/ NRC Committee on Advances in Technology and the Prevention of their Application to Next Generation Biowarfare Agents.

DAVID ACHESON, M.D., is Chief Medical Officer at the Center for Food Safety and Applied Nutrition, U.S. Food and Drug Administration. He received his medical degree at the University of London. After completing internships in general surgery and medicine, he continued his postdoctoral training in Manchester, England, as a Wellcome Trust Research Fellow. He subsequently was a Wellcome Trust Training Fellow in Infectious Diseases at the New England Medical Center and at the Wellcome Research Unit in Vellore, India. Dr. Acheson was Associate Professor of Medicine, Division of Geographic Medicine and Infectious Diseases, New England Medical Center until 2001. He then joined the faculties of the Department of Epidemiology and Preventive Medicine and Department of Microbiology and Immunology at the University of Maryland Medical School. Currently at the FDA, his research concentration is on foodborne pathogens and encompasses a mixture of molecular pathogenesis, cell biology, and epidemiology. Specifically, his research focuses on Shiga toxin-producing *E. coli* and understanding toxin interaction with intestinal epithelial cells using tissue culture models. His laboratory has also undertaken a study to examine Shiga toxin-producing *E. coli* in food animals in relation to virulence factors and antimicrobial resistance patterns. More recently, Dr. Acheson initiated a project to understand the molecular pathogenesis of *Campylobacter jejuni*. Other studies have undertaken surveillance of diarrheal disease in the community to determine causes, outcomes, and risk factors of unexplained diarrhea. Dr. Acheson has authored or coauthored more than 72 journal articles, and 42 book chapters and reviews, and is coauthor of the book *Safe Eating* (Dell Health, 1998). He is reviewer of more than 10 journals and is on the editorial board of *Infection and Immunity* and *Clinical Infectious Diseases*. Dr. Acheson is a Fellow of the Royal College of Physicians, a Fellow of the Infectious Disease Society of America, and holds several patents.

STEVEN J. BRICKNER, Ph.D., is Research Advisor, Antibacterials Chemistry, at Pfizer Global Research and Development. He received his Ph.D. in organic chemistry from Cornell University and was a National Institutes of Health (NIH) Postdoctoral Research Fellow at the University of Wisconsin–Madison. Dr. Brickner is a medicinal chemist with nearly 20 years of research experience in the pharmaceutical industry, all focused on the discovery and development of novel antibacterial agents. The inventor or coinventor on 21 U.S. patents, he has published numerous scientific papers, primarily on oxazolidinones. Prior to joining Pfizer in 1996, he led a team at Pharmacia and Upjohn that discovered and developed linezolid, the first member of a new class of antibiotics to be approved in the last 35 years.

NANCY CARTER-FOSTER, M.S.T.M., is Senior Advisor for Health Affairs for the U.S. Department of State, Assistant Secretary for Science and Health and the Secretary's Representative on HIV/AIDS. She is responsible for identifying emerging health issues and making policy recommendations for USG foreign policy concerns regarding international health, and coordinates the Department's interactions with the nongovernmental community. She is a member of the National Academy of Sciences Institute of Medicine's Forum on Infectious Diseases, and a member of the Infectious Diseases Society of America (IDSA), and the American Association of the Advancement of Science (AAAS). She has helped bring focus to global health issues in U.S. foreign policy and brought a national security focus to global health. In prior positions as Director for Congressional and Legislative Affairs for the Economic and Business Affairs Bureau of the U.S. Department of State, and Foreign Policy Advisory to the Majority WHIP U.S. House of Representatives, Trade Specialist Advisor to the House of Representatives Ways and Means Trade Subcommittee, and consultant to the

World Bank, Asia Technical Environment Division, Ms. Carter-Foster has worked on a wide variety of health, trade and environmental issues amassing in-depth knowledge and experience in policy development and program implementation.

GAIL H. CASSELL, Ph.D., is Vice President, Scientific Affairs, Distinguished Lilly Research Scholar for Infectious Diseases, Eli Lilly & Company. Previously, she was the Charles H. McCauley Professor and (since 1987) Chair, Department of Microbiology, University of Alabama Schools of Medicine and Dentistry at Birmingham, a department which, under her leadership, has ranked first in research funding from the National Institutes of Health since 1989. She is a member of the Director's Advisory Committee of the Centers for Disease Control and Prevention. Dr. Cassell is past president of the American Society for Microbiology (ASM) and is serving her third three-year term as chairman of the Public and Scientific Affairs Board of ASM. She is a former member of the National Institutes of Health Director's Advisory Committee and a former member of the Advisory Council of the National Institute of Allergy and Infectious Diseases. She has also served as an advisor on infectious diseases and indirect costs of research to the White House Office on Science and Technology and was previously chair of the Board of Scientific Counselors of the National Center for Infectious Diseases, Centers for Disease Control and Prevention. Dr. Cassell served eight years on the Bacteriology-Mycology-II Study Section and served as its chair for three years. She serves on the editorial boards of several prestigious scientific journals and has authored more than 275 articles and book chapters. She has been intimately involved in the establishment of science policy and legislation related to biomedical research and public health. Dr. Cassell has received several national and international awards and an honorary degree for her research on infectious diseases.

JESSE L. GOODMAN, M.D., M.P.H., was professor of medicine and Chief of Infectious Diseases at the University of Minnesota, and is now the Deputy Director for the U.S. Food and Drug Administration's (FDA) Center for Biologics Evaluation and Research, where he is active in a broad range of scientific, public health, and policy issues. After joining the FDA commissioner's office, he has worked closely with several centers and helped coordinate FDA's response to the antimicrobial resistance problem. He was co-chair of a recently formed federal interagency task force which developed the national Public Health Action Plan on antimicrobial resistance. He graduated from Harvard College and attended the Albert Einstein College of Medicine followed by internal medicine, hematology, oncology, and infectious diseases training at the University of Pennsylvania and University of California Los Angeles, where he was also chief medical resident. He received his master's of public health from the University of Minnesota. He has been active in community public health activities, including creating an environmental health partnership in St. Paul, Minnesota. In recent years, his laboratory's research has focused on the molecular pathogenesis of tickborne diseases. His laboratory isolated the etiological intracellular agent of the emerging tickborne infection, human granulocytic ehrlichiosis, and identified its leukocyte receptor. He has also been an active clinician and teacher and has directed or participated in major multicenter clinical studies. He is a Fellow of the Infectious Diseases Society of America and, among several honors, has been elected to the American Society for Clinical Investigation.

EDUARDO GOTUZZO, M.D., is Principal Professor and Director at the Instituto de Medicina Tropical "Alexander von Humbolt," Universidad Peruana Cayetan Heredia (UPCH), in Lima, Peru. He is also Chief of the Department of Infectious and Tropical Diseases at the Cayetano Heredia Hospital and an Adjunct Professor of Medicine at the University of Alabama–Birmingham School of Medicine. Dr. Gotuzzo has been an active member of numerous international societies such as the Latin America Society of Tropical Disease (President, 2000–2003), the Scientific Program of Infectious Diseases Society of America (2000–2003), the International Organizing Committee of the International Congress of Infectious Diseases (1994–present), the International Society for Infectious Diseases (President Elect, 1996–1998), and the Peruvian Society of Internal Medicine (President, 1991–1992). He has published more than 230 articles and chapters as well as 6 manuals and 1 book. Among the many recent honors and awards he has received, he was named an Honorary member of American Society of Tropical Medicine and Hygiene (2002), an Associated Member of National Academy of Medicine (2002), an Honorary Member of Society of Internal Medicine (2000), a Distinguished Visitor, Faculty of Medical Sciences, University of Cordoba, Argentina (1999), and the receipient of the Golden Medal for Outstanding Contribution in the field of Infectious Diseases from Trnava University, Slovakia (1998).

MARGARET A. HAMBURG, M.D., is Vice President for Biological Programs at Nuclear Threat Initiative (NTI), a charitable organization working to reduce the global threat from nuclear, biological, and chemical weapons. Dr. Hamburg is in charge of the biological program area. Before taking on her current position, Dr. Hamburg was the Assistant Secretary for Planning and Evaluation, U.S. Department of Health and Human Services, serving as a principal policy advisor to the Secretary of Health and Human Services with responsibilities including policy formulation and analysis, the development and review of regulations and legislation, budget analysis, strategic planning, and the conduct and coordination of policy research and program evaluation. Prior to this, she served for almost six years as the Commissioner of Health for the City of New York. As chief health officer in the nation's largest city, Dr. Hamburg's many accomplishments included the design and implementation of an internationally recognized tuberculosis control program that produced dramatic declines in tuberculosis cases; the development of initiatives that raised childhood immunization rates to record levels; and the creation of the first public health bioterrorism preparedness program in the nation. She completed her internship and residency in Internal Medicine at the New York Hospital/Cornell University Medical Center and is certified by the American Board of Internal Medicine. Dr. Hamburg is a graduate of Harvard College and Harvard Medical School. She currently serves on the Harvard University Board of Overseers. She has been elected to membership in the Institute of Medicine, the New York Academy of Medicine, and the Council on Foreign Relations, and is a Fellow of the American Association for the Advancement of Science and the American College of Physicians.

CAROLE A. HEILMAN, Ph.D., is Director of the Division of Microbiology and Infectious Diseases (DMID) of the National Institute of Allergy and Infectious Diseases (NIAID). Dr. Heilman received her bachelor's degree in biology from Boston University in 1972, and earned her master's degree and doctorate in microbiology from Rutgers University in 1976 and 1979, respectively. Dr. Heilman began her career at the National Institutes of Health as a postdoctoral research associate with the National Cancer Institute where she carried out research on the regulation of gene expression during cancer development. In 1986, she came to NIAID as the influenza and viral respiratory diseases program officer in DMID and, in 1988, she was appointed chief of the respiratory diseases branch where she coordinated the development of acellular pertussis vaccines. She joined the Division of AIDS as deputy director in 1997 and was responsible for developing the Innovation Grant Program for Approaches in HIV Vaccine Research. She is the recipient of several notable awards for outstanding achievement. Throughout her extramural career, Dr. Heilman has contributed articles on vaccine design and development to many scientific journals and has served as a consultant to the World Bank and WHO in this area. She is also a member of several professional societies, including the Infectious Diseases Society of America, the American Society for Microbiology, and the American Society of Virology.

DAVID L. HEYMANN, M.D., is currently the Executive Director of the World Health Organization (WHO) Communicable Diseases Cluster. From October 1995 to July 1998 he was Director of the WHO Programme on Emerging and Other Communicable Diseases Surveillance and Control. Prior to becoming director of this program, he was the chief of research activities in the Global Programme on AIDS. From 1976 to 1989, prior to joining WHO, Dr Heymann spent 13 years working as a medical epidemiologist in sub-Saharan Africa (Cameroon, Ivory Coast, the former Zaire, and Malawi) on assignment from the Centers for Disease Control and Prevention (CDC) in activities aimed at strengthening capacity in surveillance of infectious diseases and their control, with special emphasis on the childhood immunizable diseases, African hemorrhagic fevers, pox viruses, and malaria. While based in Africa, Dr. Heymann participated in the investigation of the first outbreak of Ebola in Yambuku (former Zaire) in 1976, then again investigated the second outbreak of Ebola in 1977 in Tandala, and in 1995 directed the international response to the Ebola outbreak in Kikwit. Prior to 1976, Dr. Heymann spent two years in India as a medical officer in the WHO Smallpox Eradication Programme. Dr. Heymann holds a B.A. from the Pennsylvania State University, an M.D. from Wake Forest University, and a Diploma in Tropical Medicine and Hygiene from the London School of Hygiene and Tropical Medicine, and completed practical epidemiology training in the Epidemic Intelligence Service (EIS) training program of the CDC. He has published 131 scientific articles on infectious diseases in peer-reviewed medical and scientific journals.

JAMES M. HUGHES, M.D., is the Director of the National Center for Infectious Diseases at the Centers for Disease Control and Prevention (CDC) and an Assistant Surgeon General in the Public Health Service. A board-certified physician in internal medicine, infectious diseases, and preventive medicine, Dr. Hughes received his B.A. and M.D. from Stanford University in 1966 and 1971, respectively. He completed his residency in internal medicine at the University of Washington and a fellowship in infectious diseases at the University of Virginia. Since joining CDC in 1973 as an Epidemic Intelligence Service officer, he has worked primarily on foodborne disease and infection control in health care settings. In 1992, Dr. Hughes became Director of the National Center for Infectious Diseases, which is addressing domestic and global challenges posed by emerging infectious diseases and the threat of bioterrorism. He is a member of the Institute of Medicine and a fellow of the American College of Physicians, the Infectious Diseases Society of America, and the American Association for the Advancement of Science.

LONNIE KING, D.V.M., is Dean of the College of Veterinary Medicine, Michigan State University. Dr. King's previous positions include both Associate Administrator and Administrator of the USDA Animal and Plant Health Inspection Service (APHIS) and Deputy Administrator for USDA/APHIS/Veterinary Services. Before his government career, Dr. King was in private practice. He also has experience as a field veterinary medical officer, station epidemiologist, and staff assignments involving Emergency Programs and Animal Health Information. Dr. King has also directed the American Veterinary Medical Association's Office of Governmental Relations, and is certified in the American College of Veterinary Preventive Medicine. He has served as President of the Association of American Veterinary Medicine Colleges, and currently serves as Co-Chair of the National Commission on Veterinary Economic Issues, Lead Dean at Michigan State University for food safety with responsibility for the National Food Safety and Toxicology Center, the Institute for Environmental Toxicology, and the Center for

Emerging Infectious Diseases. He is also codeveloper and course leader for Science, Politics, and Animal Health Policy. Dr. King received his B.S. and D.V.M. degrees from The Ohio State University, and his M.S. degree in epidemiology from the University of Minnesota. He has also completed the Senior Executive Program at Harvard University, and received a M.P.A. from American University. Dr. King previously served on the Committee for Opportunities in Agriculture, the Steering Committee for a Workshop on the Control and Prevention of Animal Diseases, and the Committee to Ensure Safe Food from Production to Consumption.

JOSHUA LEDERBERG, Ph.D., is Professor emeritus of Molecular Genetics and Informatics and Sackler Foundation Scholar at The Rockefeller University in New York City. His lifelong research, for which he received the Nobel Prize in 1958, has been on the genetic structure and function in microorganisms. Keenly interested in international health, Dr. Lederberg co-chaired both the Institute of Medicine Committee on Emerging Microbial Threats to Health (1990–1992) and its successor, the IOM Committee on Emerging Microbial Threats to Health in the 21st Century (2001–2003). He has been a member of the National Academy of Sciences since 1957 and is a charter member of the Institute of Medicine.

JOSEPH MALONE, M.D., is Director of the Department of Defense Global Emerging Infection System (DoD–GEIS). The author of more than 20 publications, he is also an Associate Professor at the Uniformed Services University of Health Sciences and holds the Certificate of Knowledge in Travelers' Health and Tropical Medicine from the American Society of Tropical Medicine and Hygiene. CAPT Malone has won several military awards, including the Crisis Response Service Award from the Department of Health and Human Services' U.S. Public Health Service. Dr. Malone graduated from Boston University School of Medicine in 1980. He trained in internal medicine and infectious diseases at the Naval Hospitals in San Diego and in Bethesda, MD, leading to board certification, and became a staff physician at both hospitals. His naval career has included deployment to Guantanamo Bay, Cuba, in support of Operation Safe Harbor; attachment to Surgical Team 1 during Operation Desert Shield; and directorship of the Infectious Disease Division and HIV unit at the Naval Medical Center at Portsmouth, VA. His affiliation with DoD–GEIS began in 1999 while working with the Disease Surveillance Program at U.S. Naval Medical Research Unit No. 3 in Cairo, Egypt. Later, as a member of the Centers for Disease Control and Prevention's (CDC) Epidemic Intelligence Service (EIS) program, Dr. Malone was deployed to New York City to aid the emergency public health response to the attacks of September 11, 2001. He also assisted in the public health response to documented anthrax contamination in Kansas City and was the acting state epidemiologist for the State of Missouri from February through June 2003, when he completed the CDC EIS program.

LYNN MARKS, M.D., is Senior Vice President of Infectious Diseases in the Medicine Development Center of GlaxoSmithKline. A board-certified physician in internal medicine and infectious diseases, he previously was on faculty of the Infectious Diseases department of the University of South Alabama College of Medicine. There he focused on patient care, teaching, and research on the molecular genetics of bacterial pathogenicity. He subsequently joined the anti-infectives clinical group of SmithKline Beecham, now GlaxoSmithKline, and progressed to become the global head of the Consumer Healthcare division's Medical and Regulatory group. The move to his present position represented a return to pharmaceutical research and development.

STEPHEN S. MORSE, Ph.D., is Director of the Center for Public Health Preparedness at the Mailman School of Public Health of Columbia University, and a faculty member in the Epidemiology Department. Dr. Morse recently returned to Columbia after four years in government service as Program Manager at the Defense Advanced Research Projects Agency, where he co-directed the Pathogen Countermeasures program and subsequently directed the Advanced Diagnostics program. Before coming to Columbia, he was Assistant Professor of Virology at The Rockefeller University in New York, where he remains an adjunct faculty member. Dr. Morse is the editor of two books, *Emerging Viruses* (Oxford University Press, 1993; paperback, 1996) and *The Evolutionary Biology of Viruses* (Raven Press, 1994); the former was selected by *American Scientist* as one of the "100 Top Science Books of the 20th Century." Dr. Morse serves as a Section Editor of the CDC journal *Emerging Infectious Diseases* and was formerly an Editor-in-Chief of the Pasteur Institute's journal *Research in Virology.* As the chair and principal organizer of the 1989 Conference on Emerging Viruses held by the National Institute for Allergy and Infectious Disease, National Institutes of Health, he coined the term and concept of emerging viruses and infections. He was a member of the joint Institute of Medicine (IOM)–National Academy of Sciences' Committee on Emerging Microbial Threats to Health, chaired its task force on viruses, and contributed the committee's report, *Emerging Infections* (1992). He also was a member of the IOM Committee on Xenograft Transplantation. Dr. Morse has been an adviser to the World Health Organization, the Pan-American Health Organization, the U.S. Food and Drug Administration, the Defense Threat Reduction Agency, and other federal agencies. He is a Fellow of the New York Academy of Sciences and a past Chair of its Microbiology Section. He was the founding Chair of ProMED, the nonprofit international Program to Monitor Emerging Diseases, and was an originator of ProMED-mail, an international network inaugurated by ProMED in 1994 for outbreak reporting and disease monitoring using the Internet. At present, he serves on the Steering Committee of the Institute of Medicine's Forum on Microbial Threats. Dr. Morse received his Ph.D. from the University of Wisconsin–Madison.

MICHAEL T. OSTERHOLM, Ph.D., M.P.H., is Director of the Center for Infectious Disease Research and Policy at the University of Minnesota where he is also Professor at the School of Public Health. Previously, Dr. Osterholm was the state epidemiologist and Chief of the Acute Disease Epidemiology Section for the Minnesota Department of Health. He has received numerous research awards from the National Institute of Allergy and Infectious Diseases and the Centers for Disease Control and Prevention (CDC). He served as principal investigator for the CDC-sponsored Emerging Infections Program in Minnesota. He has published more than 240 articles and abstracts on various emerging infectious disease problems and is the author of the best selling book, *Living Terrors: What America Needs to Know to Survive the Coming Bioterrorist Catastrophe.* He is past president of the Council of State and Territorial Epidemiologists. He has served on the Institute of Medicine's Committee on Food Safety, Production to Consumption and Committee on the Department of Defense Persian Gulf Syndrome Comprehensive Clinical Evaluation Program. In addition, he was a reviewer of the Institute of Medicine's report on chemical and biological terrorism.

GEORGE POSTE, Ph.D., D.V.M., is Director of the Arizona Biodesign Institute and Dell E. Webb Distinguished Professor of Biology at Arizona State University. From 1992 to 1999, he was Chief Science and Technology Officer and President, Research and Development of SmithKline Beecham. During his tenure there, he was associated with the successful registration of 29 drug, vaccine and diagnostic products. He is Chairman of diaDexus and Structural GenomiX in California and Orchid Biosciences in Princeton. He serves on the Board of Directors of AdvancePCS and Monsanto. He is an advisor on biotechnology to several venture capital funds and investment banks. In May 2003, he was appointed as Director of the Arizona Biodesign Institute at Arizona State University. This is a major new initiative combining research groups in biotechnology, nanotechnology, materials science, advanced computing and neuromorphic engineering. He is a Fellow of Pembroke College Cambridge and Distinguished Fellow at the Hoover Institution and Stanford University. He is a member of the Defense Science Board of the U.S. Department of Defense and in this capacity he chairs the Task Force on Bioterrorism. He is also a member of the National Academy of Sciences Working Group on Defense Against Bioweapons. Dr. Poste is a Board Certified Pathologist, a Fellow of the Royal Society and a Fellow of the Academy of Medical Sciences. He was awarded the rank of Commander of the British Empire by Queen Elizabeth II in 1999 for services to medicine and for the advancement of biotechnology. He has published more than 350 scientific papers, coedited 15 books on cancer, biotechnology and infectious diseases and serves on the Editorial Board of multiple technical journals. He is invited routinely to be the keynote speaker at a wide variety of academic, corporate, investment and government meetings to discuss the impact of biotechnology and genetics on healthcare and the challenges posed by bioterrorism. Dr. Poste is married with three children. His personal interests are in military history, photography, automobile racing and exploring the wilderness of the American West.

GARY A. ROSELLE, M.D., received his M.D. from Ohio State University School of Medicine in 1973. He served his residency at Northwestern University School of Medicine and his Infectious Diseases fellowship at the University of Cincinnati School of Medicine. Dr. Roselle is the Program Director for Infectious Diseases for the Department of Veterans Affairs Central Office in Washington, D.C., as well as the Chief of the Medical Service at the Cincinnati Veterans Affairs Medical Center. He is a professor of medicine in the Department of Internal Medicine, Division of Infectious Diseases at the University of Cincinnati College of Medicine. Dr. Roselle serves on several national advisory committees. In addition, he is currently heading the Emerging Pathogens Initiative for the Department of Veterans Affairs. Dr. Roselle has received commendations from the Cincinnati Medical Center Director, the Under Secretary for Health for the Department of Veterans Affairs, and the Secretary of Veterans Affairs for his work in the infectious diseases program for the Department of Veterans Affairs. He has been an invited speaker at several national and international meetings, and has published more than 80 papers and several book chapters.

JANET SHOEMAKER, is director of the American Society for Microbiology's Public Affairs Office, a position she has held since 1989. She is responsible for managing the legislative and regulatory affairs of this 42,000-member organization, the largest single biological science society in the world. She has served as principal investigator for a project funded by the National Science Foundation (NSF) to collect and disseminate data on the job market for recent doctorates in microbiology and has played a key role in American Society for Microbiology (ASM) projects, including the production of *Employment Outlook in the Microbiological Sciences* and *The Impact of Managed Care and Health System Change on Clinical Microbiology*. Previously, she held positions as Assistant Director of Public Affairs for ASM, as ASM coordinator of the U.S.–U.S.S.R. Exchange Program in Microbiology (a program sponsored and coordinated by the National Science Foundation and the U.S. Department of State), and as a freelance editor and writer. She received her baccalaureate *cum laude* from the University of Massachusetts and is a graduate of the George Washington University programs in public policy and in editing and publications. She has served as commissioner to the Commission on Professionals in Science and Technology, and as the ASM representative to the ad hoc Group for Medical Research Funding, and is a member of Women in Government Relations, the American Society of Association Executives, and the American Association for the Advancement of Science. She has coauthored published articles on research funding, biotechnology, biological weapons control, and public policy issues related to microbiology.

P. FREDERICK SPARLING, M.D., is the J. Herbert Bate Professor emeritus of Medicine, Microbiology and Immunology at the University of North Carolina (UNC) at Chapel Hill, and is Director of the North Carolina Sexually Transmitted Infections Research Center. Previously, he served as chair of the Department of Medicine and chair of the Department of Microbiology and Immunology at UNC. He was president of the Infectious Disease Society of America in 1996–1997. He was also a member of the Institute of Medicine's Committee on Microbial Threats to Health (1991–1992). Dr. Sparling's laboratory research is in the molecular biology of bacterial outer membrane proteins involved in pathogenesis, with a major emphasis on *gonococci* and *meningococci*. His current studies focus on the biochemistry and genetics of iron-scavenging mechanisms used by *gonococci* and *meningococci* and the structure and function of the gonococcal porin proteins. He is pursuing the goal of a vaccine for gonorrhea.

SPEAKERS

KATHRYN M. CARBONE, M.D., is the Acting Associate Director for Research at FDA's Center for Biologics Evaluation and Research (CBER) and leads Virus Vaccine Neurovirulence Test Development in CBER's Laboratory of Pediatric and Respiratory Viral Diseases. She is also an Associate Profesor at Johns Hopkins University School of Medicine and an Adjunct Professor of Medicine at George Washington University. Dr. Carbone graduated *magna cum laude* from Harvard–Radcliffe College in 1979 and graduated with honors from the University of Wisconsin School of Medicine in 1983. She completed internal medicine and subspecialty training in infectious diseases at Johns Hopkins Hospital, receiving her board certifications in 1986 and 1988. Upon joining the faculty of the Johns Hopkins School of Medicine in 1988, she continued studying virus infections of the brain with a special focus on multidisciplinary studies of the developing rat nervous system with Borna disease virus. She has continued these studies and also has investigated the neurovirulence of vaccines for viral diseases such as mumps since joining CBER in 1996 as Chief of the Laboratory of Pediatric and Respiratory Viral Diseases.

MICHAEL DUNNE, M.D., is Vice President of Clinical Development for Infectious Diseases at Pfizer Global Research and Development Headquarters located in New London, Connecticut. He received his M.D. from the State University of New York in Brooklyn, and completed his internal medicine training as well as fellowships in pulmonary medicine and infectious diseases at Yale New Haven Hospital. Dr. Dunne joined Pfizer in 1992. His focus in industry has included the development of antibiotics for treatment of diseases of the respiratory tract, opportunistic infections in HIV infected patients and malaria. He has also been involved in the development of antibiotics for the treatment of coronary artery disease.

MAUREEN DURKIN, Ph.D., Dr.P.H., is Associate Professor of Public Health (Epidemiology) at Columbia University's Mailman School of Public Health and Sergievsky Center, and Research Scientist at the New York State Psychiatric Institute's Epidemiology of Brain Disorders Unit. Dr. Durkin has developed methodology for and directed comparative studies of the prevalence and causes of neurodevelopmental disabilities in developing countries. Her current research pertains to international policies relevant to public health and developmental disabilities, the epidemiology and prevention of pediatric neurotrauma, and long-term outcomes of premature birth. She has published widely on these topics, presented at national and international scientific meetings, and taught graduate level courses. Dr. Durkin has served as an advisor to the World Health Organization and a consultant to numerous organizations including the United Nations Statistical Office and the National Institutes of Health.

EDUARDO L. FRANCO, M.P.H., Dr.P.H., is Professor of Epidemiology and Oncology and Director, Division of Cancer Epidemiology at McGill University's Faculty of Medicine in Montreal, Canada. He was formerly a faculty member at Université du Québec (1989–1994) and Senior Researcher and Head of Epidemiology at the Ludwig Institute for Cancer Research, Sao Paulo, Brazil (1985–1989). He received his undergraduate degree in biology (1975) from Universidade de Campinas, Brazil, and received graduate training in public health microbiology at the University of North Carolina at Chapel Hill (1981–1984). A Guest Researcher at the Centers for Disease Control in Atlanta from 1980 to 1981 and 1983 to 1984, Dr. Franco received postdoctoral training in cancer epidemiology at the International Agency for Research on Cancer in Lyon, France; at the National Cancer Institute (NCI) in Bethesda, MD; and at Louisiana State University. During the past 15 years, he has studied the molecular epidemiology and prevention of cervical cancer, upper aerodigestive tract cancers and childhood tumors, and the development of epidemiologic methods in the evaluation of screening efficacy and assessment of misclassification. He has published more than 170 scientific articles and chapters and edited two books on cancer epidemiology and prevention. Dr. Franco has held Associate Editor assignments with the *American Journal of Epidemiology* (1993–98) and with *Cancer Epidemiology, Biomarkers & Prevention* (since 1995), and as Editorial Board Member for *Epidemiology, Medical and Pediatric Oncology, Cancer Detection and Prevention*, and *Cancer Prevention & Control*. He has served on scientific and grant review panels at the National Cancer Institute, NIH; the Medical Research Council of Canada (MRC); the National Cancer Institute of Canada; the Pan American Health Organization; Health Canada; Fonds de la recherche en santé du Québec (FRSQ); and the UK Cancer Research Campaign. He has mentored more than 50 graduate students and postdoctoral fellows since 1985. In addition to teaching at McGill, he has been an instructor in several annual or sporadic cancer epidemiology courses in the United States, South America, Europe, and the Middle East. He has served as a member or chair of organizing or program committees for 12 international conferences on cancer epidemiology, papillomavirus research, and oncology. Dr. Franco has received numerous awards, including MRC Distinguished Scientist (2000), Educational Excellence at McGill University (2000), City of Montreal's "Ambassadeur" (2000), FRSQ's National Research Scholar Award (1999).

EDUARDO GOTUZZO, M.D., is Principal Professor and Director at the Instituto de Medicina Tropical "Alexander von Humbolt," Universidad Peruana Cayetan Heredia (UPCH), in Lima, Peru. He is also Chief of the Department of Infectious and Tropical Diseases at the Cayetano Heredia Hospital and an Adjunct Professor of Medicine at the University of Alabama–Birmingham School of Medicine. Dr. Gotuzzo has been an active member of numerous international societies such as the Latin America Society of Tropical Disease (President, 2000–2003), the Scientific Program of Infectious Diseases Society of America (2000–2003), the International Organizing Committee of the International Congress of Infectious Diseases (1994–present), the International Society for Infectious Diseases (President Elect, 1996–1998), and the Peruvian Society of Internal Medicine (President, 1991–1992). He has published more than 230 articles and chapters as well as 6 manuals and 1 book. Among the many recent honors and awards he has received, he was named an Honorary member of American Society of Tropical Medicine and Hygiene (2002), an Associated Member of National Academy of Medicine (2002), an Honorary Member of Society of Internal Medicine (2000), a Distinguished Visitor, Faculty of Medical Sciences, University of Cordoba, Argentina (1999), and the receeipient of the Golden Medal for Outstanding Contribution in the field of Infectious Diseases from Trnava University, Slovakia (1998).

RICHARD L. GUERRANT, M.D., is Thomas H. Hunter Professor of International Medicine and Director of the Office of International Health at the University of Virginia School of Medicine. Author of more than 350 scientific articles and reviews and numerous major textbook chapters, and editor of 6 books, Dr. Guerrant graduated from Davidson College and University of Virginia School of Medicine and was trained in internal medicine and infectious diseases at the Harvard Medical Service of the Boston City Hospital, NIH, Johns Hopkins and UVa. He has worked in the Congo, Bangladesh, and Brazil and started the Division of Geographic and International Medicine with Kellogg and Rockefeller support in 1978. Since then he has recruited outstanding faculty (including Drs. Richard Pearson, Erik Hewlett, Jonathan Ravdin, Cynthia Sears, David Bobak, and Nathan Thielman) and his group has trained more than 90 postdoctoral fellows and students who are becoming leaders in tropical medicine, including Dr. James Hughes, Director of NCID at CDC, Drs. Jonathan Ravdin, Cynthia Sears, Chris Wanke and Aldo Lima. Dr. Guerrant is holder of 8 patents on innovative approaches to the diagnosis and treatment of common gastrointestinal illnesses and was Henderson Inventor of the Year in 1997 for his new glutamine derivative-based ORNT (oral rehydration and nutrition therapy). Guerrant was named Professor Honoris Causa at UFC and received the Emilio Ribas Medal of the Brazilian Society of Infectious Diseases in 1997. He has served on several editorial and USDA and WHO advisory boards, VA and NIH Study Sections, Clark and Child Health Foundation Boards, chaired the U.S. Cholera Panel of the U.S.–Japan Cooperative Medical Science Program, and the International Affairs Committee of the Infectious Diseases Society of America.

RICHARD T. JOHNSON, M.D., is Distinguished Service Professor of Neurology, Microbiology and Neuroscience at the Johns Hopkins University School of Medicine. He has a joint appointment in the Department of Molecular Microbiology and Immunology at the Johns Hopkins University Bloomberg School of Public Health. He has studied the pathogenesis of viral infections of the nervous system in animals and humans including studies of acute meningitis and encephalitis, viral-induced malformations, demyelinating diseases, and HIV-associated neurological diseases. He has published more than 300 articles and chapters and 10 books including a single authored volume on *Viral Infections of the Nervous System* (2nd ed. 1998). He was Director of the Department of Neurology at Johns Hopkins between 1988 and 1997. Since retiring from that post, he has been the Editor of *Annals of Neurology*, served for 3 years as Founding Director of the National Neuroscience Institute of Singapore, chaired the Institute of Medicine Committee on Transmisssible Spongiform Encephalopathies: Assessment of Relevant Science, and is a Special Consultant to the National Institutes of Health on Transmissible Spongiform Encephalopathies. Dr. Johnson has been a member of the Institute of Medicine since 1987.

ALTAF LAL, Ph.D., is the Chief of Molecular Vaccine Section, Division of Parasitic Diseases, National Center for Infectious Diseases, CDC. He is also an adjunct Professor in the Biology Department, Emory University. Dr. Lal received his PhD in Chemistry from Kanpur University and did his work at the Central Drug Research Institute, Lucknow. He was a Fogarty Visiting Fellow at the National Heart Lung and Blood Institute (NHLBI) and National Institute of Allergy and Infectious Diseases (NIAID). He has been at CDC for the last 12 years; his research program focuses on conducting laboratory and field studies on parasitic diseases, with a focus on malaria. In addition to conducting studies in Atlanta-based laboratories, Dr. Lal conducts field-based studies on malaria in western Kenya and enteric parasite work in Calcutta, India. He also collaborates with investigators working on malaria in several South American, Asian, and African countries. He has published more than 175 articles and has received funding from the U.S. Agency for International Development, WHO, NIH, the National Vaccine Program Office at CDC, and the U.S. Environmental Protection Agency.

W. IAN LIPKIN, M.D., is Professor of Epidemiology at the Mailman School of Public Health, Director of the Laboratory for Immunopathogenesis and Infectious Diseases and Center for Developmental Neuroscience of Columbia University, and the Louise Turner Arnold Chair of Neurosciences and Professor of Neurology, Anatomy and Neurobiology, and Microbiology and Molecular Genetics at the University of California, Irvine. Dr. Lipkin was the first to identify an infectious agent by subtractive cloning (Borna disease virus, 1990). He also led the team that used unique molecular methods to identify the West Nile virus as the cause of the encephalitis outbreak in New York State in the fall of 1999. His laboratory investigates the role of infectious agents and immune responses in pathogenesis of acute and chronic central nervous system diseases through molecular epidemiology and animal modeling. Dr. Lipkin received a BA from Sarah Lawrence College in 1974, and an MD from Rush Medical College in 1978. His postgraduate training included Residency in Internal Medicine at the University of Washington in 1979–81, Residency in Neurology at the University of California, San Francisco in 1981–84, and Fellowship in Neurovirology and Molecular Neurobiology at The Scripps Research Institute from 1984–1990. He is a 1991 Pew Scholar and a 2001 Ellison Medical Foundation Senior Scholar in Global Infectious Disease.

WILLIAM MASON, Ph.D., Senior Member at the Fox Chase Cancer Center, joined in 1973 following a postdoctoral fellowship in retrovirology in the laboratory of Dr. Peter K. Vogt, at the University of Southern California. He began working on hepatitis B in 1980 following the discovery of duck hepatitis B virus by Dr. Jesse Summers. This early work, carried out in collaboration with Summers and with John Taylor, led to the widespread adoption of this animal model as the system for studying how these viruses replicate. One of the immediate consequences of this work was the discovery by Summers and Mason that hepatitis B viruses replicate by reverse transcription, like the retroviruses, and the development of a detailed model for this process, again with Summers and Taylor. The duck virus also served as an early and continuing model for the evaluation of antiviral therapies. Since 1990, Dr. Mason's lab has studied how hepatitis B viruses maintain a chronic infection, and the effects of antiviral agents such as lamivudine and L-FMAU on this process. This work has employed the duck model of chronic infection, as well as the woodchuck model, which had been discovered by Summers in the 1970s. Current work in Mason's laboratory is focused on the consequences of combining drug therapy with immunotherapy to stimulate the host's defenses against infected liver cells, and microarray technology to evaluate the progression of chronic infections.

PATRICK S. MOORE, M.D., M.P.H., is Professor and Codirector, KSHV Laboratory, Department of Pathology at Columbia University. Dr. Moore's primary research interest involves use of molecular biology to investigate fundamental epidemiologic problems. His laboratory is devoted to discovery and characterization of new viruses associated with chronic diseases. In collaboration with his wife and lab codirector, Dr. Yuan Chang, he discovered the newest human tumor virus, Kaposi's sarcoma-associated herpesvirus (KSHV) in 1993. Subsequent work from this laboratory demonstrated the causal association between KSHV and KS using a modern reinterpretation of Hill's criteria and employing whole KSHV genome sequencing and development of serologic and DNA-based assays. Current research efforts are devoted to identifying specific KSHV genes causing cell transformation and proliferation. Dr. Moore received his MD from the University of Utah (1985) and an MPH from University of California, Berkeley (1989). He was an Epidemic Intelligence Service (EIS) Officer in the Meningitis and Special Pathogens Branch, CDC (1987–1989), and was involved in the discovery and characterization of the 1988–1996 clone III-1 group A *N. meningitidis* pandemic of sub-Saharan Africa. He also led refugee evaluation teams in Nepal and Somalia in 1992 for CDC and was the New York City Epidemiologist in 1993.

DAVID M. MORENS, M.D., received the A.B. degree (Psychology) in 1969 and the M.D. degree in 1973, both from the University of Michigan. He is Board Certified in Pediatrics (1978) and in Preventive Medicine (1980), with fellowship training in pediatric infectious diseases. He was also trained in epidemiology in the Epidemic Intelligence Service of the U.S. Centers for Disease Control and Prevention (CDC). After joining the CDC staff, Dr. Morens served as a medical virologist studying enteroviruses and enteric gastroenteritis viruses, as Chief of CDC's Respiratory & Special Pathogens Branch, and for two years studied Lassa fever in Sierra Leone, West Africa. From 1982 to 1998, he was Professor of Tropical Medicine at the University of Hawaii, and from 1987–1998 Professor and Chairman, Epidemiology Department, School of Public Health. Dr. Morens' has studied the epidemiology of viral hemorrhagic fevers, viral pathogenesis, and the integration and role of epidemiology in biomedical science and research. His career interest for more than 25 years has been on emerging infectious diseases and on diseases of unknown etiology. In the past decade he has published and spoken on numerous aspects of the history of epidemiology and infectious diseases. Currently Dr. Morens is on University leave, working in the National Institute of Allergy and Infectious Diseases of NIH.

SIOBHÁN O'CONNOR, M.D., M.P.H., is the Assistant to the Director of the National Center for Infectious Diseases, CDC, for Infectious Causes of Chronic Diseases, and a Clinical Assistant Professor of Medicine at Emory University School of Medicine. She received a Master of Public Health from the Harvard School of Public Health in 1997, her Doctor of Medicine from the University of Texas Health Science Center at Houston in 1986, and a Bachelor of Science from the Georgia Institute of Technology. Her postdoctoral training includes both clinical rheumatology and laboratory research fellowships at Washington University in St. Louis School of Medicine/Barnes Hospital following a residency in internal medicine at the University of Texas Health Science Center at Houston. She has been board certified in internal medicine and rheumatology. Dr. O'Connor joined the CDC in 1997 to develop a collaborative research agenda on infectious etiologies of chronic diseases. Activities emphasize integrating laboratory science, epidemiology and surveillance to define causal links between recognized and novel infectious agents and chronic syndromes, translating findings into prevention strategies for the populations at risk. In this capacity, Dr. O'Connor also serves on the NIH Autoimmune Diseases Coordinating Committee, chairs several multidisciplinary and multi-agency committees on related issues and serves as a national advisor to a clinical consortium. She is a member of the Infectious Diseases Society of America, the American College of Rheumatology, and the American Society for Microbiology.

MARK A. PALLANSCH, Ph.D., is a Distinguished Consultant and Chief of the Enterovirus Section in the Respiratory and Enteric Viruses Branch at the Centers for Disease Control and Prevention, Atlanta, Georgia. Responsibilities include multiple areas of research and testing with poliovirus and the non-polio enteroviruses. Research areas include studies of natural variation and recombination, molecular epidemiology, and association of enterovirus infection with neonatal infections and chronic diseases such as juvenile-onset diabetes and myocarditis. Also responsible for enterovirus diagnostics, which includes laboratory support for epidemiological studies, characterization of enterovirus isolates, identification and strain characterization of poliovirus isolates, and development of improved diagnostic techniques and reagents. Directly involved in supporting design, technology and implementation of the poliovirus laboratory network as part of the global poliovirus eradication initiative.

DAVID PERSING, M.D., Ph.D., is Vice President of Discovery Research at Corixa Corporation, and Medical Director of the Infectious Disease Research Institute, both located in Seattle, WA. David earned his M.D.–Ph.D. from University of California, San Francisco (UCSF) in 1988. The research for his doctoral thesis in biochemistry and biophysics was conducted in the laboratories of Don Ganem and Harold Varmus at UCSF. After completing his residency in Laboratory Medicine at the Yale University School of Medicine, he joined the staff of the Mayo Clinic, where he established research programs in tickborne diseases, hepatitis viruses, and infections associated with human cancer. In 1992 he became founding director of the Clinic's Molecular Microbiology Laboratory, which became one of the preeminent molecular diagnostic laboratories of its type in the United States. In 1999, he assumed his present position in Seattle, where his focus is on innate immunity, vaccine development, and human immunogenetic influences on vaccine responses. He is principal investigator of a $3.5 million, two year research program on innate immunity funded by the Defense Advanced Research Projects Agency (DARPA), and has a long track record of extramural funding from the National Institutes of Health. David serves on a number of corporate boards and advisory councils including the Boards of Directors for Virologic and ASM resources, and science advisory boards for IDI, the Burrill and Company Life Sciences Investment Funds, and the Mayo Clinic Clinical Research Center. He has authored 213 peer-reviewed articles and book chapters, has served as Editor-in-Chief of 2 books, and is listed as an inventor on 21 issued or pending U.S. patents.

MIKHAIL PLETNIKOV, M.D., Ph.D., is Assistant Professor of Department of Psychiatry and Behavioral Sciences, The Johns Hopkins School of Medicine, Baltimore, MD. He graduated with Honors from I.M. Sechenov Moscow Medical Institute, Moscow, Russia in 1986. He completed his postgraduate training in normal physiology at PK Anokhin Institute of Normal Physiology, Moscow, Russia in 1989 and received his Ph.D. in normal physiology in 1990. He joined the laboratory of molecular neurophysiology of that institute the same year and worked there until 1996 as a team leader with a special interest in a neurobehavioral analysis of a role of the cerebellum and hippocampus in learning and memory in developing and adult rats. From 1996 to 1999, he was a postdoctoral fellow at the laboratory of Dr. Kathryn Carbone at CBER/FDA and Johns Hopkins University School of Medicine studying neurobehavioral consequences of neonatal Borna disease virus infection. He joined the faculty of the Johns Hopkins University School of Medicine in 1999 and continues pathogenesis studies of neurodevelopmental damage using the neonatal Borna disease virus infection animal model.

THOMAS C. QUINN, M.D., M.Sc., is Senior Investigator and Head of the Section on International AIDS Research in the Laboratory of Immunoregulation at the National Institute of Allergy and Infectious Diseases. Since 1981, he has been assigned to the Division of Infectious Diseases at Johns Hopkins University School of Medicine where he is a Professor of Medicine. He also has adjunct appointments in the Department of International Health, and the Department of Immunology and Molecular Microbiology in The Johns Hopkins School of Hygiene and Public Health. He currently directs the Johns Hopkins School of Medicine P3 HIV/AIDS Research Facility and the International STD Research Laboratory. Dr. Quinn's investigations have involved the study of the epidemiologic, virologic, immunologic features of HIV infection in Africa, the Caribbean, South America and Asia. In 1984, he helped establish the interagency project called "Project SIDA" in Kinshasa, Zaire which was the largest AIDS investigative project in sub-Saharan Africa. Dr. Quinn has been involved in laboratory investigations which have helped define the biological factors involved in heterosexual transmission and perinatal transmission, the natural history of HIV infections in developing countries, and the identification and characterization of unique strains of HIV-1 infection. Immunologic studies have included the changes in T-cell phenotypes and cytokines in patients with HIV infection and other endemic tropical diseases such as malaria and tuberculosis. Among his professional activities, Dr. Quinn has been an Advisor/Consultant on HIV and STDs to the World Health Organization, UNAIDS and the U.S. Food and Drug Administration. He is a member of Editorial Boards of six journals focusing on infectious diseases, AIDS and sexually transmitted diseases. He is an author of more than 600 publications on HIV, STDs and infectious diseases.

JOSEMIR W. SANDER, M.D., M.R.C.P., Ph.D., is the NSE Professor of Neurology and Clinical Epilepsy at the Institute of Neurology of University College, London. He is Honorary Consultant Neurologist at the National Hospital for Neurology and Neurosurgery in London, Queen Square and at the National Society for Epilepsy in Buckinghamshire. Dr. Sander is Head of the WHO Collaborative Centre for Research and Training in Neurosciences, London, and Director of the Clinical Trials Unit at the National Society for Epilepsy–Chalfont Centre. He qualified in the University of Parana in Brazil and after his initial medical training in Brazil, he moved to the United Kingdom where he completed his neurological training. He obtained his Ph.D. at the Faculty of Medicine of the University of London. He serves as a member of the Management Committee of the International League Against Epilepsy and is a member of numerous organisations and professional societies including the Royal Society of Medicine, The American Academy of Neurology, The American Epilepsy Society and the British Medical Association. A frequent speaker at international conferences and a member of the editorial boards of several specialist journals, Dr. Sander has published extensively on various aspects of epilepsy, particularly drug issues, patient care and epidemiology. The International League against Epilepsy and the International Bureau for Epilepsy made him an Ambassador for Epilepsy in 1993.

THOMAS M. SHINNICK, Ph.D., is Chief of the Tuberculosis/ Mycobacteriology Branch of the Division of AIDS, STD, and TB Laboratory Research at the National Center for Infectious Disease (NCID) at the U.S. Centers for Disease Control and Prevention (CDC). He also is an Adjunct Professor in the Department of Microbiology and Immunology at Emory University. The author or coauthor of more than 130 publications and editor of one book, Dr. Shinnick has focused his research on understanding the biology and genetics of the pathogenic mycobacteria, elucidating mechanisms of pathogenicity and drug resistance of *Mycobacterium tuberculosis*, and developing rapid methods for the diagnosis of mycobacterial infections. He received his bachelor of science in biochemistry from the University of Wisconsin–Madison and his doctorate in biochemistry from the Massachusetts Institute of Technology. He won the Johnson and Johnson Predoctoral Fellowship in 1977 and the Helen Hay Whitney Foundation Postdoctoral Fellowship in 1978, conducting his postdoctoral training at the Research Institute of Scripps Clinic. Subsequently, he became an assistant professor in the institute's department of molecular biology. Dr. Shinnick joined NCID in 1986 as Chief of the Hansen Disease Laboratory in the Division of Bacterial and Mycotic Diseases until 1995, when he became Chief of the Immunology and Molecular Pathogensis Section in NCID's Division of AIDS, STD, and TB Laboratory Research. The following year, he assumed his current post. Dr. Shinnick has been honored with the Arthur S. Flemming Award (1990), the PHS Special Recognition Group Award (1993), and the NCID Honor Award (1993). He has been a Fellow of the American Academy of Microbiology since 1994 and a member of the Senior Biomedical Research Service since 1997.

SUSAN E. SWEDO, M.D., is Chief of the Pediatrics and Developmental Neuropsychiatry Branch at the National Institute of Mental Health (NIMH), NIH. There she leads a clinical research team investigating the causes and treatment of pediatric and neuropsychiatric disorders such as childhood-onset anxiety disorders, affective disorders, and movement disorders such as Tourette's Syndrome. Dr. Swedo led the NIMH team that first identified a new subtype of obsessive-compulsive disorder in children, pediatric autoimmune neuropsychiatric disorders associated with strep. Not only has this work resulted in several new and prevention strategies, but it has also led to a patent on a biological marker to help identify children at risk of obsessive-compulsive disorder (OCD) and tic disorders. Dr. Swedo received her M.D. from Southern Illinois University School of Medicine and served her residency at Children's Memorial Hospital at Northwestern University in Chicago. Dr. Swedo began her career as a practicing pediatrician in Chicago, where she served as Chief of Adolescent Medicine at the McGaw Medical Center of Northwestern University. She moved to the Washington area in 1986 and joined the staff of the Child Psychiatry Branch at the National Institute of Mental Health, where she conducted research on the pharmacological treatment of childhood OCD. The recipient of numerous awards, including the American Academy of Child and Adolescent Psychiatry Award for Scientific Achievement, Dr. Swedo is the author of more than 90 professional books and articles. She is the co-author with Dr. Henrietta Leonard of *It's Not All in Your Head* for women and *Is It Just a Phase?*, a parent's guide to common childhood behavioral problems.

ROBERT YOLKEN, M.D., graduated from Harvard College and Harvard Medical School and did a residence in Pediatrics at Yale. He received Fellowship training at Cornell–New York Hospital and at the Laboratory of Infectious Diseases at the National Institutes of Health. He joined the faculty in the Department of Pediatrics in 1979 and is currently the Ted and Vada Stanley Distinguished Professor of Developmental Neurovirology in that Department. His research interests include diagnostic virology and the identification of infectious causes of chronic diseases. Since 1995 he has worked extensively on studies related to the etiology of human neuropsychiatric diseases such as schizophrenia and bipolar disorder. He is the author or coauthor of more than 200 publications in peer reviewed journals and is one of the coeditors of the *Manual of Clinical Microbiology*. He has received numerous awards including the Abbott Award for the Rapid Diagnosis of Human Diseases, the Wellcome Diagnostics Award, and the Mead Johnson Award for Pediatric Research.

FORUM STAFF

STACEY L. KNOBLER, is Director of the Forum on Microbial Threats at the Institute of Medicine (IOM). She previously served as the codirector of the IOM Board on Global Health's study, *Neurological, Psychiatric, and Developmental Disorders in Developing Countries* (2001), and as the research associate for the *Assessment of Future Scientific Needs for Live Variola Virus* (1999). Ms. Knobler is actively involved in program research and development for the Board on Global Health. Previously, she held positions as a Research Associate at the Brookings Institution's Foreign Policy Studies Program and as an Arms Control and Democratization Consultant for the Organization for Security and Cooperation in Europe in Vienna and Bosnia-Herzegovina. Ms. Knobler has also worked as a research and negotiations analyst in Israel and Palestine. She is currently a member of the CBACI Senior Working Group for Health, Security, and U.S. Global Leadership. Ms. Knobler has conducted research and coauthored published articles on biological and nuclear weapons control, foreign aid, health in developing countries, poverty and public assistance, and the Arab–Israeli peace process.

MARJAN NAJAFI, M.P.H., was the research associate for the Forum on Microbial Threats in the Board on Global Health from March 2001 to November 2003. She also worked with the IOM committee that produced *Veterans and Agent Orange: Update 2000.* Ms. Najafi received her undergraduate degrees in chemical engineering and applied mathematics from the University of Rhode Island. Subsequently, she served as a public health engineer with the Maryland Department of Environment and, later, with the Research Triangle Institute in North Carolina. After earning a master's of public health from the Bloomberg School of Public Health at Johns Hopkins University, she managed a lead-poisoning prevention program in Micronesia, funded by a grant from the U.S. Department of Health and Human Services. She also studied the effects of cellular phone radiation on human health.